FOREWORD

GIVEN the unhealthy lifestyles of most people and the extent to which we constantly abuse our bodies with social and clinical drugs, unsuitable diets and other varied stresses associated with our environment, it is not surprising that many people feel run down or even ill for much of the time.

Modern treatment therapy is quite helpless when faced with chronic diseases and is constantly reduced to providing mere palliative, rather than curative, treatment. The root cause of this inability to change can be found in the dominance of health-care services by allopathic medicine, since it sets the tone for all official attitudes towards health.

The main aim of therapies which are designated alternative or complementary is to emphasize the basic importance of each individual doing as much as possible to maintain his or her health.

Much more effort should be put into the promotion and enhancement of health, rather than waiting for people to become ill and then applying expensive medical techniques in disease management.

In this age of unprecedented technological advance, we also see unprecedented damage being done to the atmosphere, the water and the land. Human violations of the laws of nature result in the contamination of the environment and, in turn, place an increased stress on the ability of the individual to function. This, together with the fact that mankind has gradually lost the inner awareness which would have enabled the correct perception of, and respect for, the laws of nature means that we see, collectively and individually, human beings both affecting and being affected by the environment. As we deviate increasingly from the laws of nature, a vicious cycle is established which requires great insight and energy to correct.

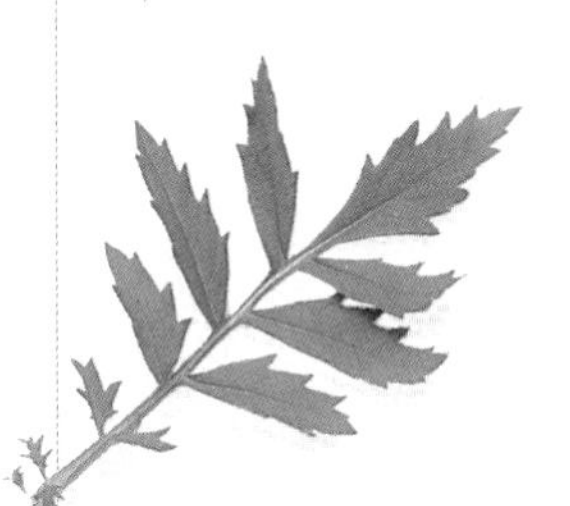

For each individual in this situation there may be a wide variety of possible responses to external stresses. Some people seem to be relatively unaffected by external or internal disturbances. They are in a state of relative balance which is maintained with minimal effort. Most people, on the other hand, experience degrees of imbalance ranging from slight to very severe. These are the people we consider diseased in the broadest use of the term. In such people the disturbance manifests itself in a highly individualistic and varied manner, but always the disturbance can be viewed as an imbalance of the organism's ability to cope with external influences.

This is where the practice of homeopathy is such a useful bridge. Many of its practitioners have been through an orthodox medical education in disease management. Homeopathic therapists are able to educate the public in the importance of a healthy lifestyle, explain the significance of our self-healing capacity and bring about the realization that health care is much more about health promotion than about the alleviation of the symptoms of the disease.

Modern medical education is a poor basis for health promotion and the great range of problems in which mind, body and environment so obviously interact. The promotion of the homeopathic philosophy is of vital importance as we become aware of the increased significance of iatrogenic illness. Dr Hammond successfully presents the benefits and philosophy of the homeopathic approach to health and the principles of an holistic view of treatment in the clearest terms.

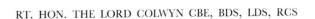

RT. HON. THE LORD COLWYN CBE, BDS, LDS, RCS

CONTENTS

PART ONE
The Theory and Philosophy of Homeopathy

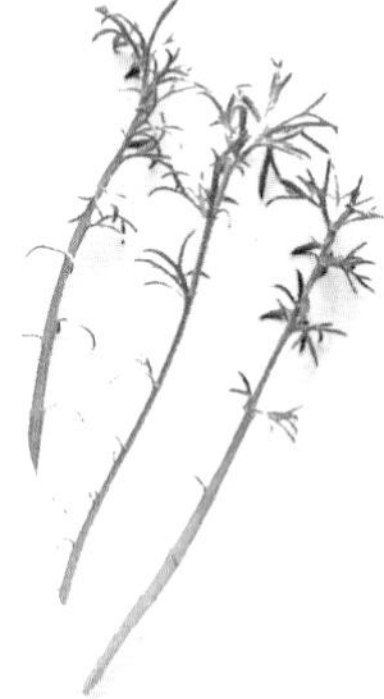

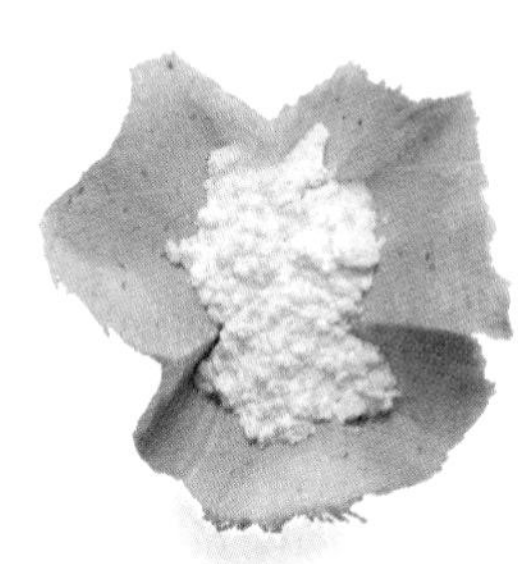

PART TWO
The Materia Medica

THE
COMPLETE
FAMILY GUIDE TO
HOMEOPATHY

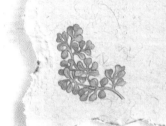

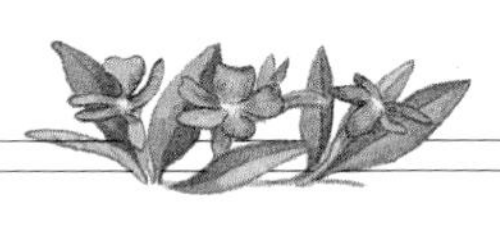

Dr Christopher Hammond
MB BS LCH

THE COMPLETE FAMILY GUIDE TO HOMEOPATHY

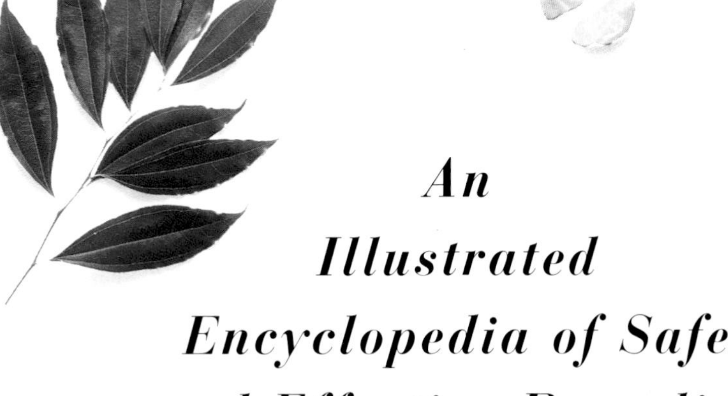

An Illustrated Encyclopedia of Safe and Effective Remedies

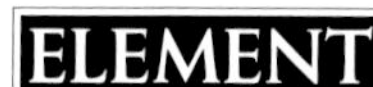

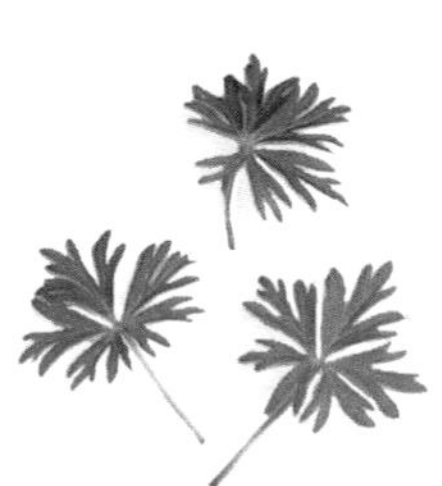

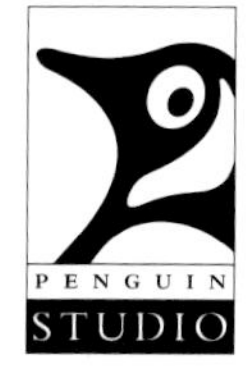

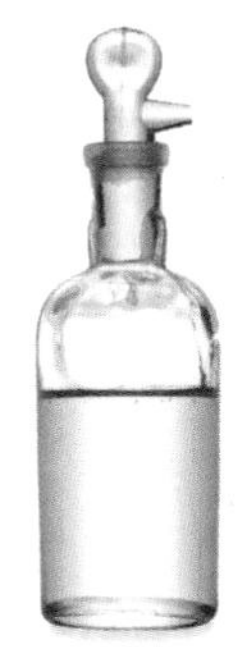

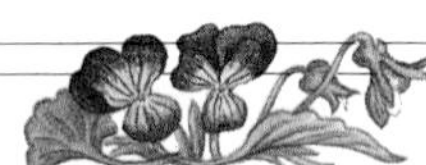

Additional text by Margaret Crowther, Carole Stephenson LCH and Rosemary Turner LCH

First published in Great Britain in 1995 by
ELEMENT BOOKS LIMITED
Shaftesbury, Dorset SP7 8BP

Published in the USA in 1995 by
PENGUIN STUDIO
Penguin Books USA Inc.
375 Hudson Street, New York, New York 10014

Published in Canada in 1995 by
PENGUIN STUDIO
Penguin Books Canada Limited
10 Alcorn Avenue, Toronto, Ontario M4V 3B2

Published in Australia in 1995 by
ELEMENT BOOKS LIMITED
for JACARANDA WILEY LIMITED
33 Park Road, Milton, Brisbane 4064

NOTE FROM THE PUBLISHER
Any information given in this book is not intended to be taken as a replacement for medical advice. Any person with a condition requiring medical attention should consult a qualified practitioner or therapist.

Designed and created for ELEMENT BOOKS by
THE BRIDGEWATER BOOK COMPANY
Art Director: Terry Jeavons
Page make-up: John Christopher
Studio photography: Guy Ryecart
Editor: Viv Croot
Picture research: Vanessa Fletcher

Origination by Graphikon
Printed and bound in Italy by Amilcare Pizzi

British Library Cataloguing in Publication
data available

Library of Congress Cataloging in Publication
data available

Element edition ISBN 1-85230-748-X
Penguin Studio edition ISBN 0-670-86157-X

PART THREE

Practical Homeopathy

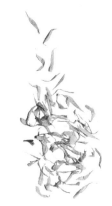

PART FOUR

The Remedy Pictures

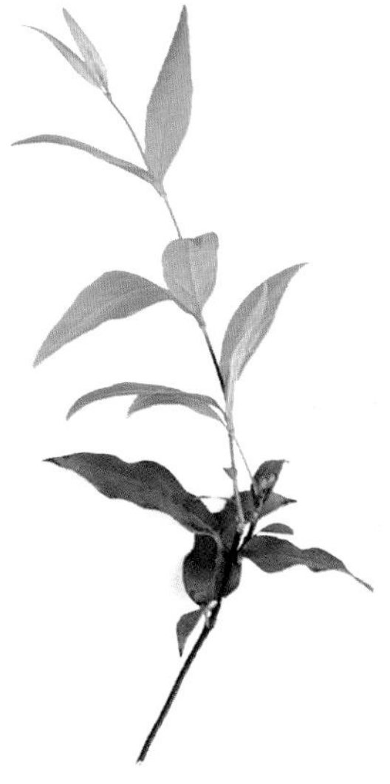

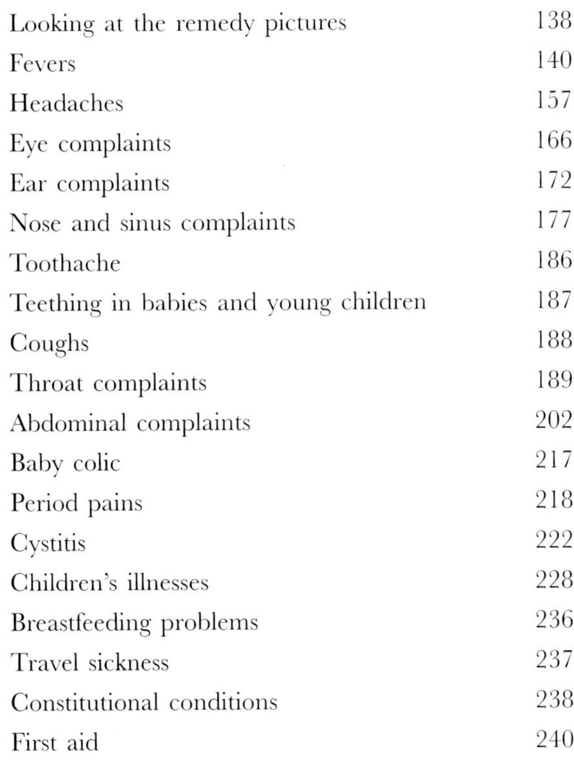

PART FIVE

Glossary and Appendix

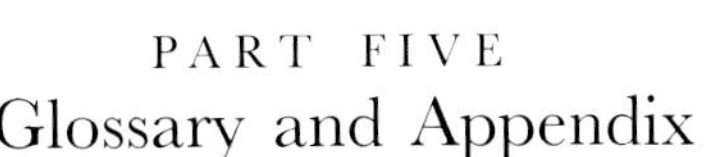

INTRODUCTION

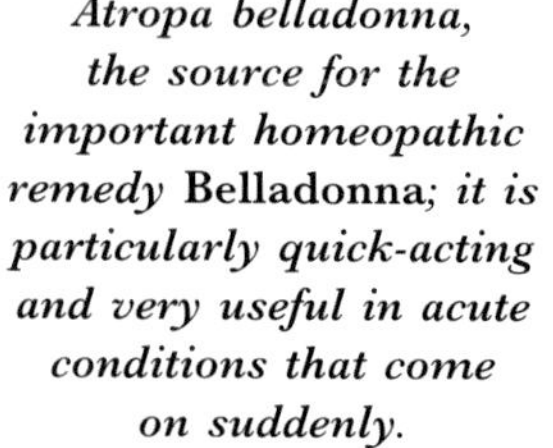

Atropa belladonna, the source for the important homeopathic remedy **Belladonna**; *it is particularly quick-acting and very useful in acute conditions that come on suddenly.*

This is a very brief overview of some of the aspects of homeopathy and a view of the world which may help to shed a little light on what is happening with a person's health. This book is designed to be used by anyone wishing to treat the common acute illnesses, in both children and adults. A complete understanding of the theory and philosophy is not necessary in order to use homeopathy effectively and safely in these types of conditions.

However a little knowledge of the history and philosophy of homeopathy may prove useful and interesting, and a brief overview of the origin, developments and tenets is given in the first part of this book. Whether or not what is suggested here reflects your view of the world is immaterial. If this book helps in the selection of remedies to assist the natural healing process then it will have achieved its purpose. This selection is not difficult and requires no academic training. The ability to observe is of far greater importance and is readily enhanced by practice.

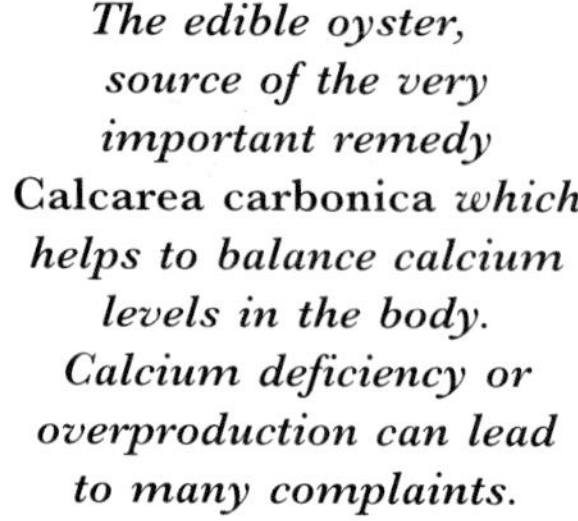

The edible oyster, source of the very important remedy **Calcarea carbonica** *which helps to balance calcium levels in the body. Calcium deficiency or overproduction can lead to many complaints.*

Causticum, *a remedy made from slaked lime and potassium bisulphate, is useful in neuromuscular problems. It is rarely used in acute cases.*

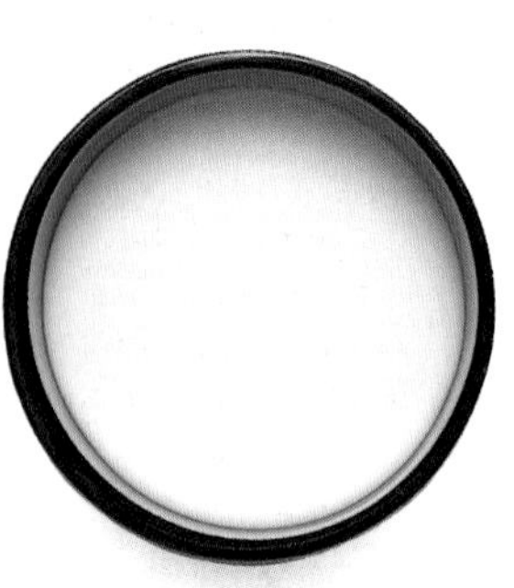

When it comes to the treatment of chronic and recurrent illnesses the situation is quite different. If the

condition is a recurrent one such as migraine or period pains, it is perfectly possible to use this book to find remedies that will give relief each time the pain occurs but it will not prevent the pain recurring next time. Curative treatment for such conditions is quite beyond the scope of this book. They reflect processes taking place much more deeply within the individual and are dependent upon many factors such as constitutional make-up, hereditability, diet, life events, lifestyle, environment and so on. Anyone requiring therapy for such conditions would be well advised to seek out an experienced practitioner in whichever constitutional therapy best suits their individual needs. Individualization is common to all the reputable therapies of which I am aware and that includes the choice of therapy itself.

There is much more to discover and there are many methods of discovery. Homeopathy is not the only practice that uses the concepts presented here and no one of repute would claim that homeopathy has all the answers or that it will suit everyone. It certainly has something of value to offer and there is only one way to find out whom it will suit; try it!

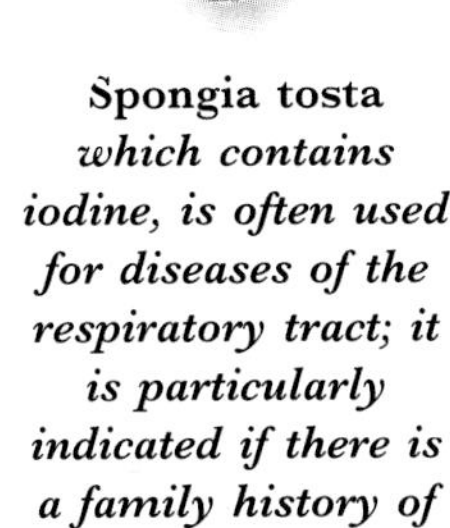

Spongia tosta *which contains iodine, is often used for diseases of the respiratory tract; it is particularly indicated if there is a family history of tuberculosis.*

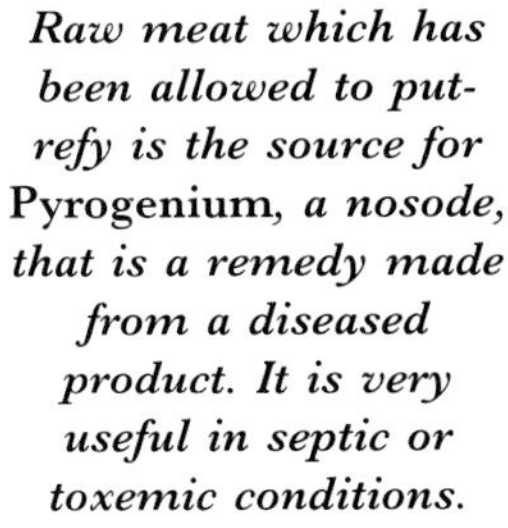

Raw meat which has been allowed to putrefy is the source for **Pyrogenium**, *a nosode, that is a remedy made from a diseased product. It is very useful in septic or toxemic conditions.*

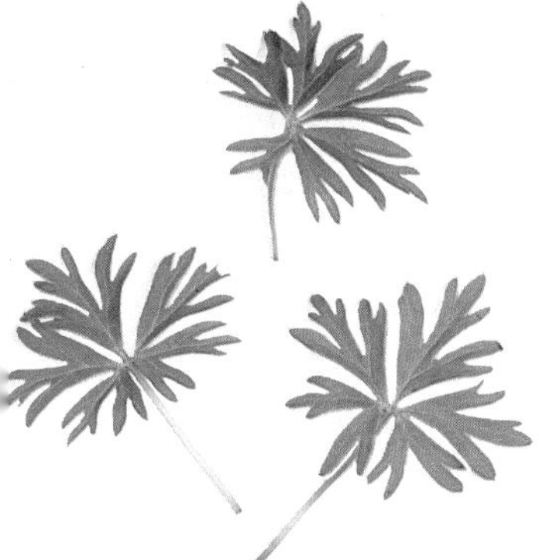

Aconitum napellus *is a short-acting remedy which is very valuable in the early stages of an illness. It is usually followed by a longer working remedy, but is an effective painkiller.*

Arnica montana, *an outstanding remedy for bruises and injuries from falling; it helps to stop bleeding, allay shock, and promote healing; it is used in a cream as a first aid remedy for bruises.*

How to use this book

The Complete Family Guide to Homeopathy has been designed to bridge the gap between the very simple and inadequate descriptions of use given with many over-the-counter homeopathic remedies and the much larger texts, the depth and complexity of which would put homeopathy quite beyond all but the most dedicated of amateurs. It has been written to help the beginner succeed in applying the homeopathic method to straightforward acute illnesses in the family; it also contains additional information which can be used as experience grows and by those who already possess some knowledge of homeopathy.

It is divided into five sections. The first part, *The Theory and History of Homeopathy* is intended as an introduction to the therapy and to Samuel Hahnemann, the German doctor who founded it. Basic principles are established and an explanation of how homeopathy works is given, together with descriptions of the making of the remedies and the principles and practice of potentization.

The second part is the *Materia Medica*, a review of all the major remedies indicated in this book, although by no means all the remedies available in homeopathy. Here is a chance to learn more about the remedies, what they are made from, the effect they have on a healthy person, the physical and mental symptoms they produce, the personality profile they typify.

The third part, *Practical Homeopathy*, introduces the art of taking a case according to the homeopathic method; how to observe the

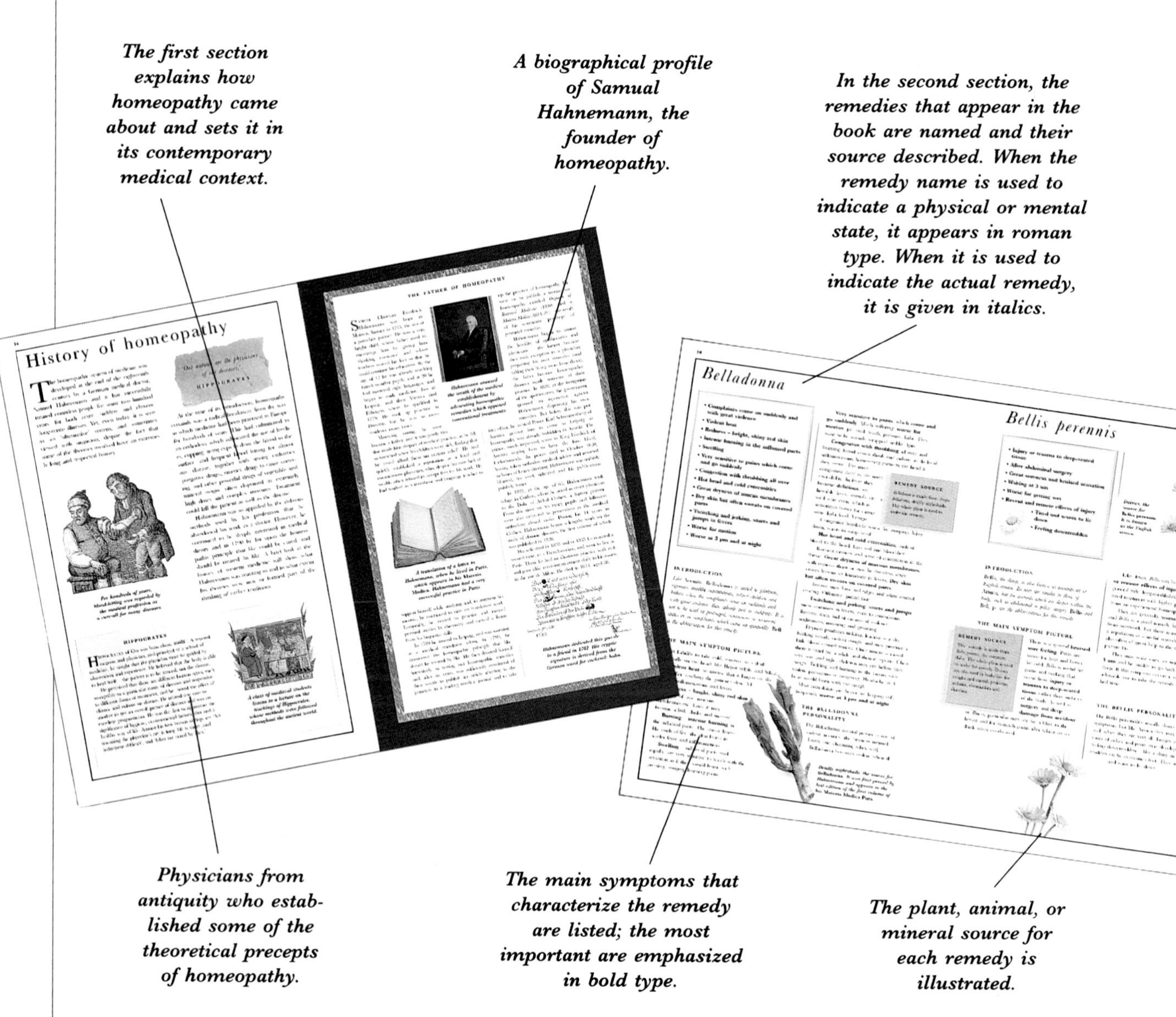

The first section explains how homeopathy came about and sets it in its contemporary medical context.

A biographical profile of Samual Hahnemann, the founder of homeopathy.

In the second section, the remedies that appear in the book are named and their source described. When the remedy name is used to indicate a physical or mental state, it appears in roman type. When it is used to indicate the actual remedy, it is given in italics.

Physicians from antiquity who established some of the theoretical precepts of homeopathy.

The main symptoms that characterize the remedy are listed; the most important are emphasized in bold type.

The plant, animal, or mineral source for each remedy is illustrated.

symptoms and take notes and how to organize the information gathered in a way that will make it easy for you to choose a remedy. Four simple case histories covering the common but distressing childhood complaint of ear ache are included to show you the way. This section also covers how to administer the remedy, what results to expect, and what to do next. A comprehensive list of recommended remedies for home use is suggested.

The fourth part, *The Remedy Pictures*, is arranged in tabular form to make it easy to match symptom with remedy. Using the symptoms you have observed during case-taking, you can look up the possible remedies in a series of charts; the charts are divided into sections dealing with complaints in various parts of the body. These charts conclude with a warning panel, advising you when to seek help, and you should always follow their advice. At the end of part four there is a section on constitutional conditions, conditions for which you should refer to a qualified homeopath. This is followed by an extensive first aid section, which shows you how to treat everyday accidents the homeopathic way and advises you on which remedies to keep handy in the home.

Finally, in the fifth part, there is a glossary which explains any medical terms outside the scope of everyday knowledge and terms which have a special relevance in homeopathy. Lastly, a section covering further reading and useful addresses listing institutions and suppliers will help you carry on your interest.

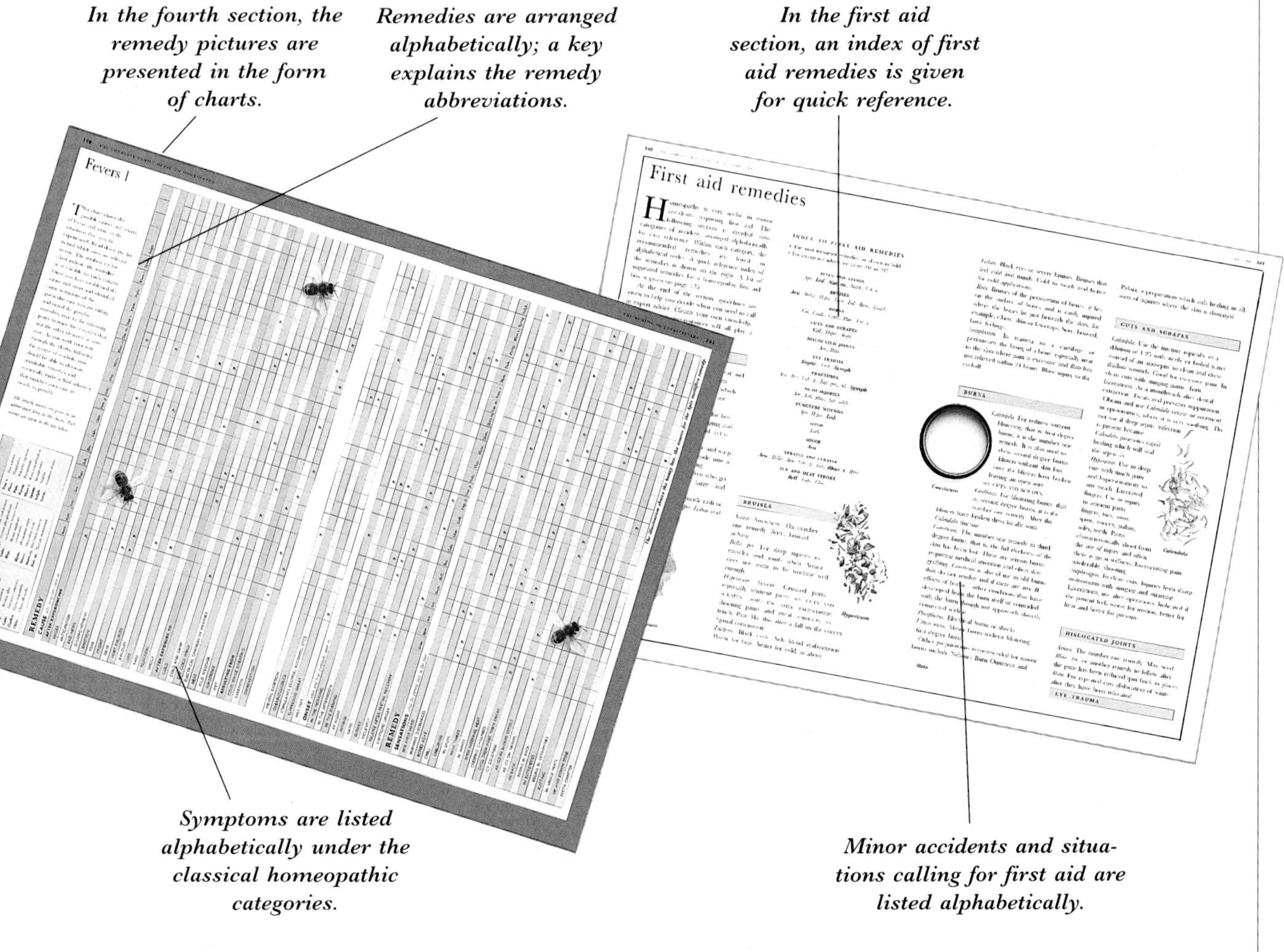

In the fourth section, the remedy pictures are presented in the form of charts.

Remedies are arranged alphabetically; a key explains the remedy abbreviations.

In the first aid section, an index of first aid remedies is given for quick reference.

Symptoms are listed alphabetically under the classical homeopathic categories.

Minor accidents and situations calling for first aid are listed alphabetically.

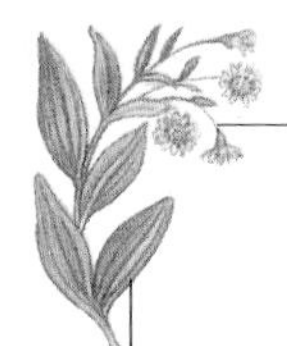

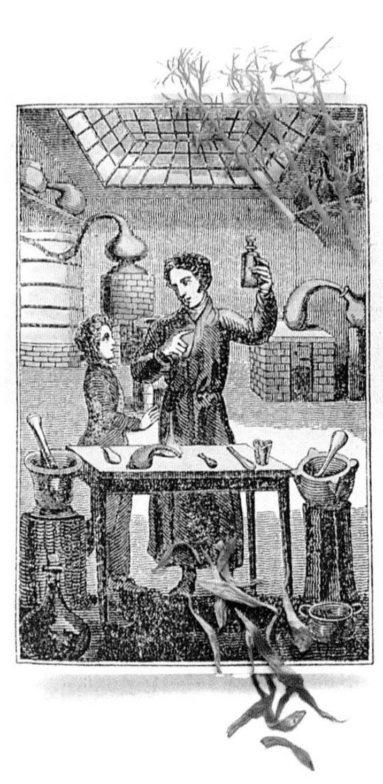

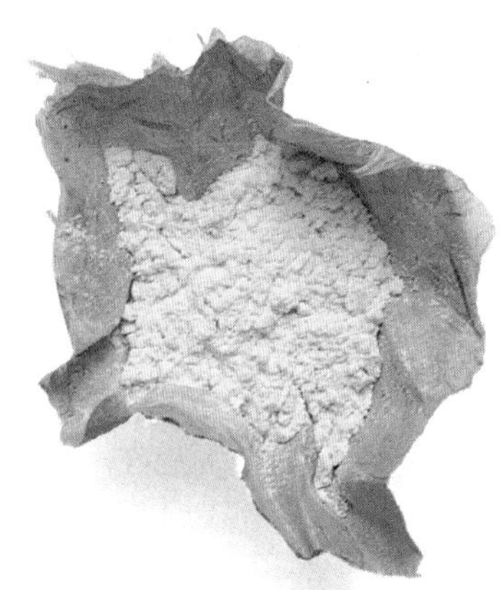

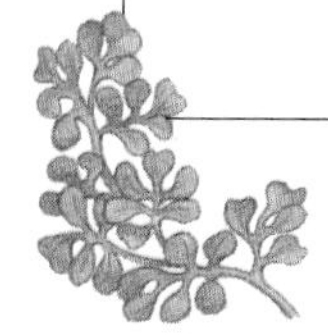

P A R T 1

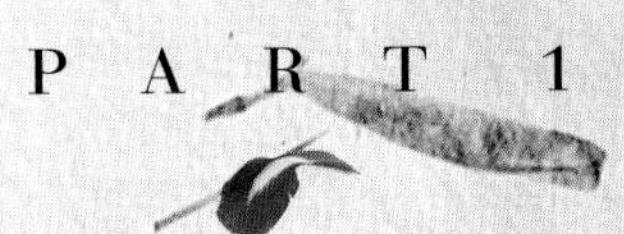

THE THEORY & PHILOSOPHY OF HOMEOPATHY

"

The highest ideal of therapy is to restore health rapidly, gently, permanently; to remove and destroy the whole disease in the shortest, surest, least harmful way, according to clearly comprehensible principles.

SAMUEL HAHNEMANN

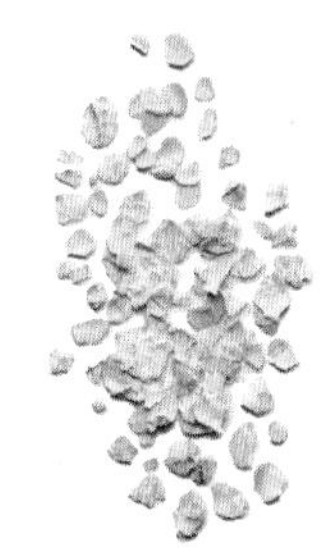

What is homeopathy?

Homeopathy is a complete system of medicine which aims to promote general health, by reinforcing the body's own natural healing capacity. Homeopathy does not have treatments for diseases. It has remedies for people with diseases.

It works in a totally different way from conventional medicine, which is known to homeopathic practitioners as allopathy. Allopathy means 'different from the suffering'; the drugs that are given work against the disease and its symptoms. Therefore drugs that are 'anti' are found, such as anti-biotics, anti-depressants, anti-inflammatory and anti-pain drugs etc. Homeopathy means 'similar to the suffering'. The remedies used to treat sick people are actually capable of producing similar symptoms in a healthy person to those present in the patient needing that remedy.

It is well known that homeopathic remedies are very dilute in their preparation though their effects cannot be explained so simply. It might be said that the remedies work at the level of energy and not of matter. The method of preparation of the remedies and how they act is

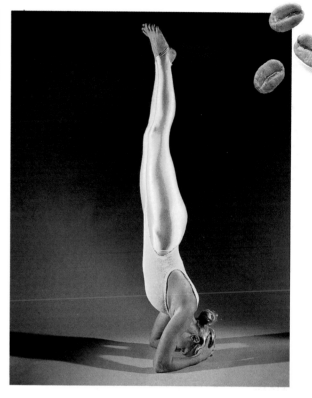

A holistic approach to health may include yoga, which is designed to promote physical and spiritual wellbeing. Many people believe it aids the body's abilities to heal itself.

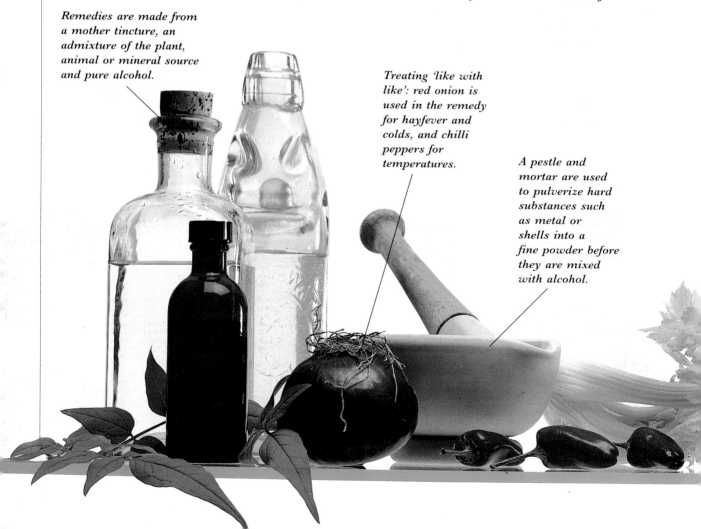

Remedies are made from a mother tincture, an admixture of the plant, animal or mineral source and pure alcohol.

Treating 'like with like': red onion is used in the remedy for hayfever and colds, and chilli peppers for temperatures.

A pestle and mortar are used to pulverize hard substances such as metal or shells into a fine powder before they are mixed with alcohol.

'Since diseases are only deviations from the healthy condition, and since they express themselves through symptoms, and since cure is equally only a change from the diseased condition back to the state of health, one sees that medicines can cure disase only if they possess the power to alter the way a person feels and functions. Indeed it is only because of this power that they are medicines.'

SAMUEL HAHNEMANN

HAHNEMANN & HOMEOPATHY

HOMEOPATHY was founded by Samuel Hahnemann. He believed the symptoms and signs of an illness are in fact attempts on the part of the organism to heal itself, so that when a substance capable of producing a similar symptom 'picture' to that of the disease is used it encourages a powerful strengthening of the defense mechanism. The physician, therefore, needs to study the totality of symptoms in order to get a full picture of the disease and prescribe the correct remedy. Often it is the symptoms that seem almost incidental, strange, rare or peculiar, that are the most valuable to the homeopathic practitioner, for they give the disease its own particular character and thus suggest the remedy.

The correct remedy, Hahnemann thought, produces a 'resonance' between the person and the substance administered as a therapeutic principle. It is thought to work rather like a similar, but stronger, disease to the one that the patient already has, which Hahnemann observed, always extinguishes the first, as two similar diseases cannot exist side by side. Homeopathic drugs thus work with the system, while allopathic drugs simply repress the symptoms and do not cure the disease.

not essential to an understanding of homeopathy. Homeopathy is about why a remedy is given, not what is given. There can be no such thing as a homeopathic remedy for colds or arthritis.

No two individuals manifest their illnesses in exactly the same way even if they are given the same disease label. It is only when a substance is matched with a patient according to the Law of Similars (see page 28) that it becomes homeopathic. When it is sitting in the medicine chest or pharmacy it is not homeopathic at all; it is just a potentized remedy.

Hahnemann, who founded the practice of homeopathy in 1790, used this ornate jar to store his remedies.

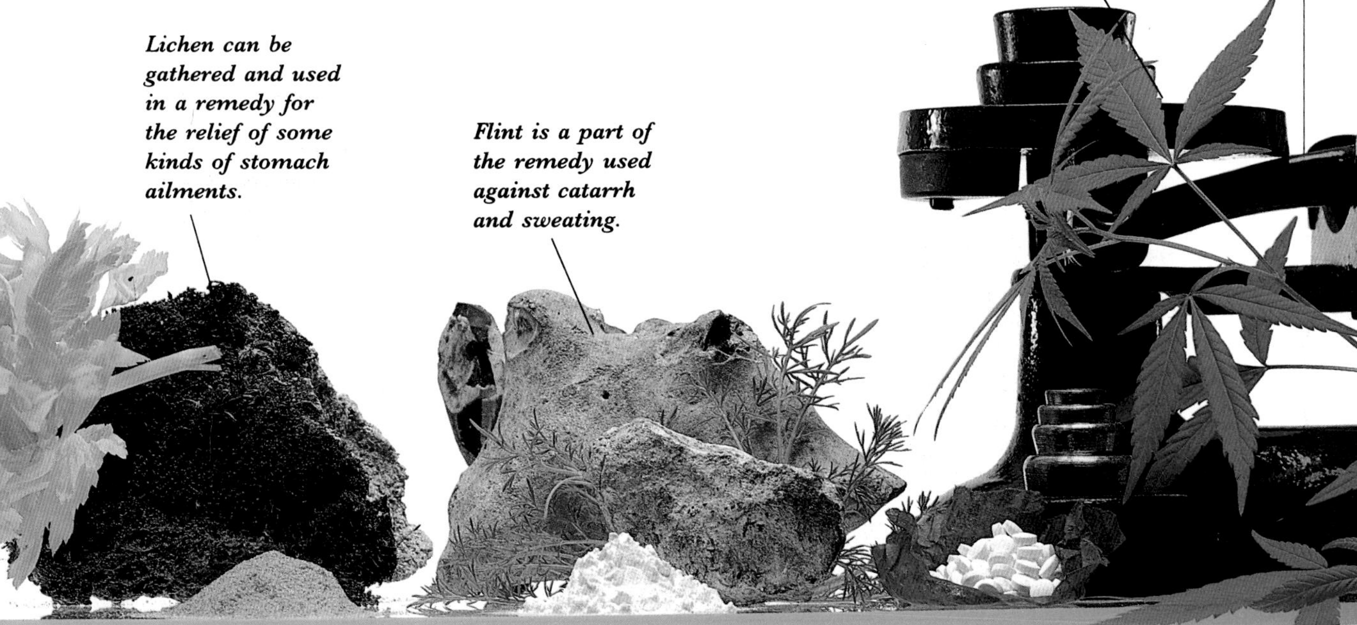

Careful measuring is vital in the work of the experienced homeopath. Each remedy requires specific quantities.

Lichen can be gathered and used in a remedy for the relief of some kinds of stomach ailments.

Flint is a part of the remedy used against catarrh and sweating.

History of homeopathy

The homeopathic system of medicine was developed at the end of the eighteenth century by a German medical doctor, Samuel Hahnemann and it has successfully treated countless people for some two hundred years, for both acute (sudden) and chronic (long-term) illnesses. Yet, even today, it is seen as an 'alternative' system, and sometimes viewed with suspicion, despite the fact that some of the theories involved have an extremely long and respected history.

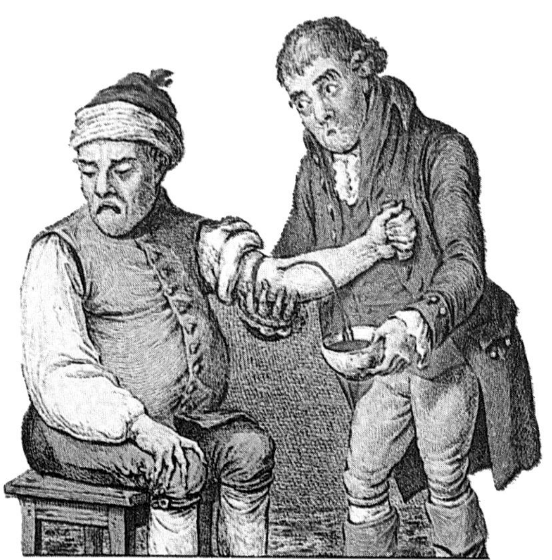

For hundreds of years, blood-letting was regarded by the medical profession as a cure-all for many diseases.

'Our natures are the physicians of our diseases.'

HIPPOCRATES

At the time of its introduction, homeopathy certainly was a radical breakaway from the way in which medicine had been practised in Europe for hundreds of years. This had culminated in an orthodoxy which advocated the use of leeches, cupping (using cups to draw the blood to the surface) and frequent blood-letting for almost any disease, together with strong cathartics (purgative drugs), emetics (drugs to cause vomiting) and other powerful drugs of vegetable and mineral origin, often dispensed in extremely high doses and complex mixtures. Treatment could kill the patient as well as the disease.

Hahnemann was so appalled by the dubious methods used by his profession that he abandoned his work as a doctor. However, he continued to be deeply interested in medical theory and in 1790 he hit upon the homeopathic principle that like could be cured (and should be treated) by like. A brief look at the history of western medicine will show what Hahnemann was reacting to and to what extent his theories were new or formed part of the thinking of earlier traditions.

HIPPOCRATES

HIPPOCRATES of Cos was born about 460BC. A revered surgeon and physician, and principal of a school of medicine, he taught that the physician must be guided by observation and experience. He believed that the body is able to heal itself – the patient is to be treated, not the disease.

He perceived that there are different human types, each susceptible to a particular range of diseases and responsive to different forms of treatment, and he noted the effect of climate and culture on disease. He related one case to another to get an overall picture of diseases and was an excellent prognostician. He was the first to appreciate the significance of hygiene, environmental factors, diet and a healthy way of life. Among his best known sayings are 'Art (meaning the physician's art) is long, life is short...and judgment difficult', and 'Likes are cured by likes.'

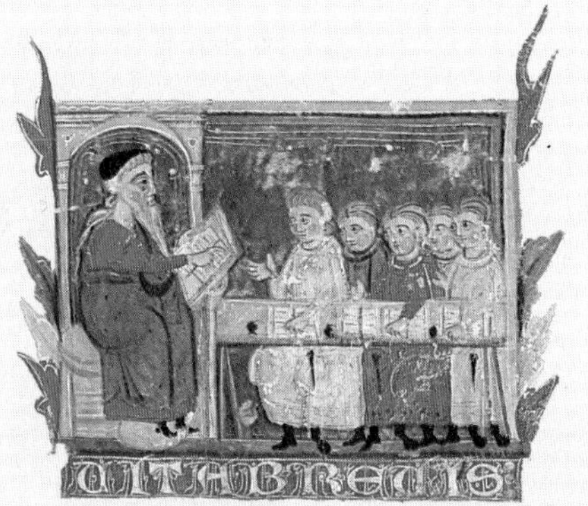

A class of medieval students listens to a lecture on the teachings of Hippocrates, whose methods were followed throughout the ancient world.

THE FATHER OF HOMEOPATHY

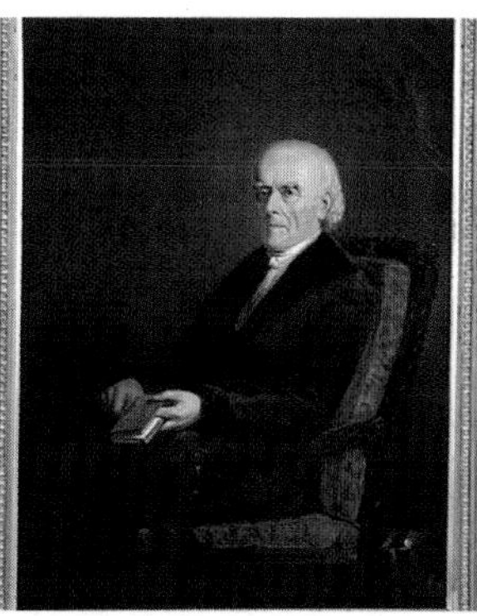

Hahnemann aroused the wrath of the medical establishment by advocating homeopathic remedies which opposed conventional treatments.

Samuel Christian Friedrich Hahnemann was born in Meissen, Saxony in 1755, the son of a porcelain painter. He was a very bright child, whose father used to encourage him by giving him 'thinking exercises' and whose teachers waived his fees so that he could continue his education. By the age of 12 he was already teaching Greek to other pupils, and at 20 he had mastered eight languages, and began to study medicine, first at Leipzig, and then Vienna and Erlangen, where he qualified in 1779. He took up practice in Dresden, but he was to move residence many times.

Marrying young, he soon became a father, and it was partly this that made him despair of medical practice, as he felt so wretched when his children were sick, finding that he 'could afford them no certain relief'. He had quickly established a reputation as a kind and conscientious physician, who, despite his own lack of wealth, often refused to accept fees for his work. He had worked as a translator and language teacher to support himself while studying and, to augment his income, he continued to take on translation work. Eventually, he ceased to practice and instead pursued studies in chemistry and earned a living from his linguistic skills.

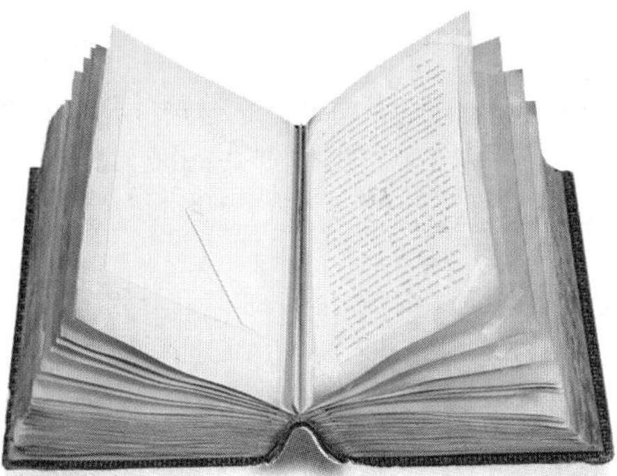

A translation of a letter to Hahnemann, when he lived in Paris, which appears in his* Materia Medica*. Hahnemann had a very successful practice in Paris.

In 1789 he moved to Leipzig, and was working as a medical translator when, in 1790, he discovered the homeopathic principle that like should be treated by like. He then devoted himself intensively to testing out homeopathic remedies and, after six years, was sufficiently convinced of their worth to publish an article alluding to the principle in a leading medical journal and to take up the practice of homeopathy. He went on to publish a treatise on homeopathy entitled *Organon of Rational Medicine* (1810) and a *Materia Medica* (1811-21) – the result of his systematic 'provings' of potential remedies.

Hahnemann began to arouse the hostility of apothecaries and physicians – the former because they took exception to a physician preparing his own remedies (and taking their living away from them), the latter because homeopathic theories made nonsense of their practice. In 1820, at the instigation of the apothecaries, the government granted an injunction against Hahnemann dispensing his own remedies. But before this was put into effect, he treated Prince Karl Schwarzenberg of Austria, getting him to come to Leipzig as homeopathy was already forbidden in Austria. The prince, much improved, wrote to King Friedrich of Austria urging him to have the ban lifted. Unfortunately, the prince died in October 1820, having taken orthodox medical advice and resorted to bouts of heavy drinking. Hahnemann was unfairly blamed, his work ridiculed and his publications publicly burnt.

In 1821, at the age of 65, Hahnemann took refuge in Cothen, where he acted as court physician to the Duke of Anhalt-Cothen, a former patient. From this time on his many pupils and followers were also subjected to persecution as the medical orthodoxy closed ranks. During his 14 years in Cothen, Hahnemann began a lengthy work on the study of chronic diseases, the first volume of which was published in 1828.

His wife died in 1830 and in 1835 he married a second time, to a Frenchwoman, and went to live in Paris. There he had an illustrious practice with rich and poor alike receiving treatment daily in his rooms in the rue de Milan. He died in 1843, aged 88.

Das Probirt man in der Gluth.
Den ob die Klinge gut.
Die Krafft der durch Gifft,
Das wenn es der Sturm Wind trifft.
Soldaten in der Schlacht.
Der Jungfern Keuschheit b der Nacht
Bei Freunden ist der Probe
Wenn wir in Höchsten nöthen s n

Meißen d. 9ten Octobr 1782.

Dem Herrn Besitzer zum Andencken schrieb dieß so gut er kan ein Freund und Diener
emann

Hahnemann dedicated this puzzle to a friend in 1782. His cryptic signature is derived from the German word for cockerel: hahn.

Greek beginnings

Until the dawn of rationalism during the fifth century BC, illnesses were thought to be visited on human beings by external, supernatural causes (a view that is still widely held in primitive societies). Those with diseases had offended the gods, or were the victims of a spell on the part of an ill-wisher or of the work of a malevolent demon. Healing could take place only if the gods were placated or the spell removed and the practice of medicine was an occult art, sacred to priests and witch doctors.

The early Greek thinkers began to see that no supernatural causes were necessary to explain the nature of human beings and the existence of disease. Hippocrates, the early Greek physician and 'father of medicine' (see page 16) developed the theory, practice and study of medicine into both an art and a science and he and members of his school were the authors of many works on the subject. In an attempt to explain human health and sickness in natural rather than supernatural terms, they adopted the philosophers' theory of the four elements, which were present in everything – earth, air, fire and water. Corresponding to these, they theorized, were the four bodily humors: blood, phlegm, black bile and yellow bile, and an imbalance in these humors made itself manifest by disease. The art of the physician lay in restoring balance.

Even if the theory of humors in itself may sound a little magical, the practice of medicine was turned into a genuinely scientific enquiry, with a study of causes and effects, and into an extremely humanistic enterprise, with the dawning of the 'bedside manner' – the doctor concerning himself with the patient's comfort.

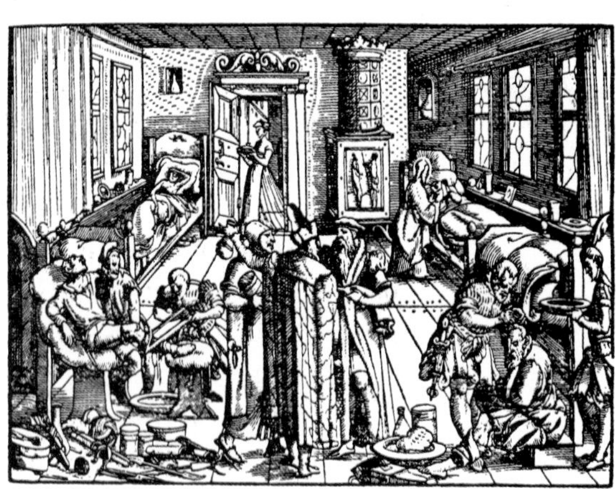

Hospital life in 1566. A surgeon performs an amputation; another treats a head injury; three physicians discuss a urine sample.

The Hippocratic way of medicine was followed throughout the ancient world, but approaches to medicine in the west began to change with the growth of Christianity. In the first century AD Erotian compiled a glossary of Hippocratic terms, and the famous physician and theorist of the second century, Galen, still considered his work to be of great importance. However, he differed from Hippocrates in many ways. While Hippocrates believed that the physician helped

PARACELSUS

Paracelsus

Phillippe Theophrastus Bombast von Hohenheim (1493-1541), who adopted the name Paracelsus, is something of a maverick in medical history. He advocated experiment and scientific study, yet he also studied alchemy and necromancy.

Some of his ideas echo those of Hippocrates or anticipate the work of Hahnemann. He maintained that what makes a man ill also cures him, and is said to have successfully cured a village of the plague by treating the inhabitants with a preparation containing traces of their own excreta. He used therapeutic herbs, guided by the doctrine of signatures (the appearance of the plant was a guide to the disease it would cure), but he also introduced 'chemical medicine' with the use of poisonous mineral substances which he prepared and refined for use as safe specific treatments.

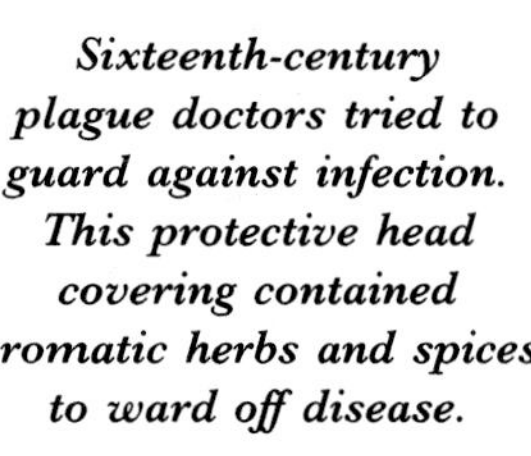

Sixteenth-century plague doctors tried to guard against infection. This protective head covering contained aromatic herbs and spices to ward off disease.

> *'All things are poison, it is the dosage that makes a thing not poison.'*
>
> **PARACELSUS**

the body to heal itself, Galen believed in applying contrary remedies to force out disease, and in the use of numerous drugs. Galen dominated medicine throughout the whole of medieval Christianity – so much so that to go against his teaching amounted to heresy – and medicine itself became increasingly dominated by dogma and superstition.

Religion preached that the human body was vile and worthless in comparison to the spirit and this led to its being held in contempt from a medical point of view also. Once again, disease came to be thought of as something that was visited from on high, and was seen as a sign of God's displeasure or a burden to be borne. The body itself, let alone the patient as a person, was of no interest to the physician – and instead the bodily excretions were examined for an insight into the nature of the disease. The Greek idea of the four bodily humors led to an increasing practice of blood-letting, in order to 'rebalance' the humors, and the production of pus, thought to be a necessary part of healing, was stimulated by re-opening and re-infecting wounds. Curing, which, in its Latin origins, meant caring, now meant driving out disease with violent treatment.

At the end of the long medieval period, the Renaissance encouraged scientific study, as well as a renewal of interest in classical learning. Yet, despite a few dissident voices, such as that of Paracelsus, superstition and harmful practice continued to dominate in medicine.

By Victorian times, there was a homeopathic hospital in London. This scene shows Christmas in the children's ward, with nurses gathered round the piano.

With the advancing spirit of investigation the ideas of the French philosopher René Descartes (1596-1650) and other rationalist thinkers gradually helped to sweep away medieval notions and to advance medical theory but to some extent also introduced new dogma. The study of the human body was limited by the fact that Christianity did not allow dissection, and investigations thus sometimes came up with misleading conclusions. The theory known as dualism, based on the Cartesian idea of the mind being separate from, but seated in the body influenced medicine to concentrate on the curing of the body alone, discouraging the return to the caring of the patient as a person, and there was still no understanding of hygiene.

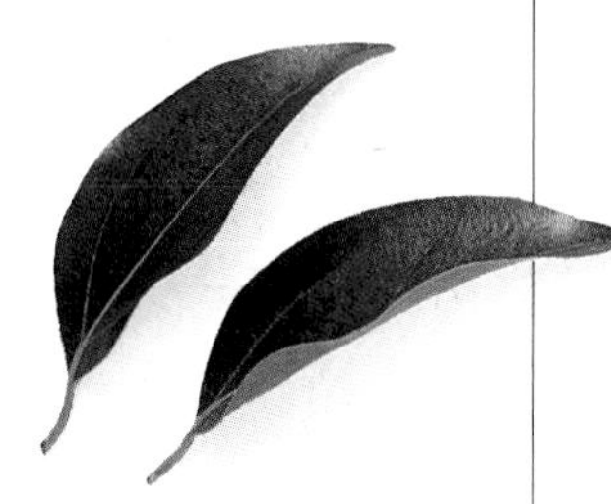

Leaves from the Camphor tree. Plants that had long been well-known for their herbal properties were potentized and tested by Hahnemann and his followers to find out whether they had any homeopathic virtue.

Hahnemann's approach

This was the tradition that Hahnemann inherited when he qualified as a physician in 1779. In practice, he quickly saw that such treatments as blood-letting weakened the body's powers of recovery and had no convincing theoretical basis, while the multiple use of strong drugs, often again without theoretical or empirical justification, caused bodily harm. He therefore abandoned the practice of medicine for fear, he said, of actually causing injury, and took to working as a translator. And while translating Scot Cullen's edition of *Materia Medica*, he received the inspiration that led to the discovery of the principles of homeopathy.

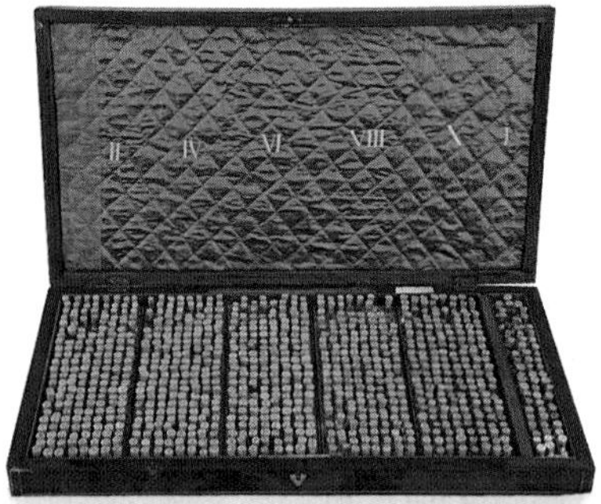

Hahnemann used this wooden case to store hundreds of remedies in small glass vials. He first tested many of the preparations on himself.

The new theoretical approach to therapy, advocated by Hahnemann's contemporary John Brown (1735-88), was that disease persisted through lack of stimulation, and that only 'heroic' doses of drugs could stimulate the body back to health; Hahnemann's ideas are in complete opposition to this. Drugs, or remedies, should be used gently to stimulate the restorative forces of nature, and without provoking harmful side-effects which cause ultimate injury. The smallest possible doses should be given at the most widely spaced intervals possible, and of only one drug at a time, so that the patient's system is not overwhelmed by complexity.

The word 'homeopathy', invented by Hahnemann to describe his system of medicine, is derived from the Greek for 'similar suffering' (*homois pathos*). The theory that underlies it is that substances which would cause symptoms of disease in a healthy person will cure a person who already exhibits the same symptoms. It came about because one of the substances referred to in Cullen's work, Peruvian bark (*Cinchona offinalis*), which is the source of quinine, was used for the treatment of malaria (then known as intermittent fever). Cullen said the substance worked 'because it was bitter', but Hahnemann was dissatisfied with this account and decided to test the bark on himself. Meeting his expectations, the symptoms of the fever occurred. Like could cure like. This was a part of Hippocrates' teaching and sprang from the notion that symptoms could be an indication that the body was struggling to overthrow a disease so it would be helped if the symptoms were encouraged. Hippocrates had been translated in Latin as saying '*Similia similibus curantur*', or 'Likes are cured by likes'. Interestingly Hahnemann, a skillful linguist, slightly reformulated this to say '*Similia similibus curentur*' or 'Let likes be cured by likes'.

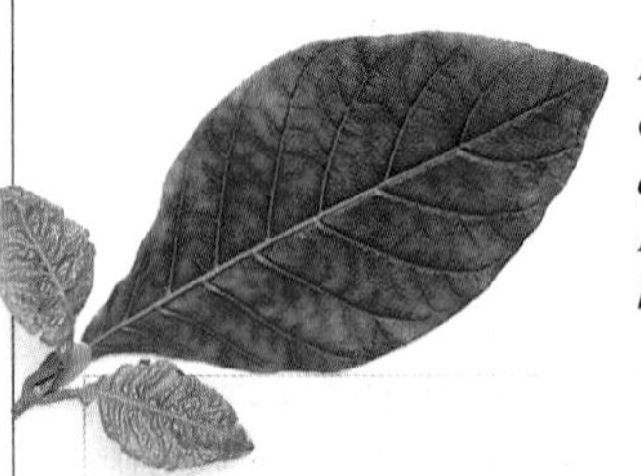

Leaves from* Cinchona officinalis, *the quina quina tree, which inspired Hahnemann to develop his theory of homeopathy.

An ayurvedic treatise on the art of healing. Ayurveda is a traditional Hindu system of medicine which embraces many of the principles of homeopathy.

SUCCESS ON A GRAND SCALE

THROUGHOUT his life Hahnemann had many grateful patients, both poor and aristocratic, but in two notable cases he brought homeopathy to wider fame in the treatment of epidemics.

The first was the typhus epidemic that attacked Napoleon's defeated troops after the Battle of Leipzig in 1813; Hahnemann treated 180 men and only one died. The second was 20 years later, when he successfully treated cholera patients during a violent outbreak of the disease.

After his death there were similar successes in Cincinnati in 1849 when only three per cent of homeopathic patients died during a cholera epidemic, compared to up to 70 percent receiving allopathic treatment. Again, in London in 1854, the London Homeopathic Hospital had a 16.4 percent death rate during a cholera epidemic, while at other hospitals the rate was 51.8 percent.

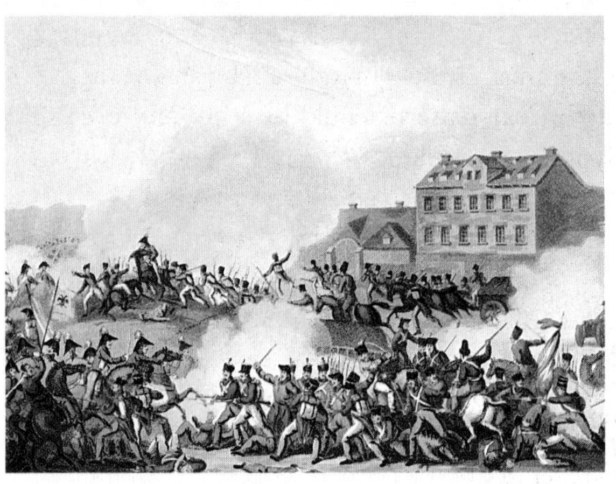

After the Battle of Leipzig, Hahnemann successfully treated many of the soldiers who fell victim to a typhus epidemic.

> *'...everything must be the pure language of nature carefully and honestly interrogated.'*
>
> SAMUEL HAHNEMANN

Proving the theory

Hahnemann had thus provided a theoretical basis for a known cure. In theory, cures could therefore be found for many symptoms, once he had discovered a substance that was capable of causing the same symptoms in a healthy person. In true scientific spirit he bravely prepared to experiment by testing the effects of various substances on himself, and such was his zeal that he found many willing volunteers, not just among his family but also among like-minded young practitioners anxious to find safer and more rational remedies. These experiments were known as provings (which simply means tests) and the first set of provings was conducted over about six years. Minute quantities of many substances were self-administered by the provers, and all symptoms provoked were carefully recorded in great detail. Any change whatsoever in the health and functioning of the body, including mental changes, the circumstances in which they arose, and even the time of day, were noted. At the same time an exhaustive enquiry was made into recorded cases of poisoning, taken from medical sources from various countries and dating back over several centuries. As the mass of information acquired was assimilated, clear patterns could be seen, and eventually it was possible to test substances as curatives on patients, with remarkable success.

THE VITAL FORCE

MOST cultures have developed the notion of some sort of vital principle which animates and regulates us. In western thought the idea dates back to the early Greek thinkers, and the physician Galen developed their ideas in the second century, stating that the world spirit or breath of life, *pneuma*, was inhaled from the air and circulated through the body to be converted into vital spirit on encountering the body's natural spirit in the heart.

From the east come the Hindu Yoga idea of *prana*, the vitalizing energy behind all life, described as the breath of life, the life principle, vital force or absolute energy, and the Chinese notion of *ch'i*, the flow of energy which circulates our bodies and which is stimulated and regulated by the Chinese in acupuncture.

Hahnemann came to the view that it is the vital principle that is acted upon by homeopathic remedies to restore the body to health.

The Legacy

Later in the eighteenth century, the discovery of bacteria seemed to confirm the theory that disease was caused by forces outside the body (albeit no longer demons) and again led to the notion of treating disease by driving out its causes from the body, with little to say for the idea of treating the whole person or encouraging the body's own healing powers. In the main, this approach dominated medicine and homeopathy, although still adhered to by many followers, took a back seat. However, it is now becoming clear that microbes can become resistant to antibodies, and that orthodox treatment often has serious side effects, and there is a new interest in homeopathy as a gentle and effective way of treating many kinds of disease.

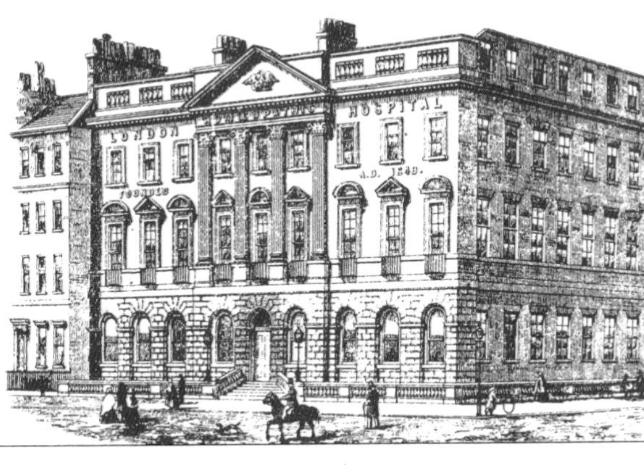

In 1849, Frederick Quin founded the London Homeopathic Hospital in Great Ormond Street.

How homeopathy works

So how does homeopathy work? Before attempting to answer that question it is necessary to understand a little about the function of disease in our lives.

Gentle and enjoyable exercise enhances the vital force that flows through our bodies. Exercise is a way to keep the body fit enough to fight off disease.

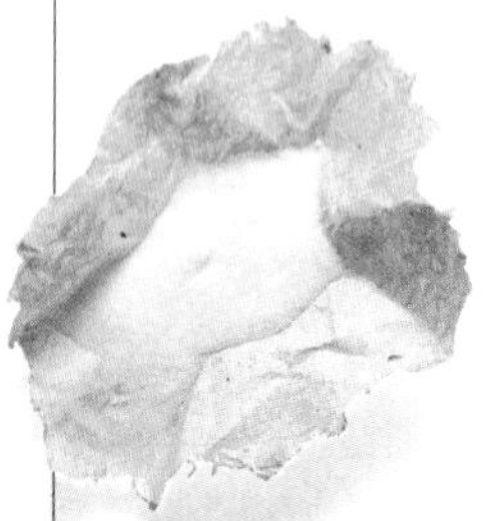

Kali bichromichum, *a remedy for people whose symptoms include chronic nasal catarrh.*

Does disease have a function?

It is often useful, when explaining a very large concept, to start at the beginning. In this case let us consider the healthy child and the illnesses that commonly occur in childhood. Healthy children have lots of energy as a rule, so much so that they can wear out their poor unhealthy parents! When they get ill, what sort of illnesses do they get? They mostly tend to get sick rapidly with a very high fever, a vigorous illness which puts them in bed. Then in a matter of days, or even in one day, they are up and about again eating us out of house and home. At least, this is the tendency in the beginning with most very young children and certainly with lively, healthy ones.

So what is going on in illness? Sometimes an observant parent will notice something that will give us a clue; after a child recovers from one of those high fevers that 'lay it very low' for a short time, it is sometimes seen that the child is more 'well' than before it became 'ill', provided the illness has not been inappropriately treated or interfered with in some way. Often this is very subtle. There may be an improvement in the child's already abundant energy or that nebulous sense of well being that we all know about but find so hard to put into words. This may show itself by an improvement in the child's behavior or in the resolution of some lingering problem, such as the slight cough or persistently runny nose. Frequently this improvement is missed or does not occur because of some form of interference. If you have healthy young children, observe them closely and see what you can find out about their responses for yourself.

What happens as we grow up? There is a tendency for illnesses to become more prolonged, less intense and for the recovery to be slower. Eventually the recovery becomes incomplete and we can see the gradual

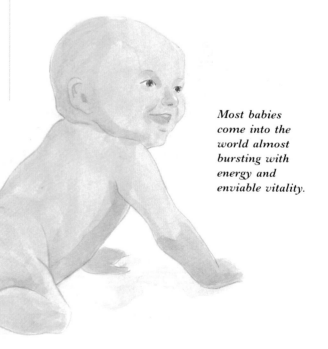

Most babies come into the world almost bursting with energy and enviable vitality.

emergence of chronic disease. From this progression it becomes possible to consider chronic diseases either as acute illnesses from which we have not been able to recover fully or as arising from the individual having insufficient 'energy', for whatever reason, to develop an acute illness and be done with it! Of course this can start in the very young, though it is much more rare.

Is chronic disease inevitable?

Why does this happen? What has gone wrong? Is it natural for man to slowly degenerate in this way? Just because it is so common that it is regarded as 'normal' to expect chronic ill health with advancing years does that mean that it is the way things have to be or, indeed, should be?

Occasionally we hear of people of very advanced years who appear and act as if they were in their prime, both mentally and physically. Plainly not everyone has to be subject to chronic disease. Is it not possible that these few exceptional individuals are, in fact, the normal ones and the rest of us have somewhere deviated from this path of health?

For me, it makes much more sense to look at the world from the point of view that things should be perfect. If they are not, something has interfered with the natural state and thrown things out of balance. This is of direct importance to the view of health and the function of disease in homeopathy.

Already we have looked at the healthy state of the majority of children when they enter this world and how their health tends to deteriorate slowly with time. This need not be considered 'normal' or inevitable.

Physical wear and tear on a middle-aged body need not diminish the vital force.

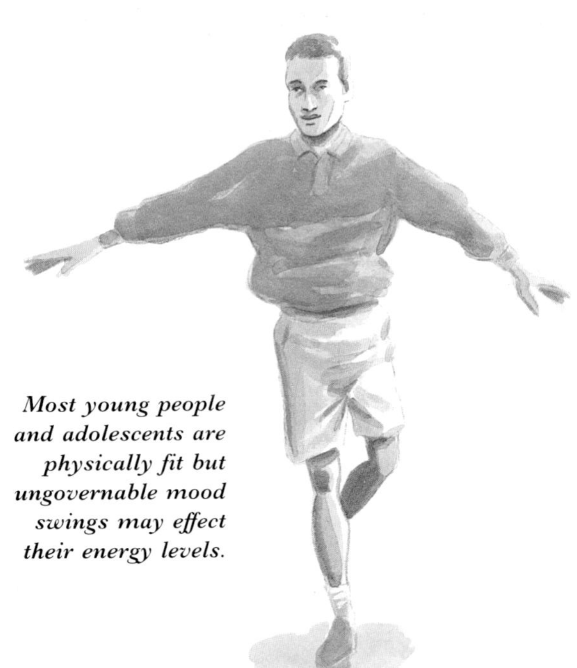

Most young people and adolescents are physically fit but ungovernable mood swings may effect their energy levels.

When does disease begin?

This is the first point to consider. Let us look at an example of acute illness that would naturally resolve in time. We commonly think of an illness as starting when the symptoms commence, like the lethargy and runny nose at the beginning of a cold. To understand homeopathy we must consider a little more deeply and look at the situation afresh.

Consider a crowded bus in the rush hour. Right in the center is one person with a streaming cold who is sneezing his head off. What happens next? During the following few days a number of people on the bus will go down with a cold and will likely blame the poor soul who was suffering on his journey home. But look a little more deeply and you will see that something else has happened too; if a number of people have gone down with the cold, does it not mean that a number of people have *not* gone down with the cold? So why, if the bugs that the sneezing man spread about the bus were the cause of the illness, did not everyone get a cold? What have we overlooked in blaming the man or his bugs for the cold?

It is, of course, quite obvious once we stop to think about it that the important difference between those that produced the cold and those that did not is that one group was susceptible to it whilst the other one was not. Plainly the dose of bugs is a factor too.

Disease and susceptibility

In order to become ill one has to be susceptible to that illness. If a person is not susceptible to an illness then he (or she) simply will not develop it. So when did all those people on the bus who went down with a cold become ill? When did the illness actually begin? We commonly think of the illness as the symptoms but perhaps we should take into consideration the individual's susceptibility because, as we have just seen, it is essential to the process of producing an illness that he or she be susceptible to it. With that in mind, how can we reasonably leave it out of our picture of disease?

When we consider the essential role of susceptibility it becomes plain that the people who caught a cold in the bus were 'ill' before they ever stepped onto it, for if they had been healthy they would never have picked up the bug in the first place. How long they had been 'carrying' their susceptibility to that cold around with them just waiting to meet up with the right bugs will depend upon the individual circumstances of each of them.

At this point there is a need to distinguish between two uses of the word 'disease' (or 'illness'). Commonly we consider a disease to be the symptoms that we experience when ill but if we are to take the susceptibility into account then we need a word to include it in this larger view of disease.

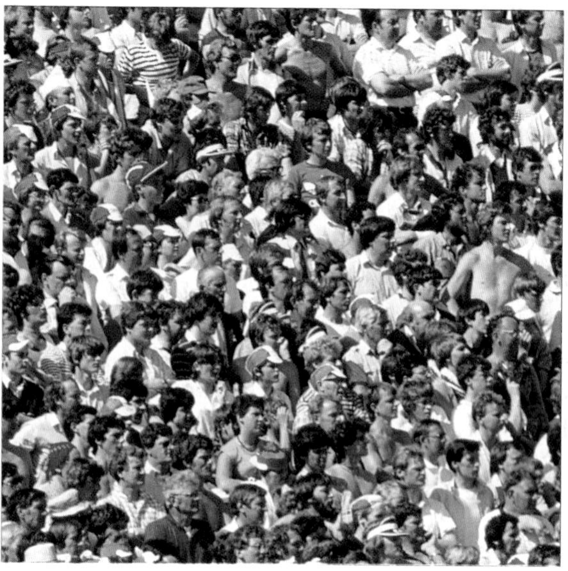

Some people seem to be more susceptible to illnesses than others. Not everyone who is exposed to a flu-ravaged stranger will succumb to the same bug. Stress may be a contributory factor.

Unfortunately, we have no such word in the English language. When the word 'disease' is used in the field of homeopathy it often should be understood to include the susceptibility and this should be apparent from the context.

Consider the susceptibility as the soil in which the seeds of disease are sown. If the soil is not right then the seeds will not grow. The seeds are all the external influences that tend to throw us out of balance and they may affect us on any level of our being; on the physical level it may be something simple like being exposed to a cold wind, getting soaked in the rain or even some form of trauma. They will all tend to put a stress on the system and depending on our health or susceptibility we will be affected to a greater or a lesser degree. On the emotional level, stresses come in many different forms; such as problems in relationships, or with family. On the mental level we may experience stresses from business problems and financial worries, the pressure of examinations and so on. Frequently the stresses involve a combination of these different levels.

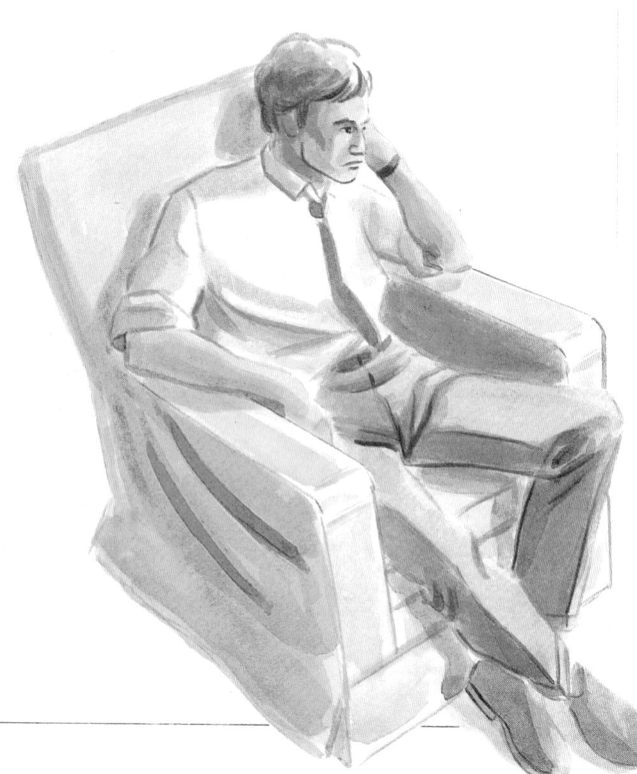

The mental stress brought on by financial worry or emotional problems can be as debilitating to the body as any more physical illness.

Natural healing powers

Our natural healing or life powers will cope with many of these stresses without ever producing any symptoms. It is as if our vitality is sufficient to stop those apparently unhelpful influences from having any effect. A point may be reached when the external stresses on any level become so great that in order to defend, repair and maintain order in the system the healing powers produce symptoms and signs of what we call an illness or disease. If our vitality is low then our susceptibility is high.

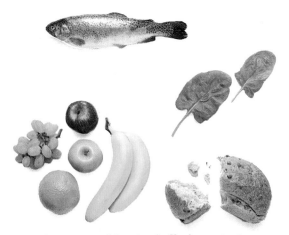

Correct nutrition is vitally important. A balanced diet which is low in fat, high in fiber, and rich in fruit and vegetables, provides the building blocks for good health.

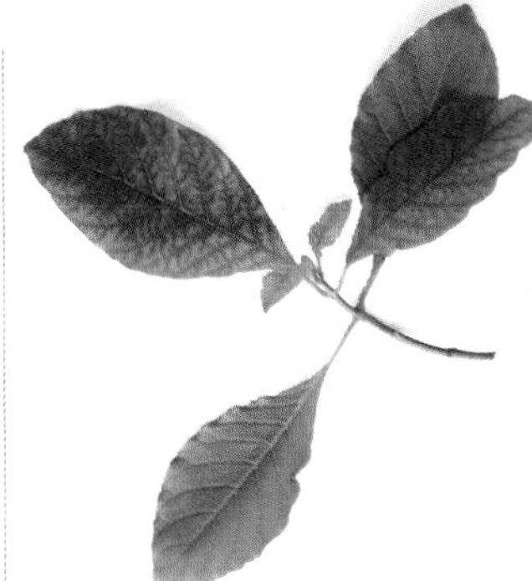

According to homeopathic thinking, quinine was such a spectacular success as an allopathic remedy for malaria because it produced the same symptoms as the disease in a healthy person. These are leaves from the quinine tree.

The body has an organizing intelligence that orders it and runs all the processes and functions of the parts and integrates them into the whole. It operates through the agencies of the different control systems such as the autonomic nervous system, hormonal system, immune system etc. Without this intelligence the body would rapidly cease to exist. This same intelligence is concerned with the natural healing power of the body. Is it sensible to consider that this natural intelligence, or healing power, would produce a situation that was without a purpose, for which no reason existed and which was harmful to the person when considered as a whole? It may cause damage to a part of the person but we should not lose sight of the whole person if we wish to understand what is going on.

ACUPUNCTURE

ACUPUNCTURE is an energy medicine which has an affinity with homeopathy. Both work on an energy or dynamic plane which exists alongside the physical and material plane. This energy has been described as that which makes the difference between a dead body and a living one; both have identical physical and chemical make-up, but when the vital force or life energy departs, the body stops functioning. When this force is reduced in effectiveness, the material constituents of the body are damaged, resulting in illness. By boosting the vital force, the body is able to rebalance its chemical and physical particles and health is restored. No amount of tinkering with the chemical elements can heal effectively and permanently unless the energy field holding them together is also repaired. The physical effects of energy disorders manifest as symptoms. In acupuncture, the energy, or *ch'i*, is considered to flow along pathways in the body called meridians. Needles are used to stimulate or slow down the flow of *ch'i* along the meridians as necessary. The art and skill of homeopathy is in the accurate matching up of the subtle energy patterns of the remedies with those of the diseased patient.

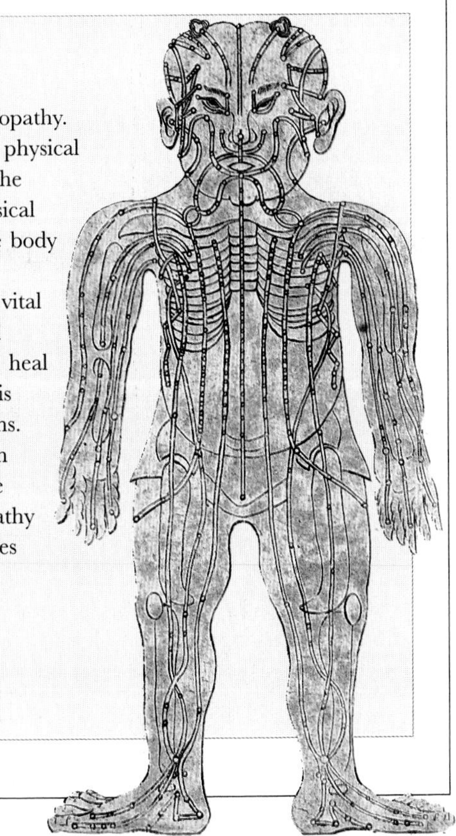

Acupuncture is an alternative medicine for many ailments. This seventeenth-century drawing shows the points at which acupuncture needles may be inserted.

What symptoms tell us

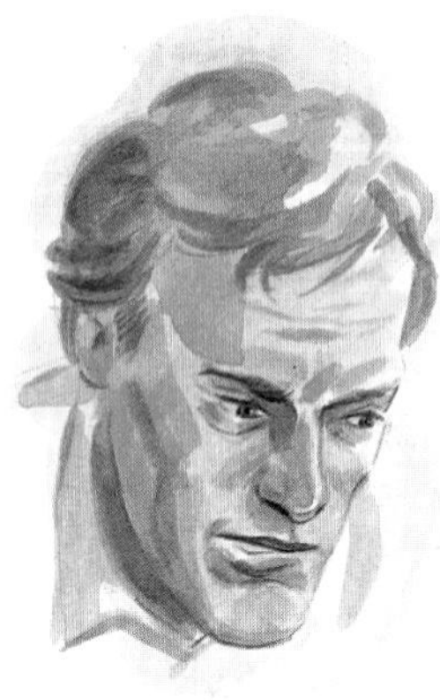

Homeopathy takes as much note of mental symptoms of distress as the physical ones. Many mental symptoms are typical of certain remedies.

What, then, is the purpose of disease symptoms? Is it not likely that the healing powers are continually trying to maintain order in the system but once the external stresses reach a certain level this can no longer be done 'passively'? The very attempt to keep a balance produces outward signs which we generally find uncomfortable and so call disease; which is literally a lack of ease or dis-ease. Viewed in this way the symptoms and signs of disease appear entirely different. They are no longer the inconvenient, unwanted, useless and 'why did I have to get it now?' things that they are commonly thought to be but they are actually the manifestation of each person's attempt to get well, to maintain order and balance in the system. They are the external effect of the internal fight to get well, recover and heal. They are not a part of becoming ill, which went on, generally unnoticed, beforehand, but are an important part of the body's healing process.

Now it becomes a little clearer why, in a young healthy child where 'disease' serves its function in its most simple and natural form, it has been observed that the child is more well after an acute ailment has resolved than she or he was before it started. It also becomes quite understandable why people tend to become ill when there are a lot of stresses going on in their lives and especially at times of life crises such as griefs, changes in work and divorce. Quite simply, these are times when there is more healing to be done, more effort is required by the natural healing powers to maintain order or, to put it slightly differently, it is no longer possible for a balance and harmony to be sustained without the production of symptoms of disease.

A further question may have arisen; why is the fertile soil or the susceptibility present in the first place? What gave rise to it? This is connected to questions about why some people are born with poor health and touches on some very deep aspects of philosophy which go

BOUNCING BACK

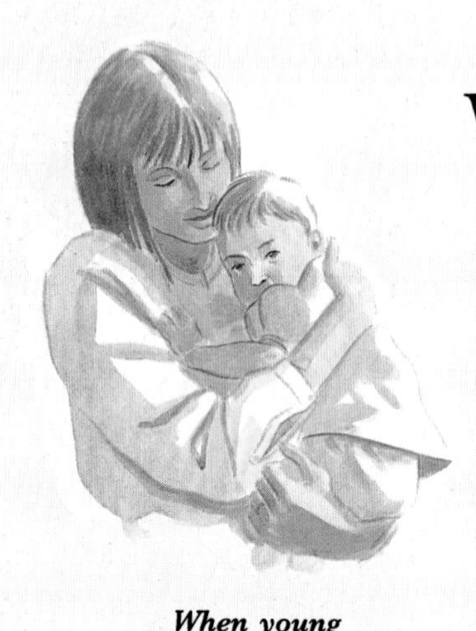

When young children fall ill, their mental and physical symptoms are easy to see.

When young children become ill, they do so frighteningly quickly; however, they often recover just as rapidly, and are up and running again very soon after any treatment. This may be because their energy levels are high and their vital force unencumbered. It is also reasonably easy to select the right remedy for a child, (especially your own, who you know well). Children are often easier to prescribe for homeopathically than adults, because they exhibit very clear remedy states. This is especially true for children too young to speak. You can take the case without verbal information from them, by observing their behavior carefully – how they play, how they sit, whether they are tearful or silent. Homeopathy works well on children as it does not interfere with their energy levels but works with them so that they can recover their healthy state as soon as possible.

When they recover, they become once again 'a picture of health'.

beyond the scope of this book. Suffice it to say that some people are better built at the beginning. They are constructed with few weaknesses and have a sound, strong constitution. These are the people who are often quoted as enjoying good health to a ripe old age despite smoking, drinking and never taking any exercise. These days there are not many of them around.

The key to homeopathic cure

How does homeopathy fit into this picture of disease? Once it is understood that the symptoms of disease are actually a good thing in that they are the highly characteristic outward indication of the healing and balancing process that is going on inside each individual person, then to give a medicine that is capable of mimicking and bringing about that same process suddenly seems to be a good idea; both totally reasonable and logical.

The key to homeopathy is that no two people suffer from the same disease. We each have our own highly individual ways of reacting to the stresses of life and of maintaining our inner harmony. Certainly there are broad similarities and a degree of categorization is possible but with detailed analysis there are always differences. After all, no two people are exactly the same. Take as an example a simple sore throat. Let us assume that we have selected 20 cases who all have the same bugs growing in their throats. The usual view is that they are all suffering from the same disease and yet it is plain that there are marked differences between the reaction of one patient to that of another. For instance, one may find marked relief from taking warm drinks which would make another feel much worse; one may have a high fever and sweats while another has no fever at all; one may be hot and want to be uncovered and in the fresh air while another is hot yet wants to be covered up to his chin; one may wish to continue his work while another might only wish to lie down and die, and so on.

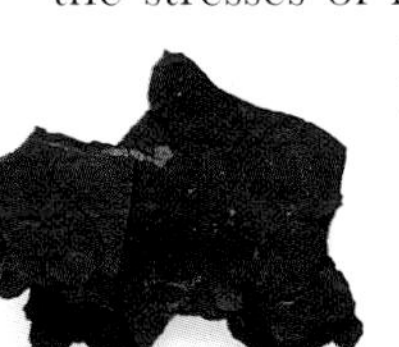

Carbo vegetabilis *may help in a sore throat case which is the result of a a cold spreading down from the nose.*

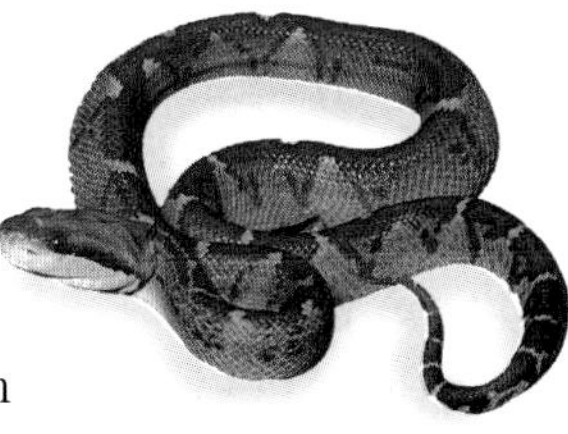

Lachesis *might be the remedy if the throat is sore but there is no inflammation and it feels as if a fishbone is stuck in the throat.*

These differences are an indication of the unique way in which each individual is responding to the circumstances in which he or she finds themself and of the state of that person as a whole, that is they show how his or her healing powers are operating at that time.

Now, if a medicine is given to a healthy person and it causes them to produce a particular reaction, a set of symptoms, then these are the healing responses that this particular medicine brings about. To put it another way, bearing in mind that symptoms are part of the healing process and not the disease process, then particular medicines will bring about particular healing responses, that is, symptoms.

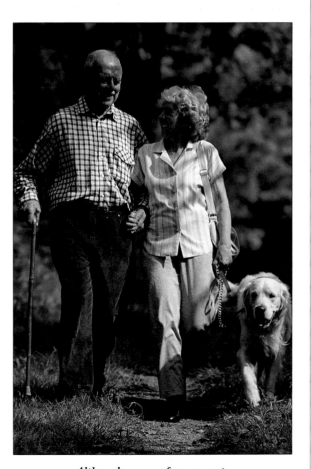

Although some of us seem to be programmed to suffer more illness than others, it's never too late to adopt a holistic approach to our own health.

Like cures like

It now makes perfect sense to give a remedy that is capable of bringing about the same or very similar healing responses, that is symptoms, to the healing response which is occurring in the patient as shown by the individual symptoms. Hence we have the Law of Similars which is very ancient and predates the formulation of homeopathy in the eighteenth century. It was known to Paracelsus in the fifteenth century, it can be found in the fourth century BC in Hippocratic writings and is one of the principles of treatment in Ayurvedic Medicine which was written down over 5,000 years ago. It states 'that which can cause a disease can also cure it' or 'like cures like'. It is interesting that examples of this law in operation are found in many different areas. In the field of cancer therapy it is well known that irradiation can cause tumors and yet they can also be treated by radiation and many of the drugs used in chemotherapy for tumors can also cause tumors. Digitoxin can cause heart irregularities, or arrhythmias, but it is also very useful in the treatment of certain arrhythmias.

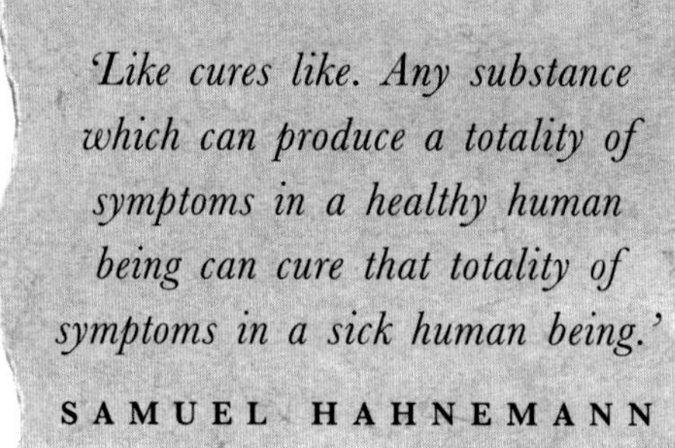
'Like cures like. Any substance which can produce a totality of symptoms in a healthy human being can cure that totality of symptoms in a sick human being.'

SAMUEL HAHNEMANN

Many of these seemingly contradictory properties of the agents are related to dose. The healthier a person is, the higher the dose necessary to throw that person out of balance, as shown by the appearance of symptoms and signs. In disease, even a small stimulus, if it is aligned with the healing process of the individual, will have an effect. Nevertheless, a higher dose or one not sufficiently matched to the individual will still tend to overstimulate and may then cause what are

THE LAW OF SIMILARS

The Law of Similars was Hahnemann's second principle, formulated in 1796. His paper, 'An Experiment Concerning a New Principle for Determining the Medicinal Powers of Drugs', described this principle, which was based on the testing of drugs on healthy human subjects.

HAHNEMANN CONCLUDED:

Every active principle provokes its own kind of disease, as it were, in the human organism. We should imitate nature, for she often cures a chronic disease with another that comes in new. When it is a question of curing a particular disease (especially chronic disease), we should therefore use a drug which is capable of provoking another, artificial disease that resembles the original disease as closely as possible. SIMILIA SIMILIBUS.

The Law of Similars was put more succinctly in the *Organon of Practical Medicine:*

To achieve a gentle and lasting cure, always choose a drug capable of provoking a disease similar (homion pathos) *to the one it is to cure.*

The patient's symptoms are matched against symptoms produced by the drug action on healthy subjects. When the picture fits, that remedy is chosen.

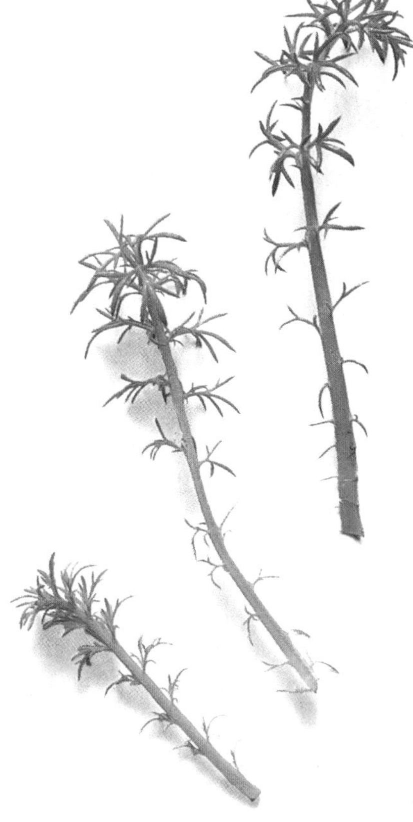
Chamomilla ***is a remedy made from wild chamomile. It is indicated for temper tantrums, especially in children.***

PASTEUR AND VACCINATION

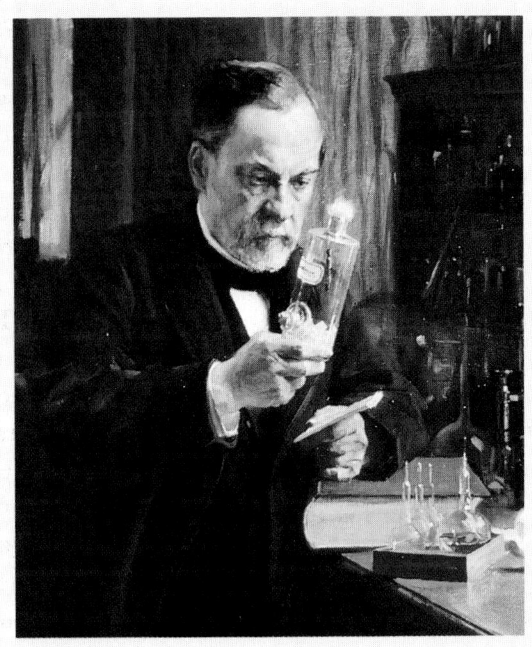

Louis Pasteur (1822-95) pioneered vaccination as a prevention for disease. Many people think that vaccination is a homeopathic action, but this is not the case. Vaccination infects a person with tiny amounts of the actual disease whereas homeopathy prescribes a remedy to produce the same symptoms of the disease. Vaccination takes no account of the individual state, giving everyone the same remedy, whereas homeopathy is predicated on the study of the individual. That is why different people react differently to vaccination. Homeopathy can be very helpful to counteract the side-effects of orthodox vaccination, especially the catarrhal problems and 'glue ear' suffered by many children as a result of the polio-diphtheria-tetanus vaccinations they are routinely given throughout childhood.

Louis Pasteur, the French chemist and bacteriologist, devised methods of immunization against anthrax and rabies.

usually called side-effects. The closer the stimulus or medicine is aligned to the healing in the patient the lower the dose of drug needed; they are more susceptible to it. The unwanted effects, which are an indication of the mismatch between the powers of the drug and those of the patient either in quality (the type of medicine used) or in quantity (the dose administered), are fewer.

Silica ***is a remedy made from silicon, which is also used in the electronics industry to make silicon chips. Silicon is chosen because it is particularly inert;*** **Silica** ***the remedy is indicated for people with no mental or physical energy, who prefer inertia to action.***

This explains a phenomenon frequently observed in homeopathy; often after the administration of the indicated remedy there is a brief and mild worsening of the symptoms followed by their gradual resolution. This is due to the stimulus of the remedy causing the healing powers to respond. In principle if the dose were to exactly meet the requirements of the patient there would be no observable reaction before the resolution took place. In practice this rarely happens and a mild reaction is commonly produced.

It can be seen that the correct dose of the correct medicine will aid a person's healing. Give too much and it may bring about the very conditions it is capable of curing.

'Through the like, disease is produced and through the application of the like it is cured'

HIPPOCRATES

Making the remedies

All kinds of substances are used to create homeopathic remedies: plants, animals, minerals and even diseased tissue. Over 2,000 have been proved to date and their drug pictures noted.

Remedies made from plants may be made from the whole plant or just a part of it, such as the flower or root. Plants used as homeopathic remedy sources include any which are also well known in their unpotentized state as herbal remedies, such as Hypericum and Calendula.

Other remedies come from animals, and often the most deadly beasts produce the most powerful healing remedies, such as those from the tarantula spider and the rattlesnake.

Minerals, of which one of the most frequently used is common salt, and metals such as gold, iron, and copper also have an important place in the *Materia Medica*. There is an additional group of remedies made from chemical compounds known as tissue salts.

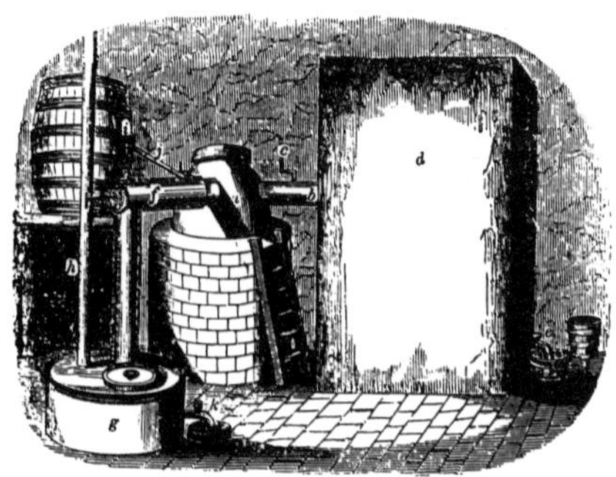

Sulphur is the source of a very important homeopathic remedy. This early engraving shows the apparatus for purifying crude sulphur by distillation.

In the process of manufacturing homeopathic remedies from plants or organic matter, the first step is to create a mother tincture. This is usually done by extracting the juices of the plant and adding them to equal amounts of alcohol. After 24 hours, solid particles have settled out and the liquid is decanted and stored away from sunlight. Organic matter is infused in alcohol for days or weeks and the result is strained into a storage jar.

Where the original substance is insoluble, such as lead, a method known as trituration is used. Here a portion of the substance is ground together

A pestle and mortar is used to grind up insoluble or inorganic remedy sources so that they can be dissolved in alcohol. The process is called trituration.

MAKE YOUR OWN REMEDY

NATRUM MURIATICUM is a remedy you can make for yourself at home provided you have the time and the patience. By making it yourself by hand you will be adding your own subtle energy to the remedy which will give it an extra element when you use it.

- In a wine glass place 5ml (1tsp) of rock salt and fill the glass with spring water. Stir well with a plastic (not metal) spoon until all the salt has dissolved. This is your mother tincture.
- Take 5ml (1tsp) of mother tincture and place in a screw top bottle, then add 45ml (3tbsp) of spring water. Make sure the lid is firmly screwed on and holding the bottle by the neck, tap the base of the bottle firmly on a thick book or hard cushion 20 times. This will give you a 1x potency.
- Discard all but 5ml (1tsp) of the resulting liquid. Return to the bottle and add a further 45ml (3tbsp) of spring water. Carry out a further 20 succussions as before. This will give a 2x potency.
- Repeat this process four more times, each time take 5ml (1tsp) of the original liquid, add 45ml (3tbsp) of spring water and succuss 20 times. The result is a 6x potency of *Natrum muriaticum.*
- To store your remedy mix it with alcohol in the proportion of 10% remedy to 90% vodka and keep in a dark glass bottle. This remedy will be very strong. To use it, add one drop to a glass of water.

NATRUM MURIATICUM

YOU WILL NEED:

- *Pure rock salt*
- *Spring water*
- *Plastic spoon*
- *Small screw top jar*
- *Alcohol*

(Vodka is recommended)

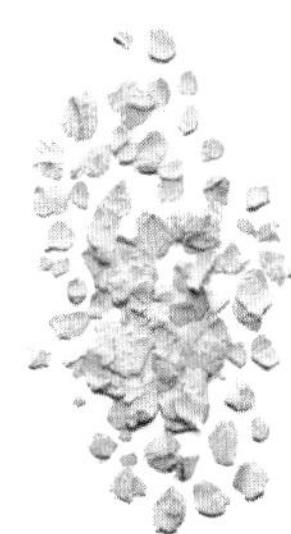

Grain cereals contain magnesium phosphate, the source of* Magnesia phosphorica *which is one of a group of remedies known as tissue salts.

NOSODES

NOSODES are homeopathic remedies made from a disease product. Hahnemann's first nosode was made from a scabies vesicle, and was called psorinum (after the Greek *psora*, meaning itch). Later homeopaths potentized other nosodes, including *tuberculinum* (from tubercular tissue), *Carcinosin* (a nosode of cancer) and *Medorrhinum* (from gonorrheal discharge). Nosodes are indicated for constitutional remedies and should only be prescribed by a homeopathic practitioner.

with lactose (milk sugar) powder. This is extremely time consuming and very laborious, for example the grinding process required to produce a 3c potency (see pages 34-5) of an insoluble substance can take nine hours when done by hand, so modern pharmacies which produce remedies in bulk and to very high potencies, have machines to do the hard work. Once the substance is ground to the 3c potency, it is soluble in alcohol.

Remedies are prepared in the form of tinctures, granules, powders, tablets (where the liquid has been infused over bland tablets so they acquire the potentized remedy) and in some first aid remedies, as creams for external use.

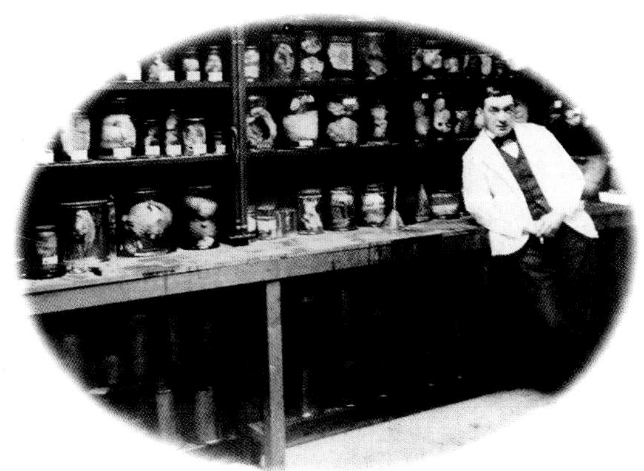

Not a shopkeeper in front of his shelves, but the London Homeopathic Hospital's collection of pickled organs!

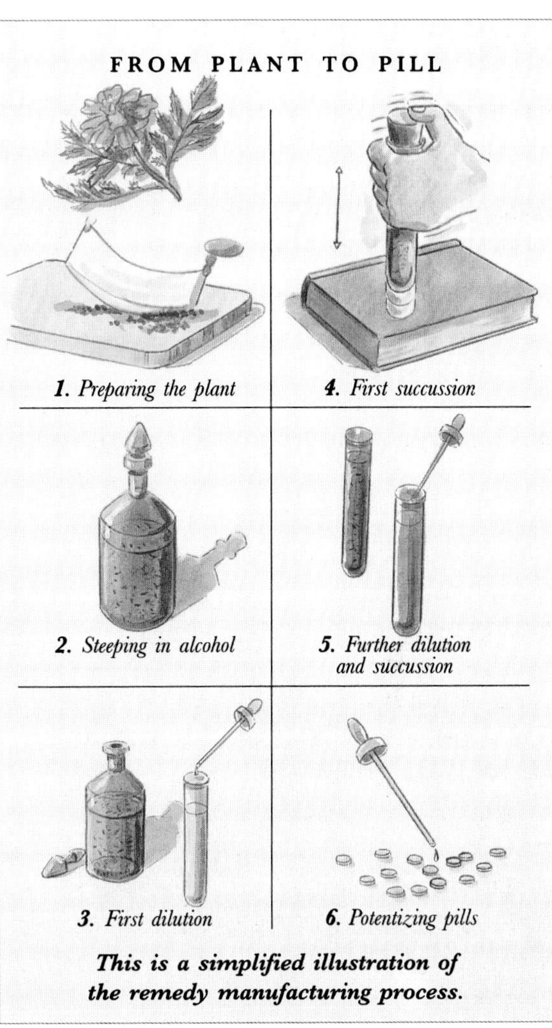

This is a simplified illustration of the remedy manufacturing process.

Hahnemann considered that homeopaths should prepare their own remedies themselves, or obtain them from pharmacists who were themselves homeopathic practitioners. Today, many homeopaths make their own most commonly prescribed remedies. There is some evidence to show that hand-prepared remedies are more dynamic, that is, work better on the energy plane, than machine made potencies.

Releasing the healing energy

Because homeopathy uses the energy of substances rather than their chemical properties, a system had to be discovered that would release this energy and make it available for assimilation into the body.

This system is called potentization, and it is the result of repeated dilution and succussion (vibration) of the mother tincture until the material content of the remedy disappears and only the energy pattern remains.

Potentization

Hahnemann discovered the principle of potentization – central to homeopathy – when he was conducting clinical trials to prove (test) his remedies. Clearly, strong poisons could not be administered in dangerous doses to test their effects. Hahnemann therefore experimented with finding the minimum dose for his provings, an approach in sympathy with his idea that substances should be used curatively in the smallest possible amounts at which they were still effective, since they were to stimulate the body's healing powers rather than attack a disease. It was found that tiny quantities of the substance being tested could have effective results, and indeed that some provers had a greater response when the substance was greatly diluted.

Less is more

In his first series of provings, Hahnemann administered the remedies in the form of a tincture. It soon became clear that the remedies were more potent when they were diluted. If one part of the tincture was added to 99 parts of alcohol, its powers, if anything, seemed enhanced. This is what is known as potentization. To ensure that the tincture was thoroughly mixed during dilution, the phial was rhythmically shaken and Hahnemann found that this increased the effectiveness of the remedy. This shaking is known as succussion. Chemically, progressive dilution soon results in not one single molecule of the original substance remaining in the remedy, and one might expect that at this point the remedy would have no effect, yet the opposite seemed to be true – remedies subjected to repeated dilution and succussion were more powerful than the original tinctures from which they had been prepared.

POTENCIES AND THEIR DILUTIONS

DECIMAL SCALE		CENTESIMAL SCALE	
DILUTION	POTENCY	DILUTION	POTENCY
$\frac{1}{10}$	1X	$\frac{1}{10}$	1C
$\frac{1}{10^2}$	2X	$\frac{1}{10^4}$	2C
$\frac{1}{10^3}$	3X	$\frac{1}{10^6}$	3C
$\frac{1}{10^6}$	6X	$\frac{1}{10^{12}}$	6C
$\frac{1}{10^9}$	9X	$\frac{1}{10^{18}}$	9C
$\frac{1}{10^{12}}$	12X	$\frac{1}{10^{24}}$	12C

THE CHART shows the decimal and centesimal scale of potencies, indicating how many dilutions it takes to produce a certain potency. In the decimal scale, one part of the mother tincture (and subsequent dilutions) is diluted in nine parts of alcohol or water, and the potencies are diluted ten times each time; in the centesimal scale, one part of the mother tincture (and subsequent dilutions) is diluted in 99 parts alcohol or water and the potencies are diluted 100 times each time. Most classical homeopaths prefer the centesimal scale, as did Hahnemann himself for most of his life.

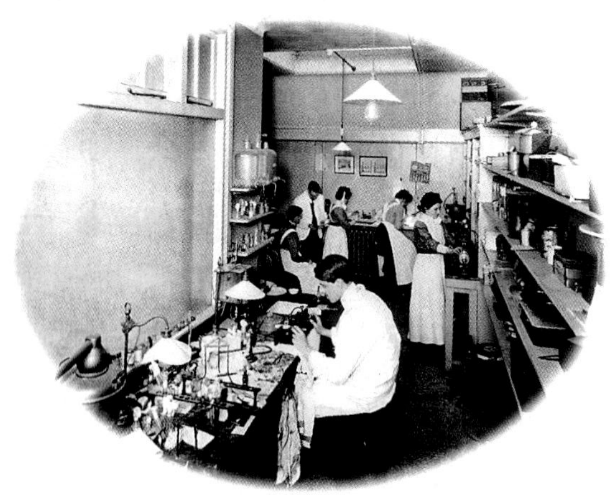

Preparing remedies in the laboratory of the London Homeopathic Hospital.

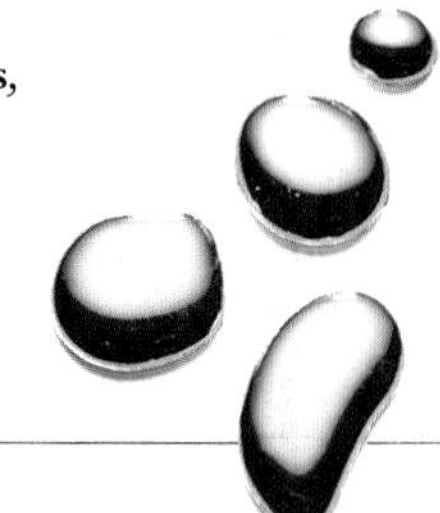

Bicyanide of mercury, the source for **Mercurius cyanatus**, *is extremely poisonous itself, but when it is potentized its energy is released while its poison is discarded.*

KENT'S CENTESIMAL PROGRESSION

6C, 12C, 30C, 200C, M, 10M, CM

ABOVE you can see a centesimal scale progression devised by Dr James Tyler Kent, an American homeopath, who practiced in Chicago in the nineteenth century. The centesimal scale was already established, but Kent favored remedies made to these specific potencies only. He found they were useful in the treatment of psychosomatic disorders among others. In the scale, M means 1,000 dilutions and succussions, 10M is 10,000 and CM is 100,000. The more a remedy is diluted and succussed, the more powerful it becomes. Towards the end of his life, Hahnemann developed a millesimal scale, in which the remedy was diluted by one part to 49,999 for each potency, producing very high potencies indeed.

Scales of potency

Although any potency can be created, homoeopaths generally work according to a scale which has been found to give harmonious progress to treatment. The most commonly used scales are the centesimal (c) and decimal (x). Remedies are sold with their potency clearly marked – for example *Pulsatilla* 6x, *Ant. crud.* 30c. Where neither an x or a c is given against the number the remedy will be a c.

The centesimal scale is named after the Latin for 100 because one part of the mother tincture is mixed with 99 parts of double-distilled water or alcohol and succussed to create 1c. One part of this dilution is then mixed with a further 99 parts water/alcohol and succussed to create a 2c. When this process has been repeated six times the 6c potency is reached, which is the lowest potency at which remedies are commonly sold and used.

Where trituration is used the process involves grinding one part of the substance with 99 parts of lactose powder to produce a 1c potency. One part of the resulting powder is then added to a further 99 parts lactose powder and ground to create a 2c potency. After 3c the substance becomes soluble and further potencies are produced in the usual manner by dilution and succussion.

When the process has been repeated 30 times the 30c potency is achieved. This potency is also sold over the counter but higher potencies have to be obtained direct from a reputable homeopathic pharmacy and should not be used by anyone who has not had a certain amount of professional training in homeopathy, because they can bring about strong and dramatic reactions.

As a general guide lower potencies are suited to conditions with much physical pathology and higher potencies are indicated where there is a marked mental and emotional picture. Because higher potencies penetrate deeper within the individual, it becomes more important to match the remedy accurately. Generally, dosage of higher potencies is not repeated as frequently as that of lower potencies.

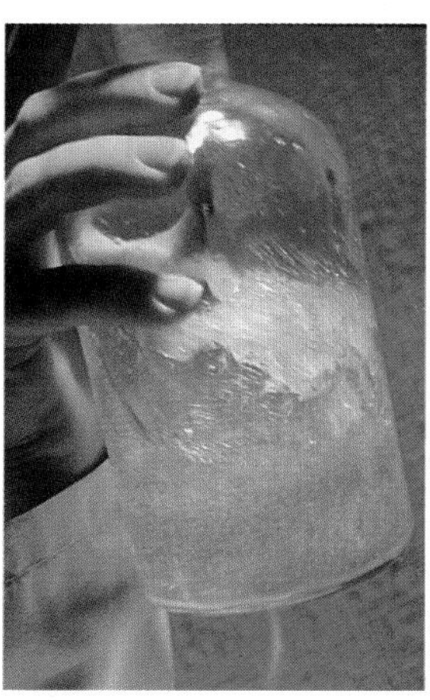

Succussion is the mixing of an original tincture with a neutral liquid, to form different potencies of the remedy. Now carried out by machine, this process of rhythmic shaking may take up to 12 weeks.

HOMEOPATHY AND ANIMALS

A 1984 experiment carried out on pigs attempted to reduce stillbirths amongst sows by using a homeopathic remedy. Stillbirths were successfully reduced by ten percent. Many domestic animals have also been shown to respond to homeopathic remedies.

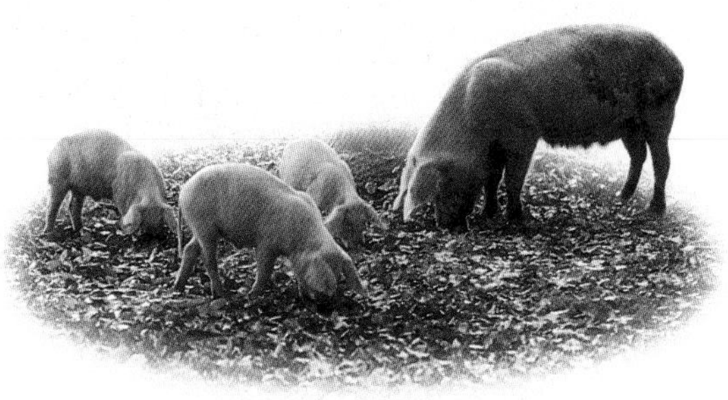

Testing the remedies

How is the capability of each remedy known? How is the picture which determines its use ascertained? Very simply by giving the remedy to a group of healthy people in a carefully controlled and closely monitored fashion. All the changes and symptoms that arise are noted and studied to detect patterns and trends that are characteristic and commonly occur. These are likely to be of great importance when prescribing the remedy for a patient. This process is called a proving of the remedy and strict criteria are laid down in order to ensure that the true action of the remedy is brought out and not any interferences from other sources. A properly conducted proving may last for many months.

Once the proving picture is obtained then enough is known about the remedy to start using it in practice. Subsequently, when the remedy is given to treat sick people, other

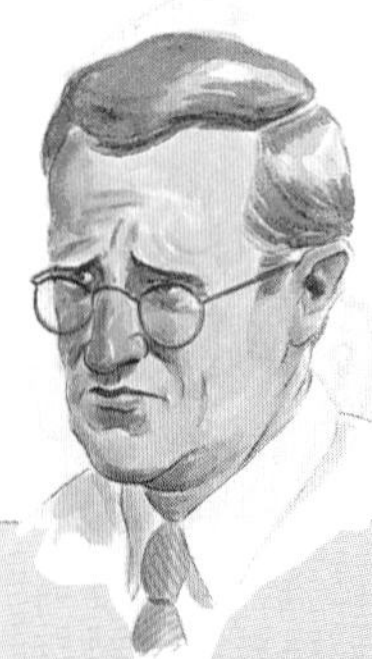

BRYONIA ALBA

BRYONIA was one of the early remedies proved by Hahnemann and the results were published in the second volume of his *Materia Medica Pura*. It already had a reputation in folk medicine, and it had been noted by the herbalist Nicolas Culpeper and used by physicians Dioscorides and Galen, which may have prompted Hahnemann to choose it. In the healthy person, *Bryonia* produces inertia, vertigo, frontal headache, hot eyes that feel full of dust, dryness in nose and throat, early morning diarrhea, and stitching, tearing pains in the chest, neck, back, and limbs. Cold and cool drinks make them feel better, heat makes things worse. Muscular effort is impossible, lying still brings relief. The typical Bryonia patient finds comfort in immobility, in holding everything in. See pages 52 to 53 for more information.

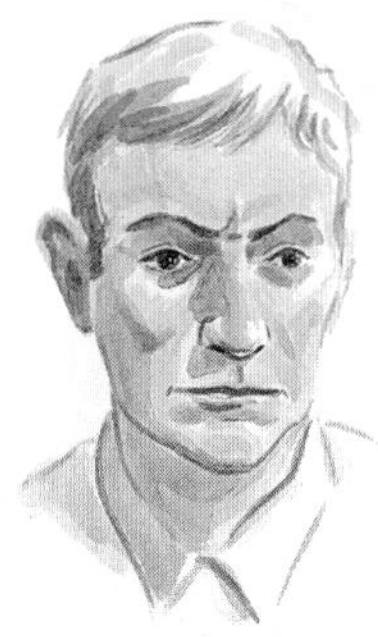

HYOSCYAMUS NIGER

HYOSCYAMUS was proved by Hahnemann and the results published in the fourth volume of his *Materia Medica Pura*. Its properties were noted by Pliny. In the healthy person, *Hyoscyamus* produces giddiness, tinnitus and disturbed vision, with spots before the eyes or objects suddenly appearing enormous, a dry cough with thick catarrh, tender abdomen, constipation, cramps, and uncertain gait. Lying down or being touched makes things worse, walking about or sitting up makes things better. All symptoms are worse at night. The typical Hyoscyamus patient may suffer from delusions and hallucinations, mutter irrationally, stagger about and pluck compulsively at bedcovers or clothes. See page 78 for more information.

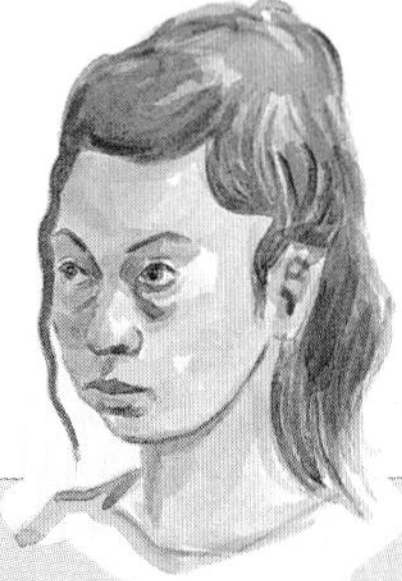

NATRUM MURIATICUM

NATRUM MURIATICUM was proved by Hahnemann and the results published in the first edition of his *Chronic Diseases*. In the healthy person, *Natrum muriaticum* produces migraine-like headaches with nausea, the sensation of grit in the eyes, 'crackling in the ears' when eating, recurrent colds, tightness in the lungs, mouth ulcers, low backache, heavy leaden feet, skin problems (acne, eczema, boils, warts). Extreme heat, hot, stuffy rooms and physical exertion make things worse, and symptoms are aggravated during the menstrual period. Open air, washing in cold water and very gentle exercise brings relief. The typical Natrum muriaticum patient may suffer from excessive mood swings, hypersensitivity and shun sympathy. See page 95 for more information.

> *...when remedies cure they do so only through their ability to alter human health by causing characteristic symptoms,*
>
> SAMUEL HAHNEMANN

symptoms that had not been brought out in the proving are noted to be cured by the remedy and if this happens repeatedly then those symptoms are added to the picture of that remedy.

So gradually a fuller understanding of the actions of the remedies is obtained, enabling them to be used with greater accuracy. This process has continued from one generation of homeopaths to the next so that instead of the new discoveries sweeping away all the previous ideas, as commonly occurs in many 'scientific' studies, the knowledge of the remedies, known as the *Materia Medica*, is continually being added to, developed and refined.

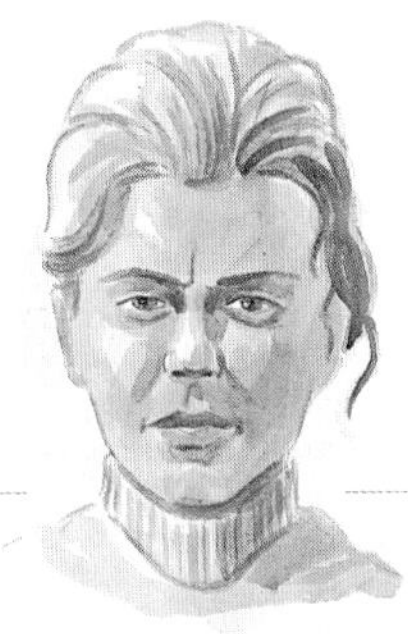

NUX VOMICA

NUX VOMICA was proved by Hahnemann and the results published in the third edition of his *Materia Medica Pura*. In the healthy person, *Nux vomica* produces sudden bouts of exhaustion, heavy painful limbs, momentary blackouts, 'hangover headaches', dry tickling cough, sudden hot flushes while eating, muscular spasms and night cramps. Everything is worse in cold, dry weather, after eating and early in the morning. Wet weather and lying down make things better, as does vomiting, and evenings are the best time of day. The typical Nux vomica patient feels the cold badly, is fussy, tense and overanxious and given to peevish outbursts. See page 98 for more information.

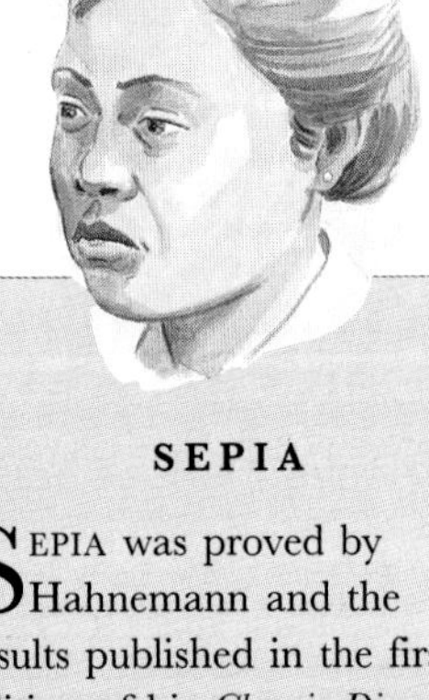

SEPIA

SEPIA was proved by Hahnemann and the results published in the first edition of his *Chronic Diseases*. In the healthy person, *Sepia* produces extreme tiredness, pins and needles, cold feet or hands, cramps and flushes, sick headaches, a hacking cough, bouts of faintness, menstrual problems in women, weakness in the limbs (especially knees), low back pain and itchy skin rashes. Warmth, vigorous exercise and food make things better; cold, dull weather, menstrual periods and evening make things worse. The typical Sepia patient feels immensely sad, tearful, exhausted and apathetic, unable to cope. See page 109 for more information.

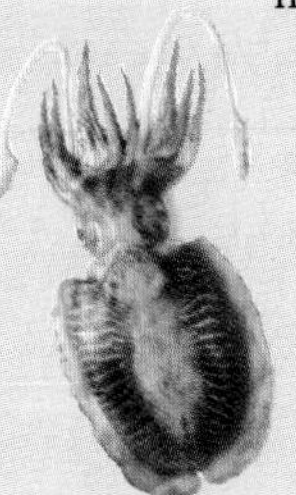

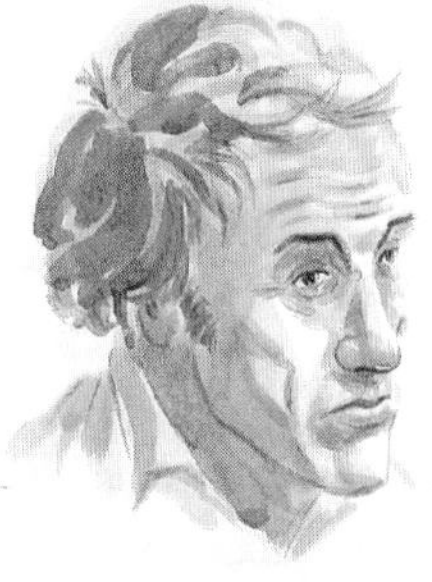

SULPHUR

SULPHUR was proved by Hahnemann and the results published in the fourth edition of his *Materia Medica Pura*. In the healthy person, *Sulphur* produces dizziness, dryness in the scalp and hair loss, sick headaches, sticky discharge from the eyes, oversensitive hearing, dry, sore throat, asthmatic attacks, heartburn, indigestion, kidney pains, backache, night cramps, itchy skin or eruptions such as boils. Heat makes things worse as does severe cold; there is sensitivity to water; standing still and stooping aggravate. The typical Sulphur patient feels contemptuous of others, is inconsiderate, self-centered and quick tempered; they may also be hypochondriacal, self-pitying and always hungry. See pages 114 to 115 for more information.

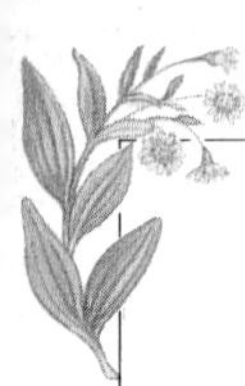
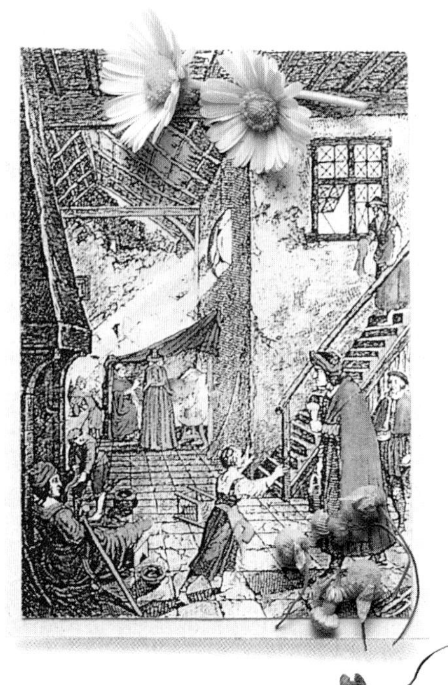
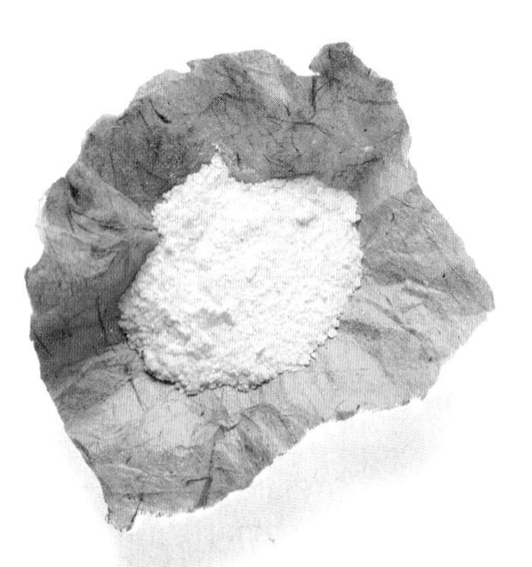
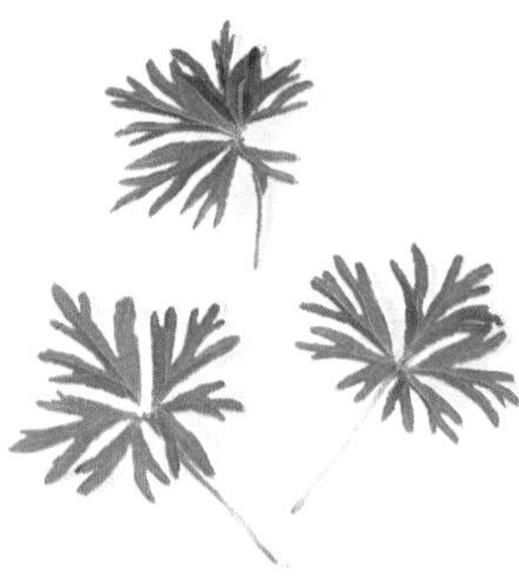
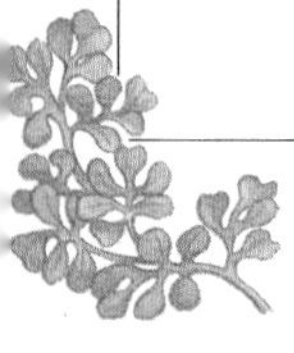

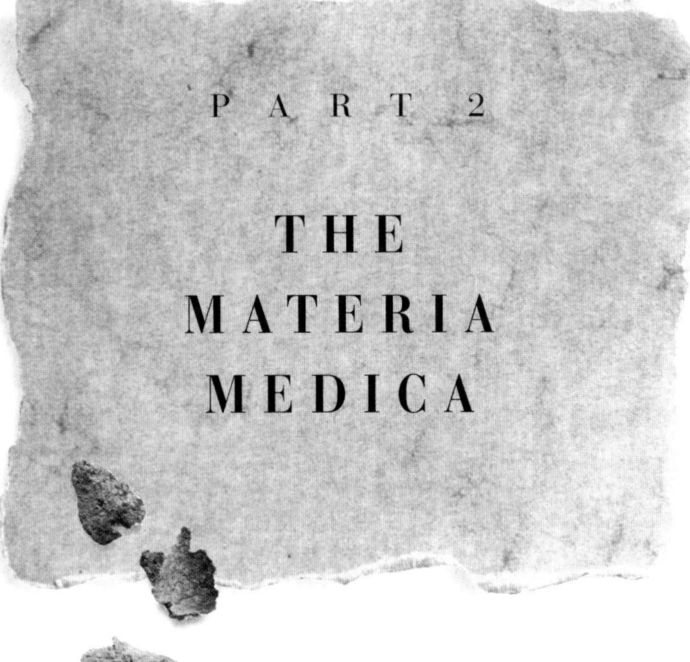

PART 2

THE MATERIA MEDICA

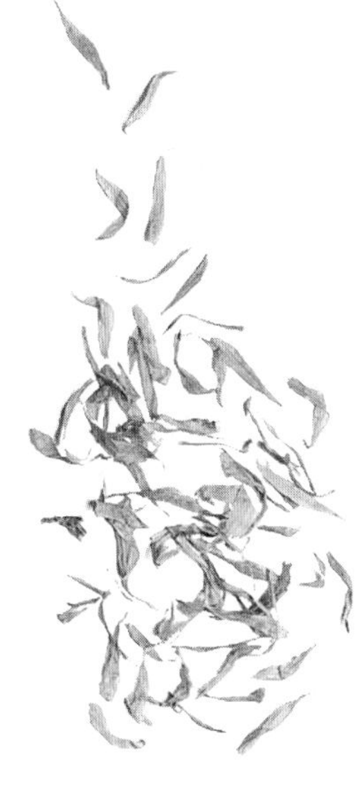

INTRODUCTION

Many remedies are made from exotic sources. The tarantula spider is asphixiated and pickled in alcohol to make the Tarantula hispania *remedy, indicated for mania and hyperactivity.*

A materia medica *describes the science and properties of substances used in medicine; it is not exclusive to homeopathy. However, an allopathic* materia medica *describes the effect of drugs on a disease, with the sick patient as the experimental laboratory; in contrast, the homeopathic* materia medica *describes what state the potentized remedy brings about in a healthy person. The symptoms brought on by the remedy in a healthy person mirror the symptoms presented spontaneously by a person in the diseased state.*

All the symptoms of the state are noted, physical, mental and peculiar. In homeopathy, this is an open-ended process. New symptoms are not seen as contradictory or thought to invalidate the remedy.

The fatally poisonous toadstool, fly agaric, is the source for the Agaricus muscarius *remedy.*

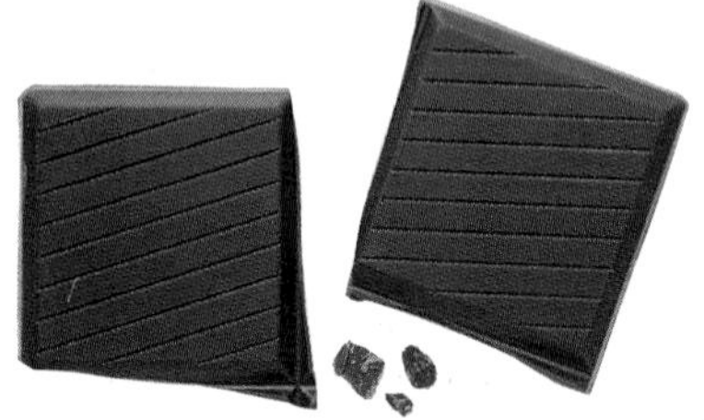

One of the remedies now being proved is made from chocolate; it is said to help chocaholic excess.

If more provings and research indicate additional or different symptoms, they are simply added to the existing picture of the state. Hahnemann, the founder of homeopathy, set out his provings in Materia Medica Pura *(titled in German* Reine Arzneimittellehre*), published in six volumes between 1825 and 1827, and in the five-part work* Chronic Diseases *(1828 to 1839).*

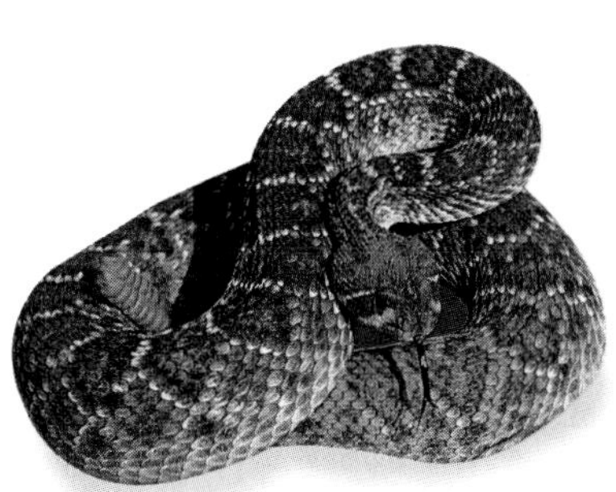

The North American rattlesnake is the source for the Crotalis horridus *remedy for nervous shock and malignant septic conditions. The mother tincture is made from the venom.*

This illustrated materia medica *describes all the remedies indicated in this book with the exception of some specifics for breastfeeding problems. It is by no means exhaustive. There are some 2,000 homeopathic remedies to date, made from a wide variety of sources, and more are being proved all the time. For example, work is being done on potentized remedies made from chocolate and human milk.*

The remedies are listed in alphabetical order so that when you have chosen a remedy for the case you are treating, you can easily find out more about it. For each remedy, the full name is given together with any abbreviations you may come across. Under the heading The Main Symptom Picture, *all the major symptoms are shown, listed from the head downwards, in the classical homeopathic style; the most important are emphasized in bold type. The personality of each remedy, the mental state, is briefly outlined in a self-contained paragraph, and some information on the remedy source is given. The text is written in an informal, note-taking style, just as you might jot down your own observations when taking a case and formal and medical terms are kept to a minimum. Medical terms outside normal vocabulary and particular homeopathic terms for pain are explained in the Glossary.*

Gold, the source for the Aurum *remedy. This was the remedy indicated for the defenestrating plutocrats of the great Wall Street crash of the 1920s.*

Aconitum napellus

- **Suddenness and intensity**
- **Exposure to cold, especially very cold dry weather and then ill the same day**
- **Great excitement of the circulation**
- **Fear**
- **Awful anxiety, anguish, great restlessness**
- **Oversensitivity and burning pains**
- **Great thirst for cold water**
- **Bright red in its inflammations**

INTRODUCTION

Suddenness and intensity mark out Aconite. A great storm that suddenly appears and is soon over. If the condition lingers or does not have much intensity, it is not Aconite. Aconite is not feeble! Vigorous, robust, healthy, rugged outdoor types, and energetic children are typical of this remedy picture. Aconite *and* Acon. *are the abbreviations for this remedy.*

THE MAIN SYMPTOM PICTURE

There is sudden, violent illness, a raging fever, often precipitated by a period of considerable **exposure to cold, especially very cold dry weather; illness occurs the same day**. *Aconite* can also come in for gastric complaints following intensely hot weather. Illnesses may follow a fright, especially in children.

REMEDY SOURCE

Aconite is made from *Aconitum napellus*, also known as monk's-hood or wolf's-bane. It grows in damp, shady places in hilly areas, bursting into vigorous bloom in high summer. *Aconite* is extremely poisonous and should not be touched or eaten. The whole plant is used to prepare the remedy.

There is great **excitement of the circulation**; a full, fast pulse; great nervousness and excitement without much delirium. **Awful anxiety, fear, anguish, great restlessness** with the **suddenness and violence** of the illness.

Marked congestion of the head and the person is hot. The remedy is often needed in the first stage of high-grade inflammations, fevers and congestions with great anxiety, heat and restlessness; the patient tosses about, throws off the covers. The skin and the senses are **oversensitive and burning** pains are characteristic but there may also be stinging, stabbing, tearing, cutting pains with numbness, tingling and crawling. **Intense pains,** neuralgic pains, person cannot bear to be touched, worse at night and especially in the evening.

Aconite, the source for **Aconitum napellus.** *It was first proved by Hahnemann and appears in the first volume of his* **Materia Medica Pura.**

There is great **dryness** and with it **great thirst for cold water**. Characteristically the skin is dry and hot with no sweat. Worse in a warm room and under warm covers, better uncovered.

Violent headaches which may be from exposure to a dry, cold wind that has stopped a nasal catarrh from flowing.

There may be **photophobia** in fever with small contracted pupils.

Aconite is **bright red in its inflammations**, congested face etc., though may turn pale on rising up. It is not dusky or mottled and it has no results of inflammation such as suppuration, or thick green or yellow purulent discharges. There is continued fever; Aconite is over quickly, in a night.

Everything may taste bitter, except water. Patients may crave bitter things in a fever. There is a burning, smarting and dryness of the throat with great redness and may be swelling.

Violent, sudden nausea and vomiting.

Patient may go to sleep. The larynx becomes dry and he or she may wake with spasms in the throat thinking he or she will choke. Croupy, choking, violent, dry cough with hoarse barking coming on in the night after being chilled in the day; intense febrile excitement. Suffocating cough. **Croup arising after exposure to cold, dry air**. Dry mucous membranes. A short dry cough, maybe a little watery mucus.

Other remedies will be needed if *Aconite* does not suffice and the condition lingers.

THE ACONITE PERSONALITY

The person who needs *Aconite* is in a state of fear, panic and ungovernable impatience. The fear may be of death, crowds or of vague unnameable horrors; of course, the Aconite state may be precipitated by a real threat. The person is easily startled, and may be agitated. There is a great aversion to being touched.

Allium cepa

- **Complaints often from cold, damp, penetrating winds**
- **Principally of use in colds and coughs**
- **Copious watering of the eyes, bland watery discharge**
- **Watery nasal discharge which is acrid and excoriates the skin**
- **Worse for warmth, and in the evenings**

INTRODUCTION

Allium is the remedy often indicated at the early, 'streaming' stage of a cold, when the sufferer looks as if he or she has been peeling onions on an industrial scale. It may also be useful for some hay fevers, but careful case-taking is necessary in all hay fever situations as it would be more effective to find out exactly what triggers the attacks. Allium *and* All. c. *are the abbreviations for this remedy.*

THE MAIN SYMPTOM PICTURE

Complaints often from cold, damp penetrating winds and this remedy is **principally of use in colds and coughs**.

Copious watering of the eyes producing bland, watery nasal discharge which is acrid and excoriates the skin of the nose and upper lip are the strong characteristics of this remedy. All phases of the cold are **worse for warmth** except the tickling in the larynx which can be worse for drawing in cold air.

Worse in the evenings too. Coryza worse indoors, better in the open air.

Rawness of the mucous membranes. Tearing, painful larynx with each cough. Nose drips and burns with a sore upper lip and wings of the nose, red and raw. **Sneezing** comes early and with increasing frequency. Watery nasal discharge and obstruction goes from left to right nostril.

Much **congestion**; full, congestive headache often; fullness in the nose, may be throbbing and burning and sometimes nosebleeds.

Dull frontal headache, occipital headache; pains in the jaws go to the head. Severe headache sometimes, and the eyes cannot stand the light. Tearing, bursting and throbbing headaches. Headaches worse in a warm room, better in the open air, as is coryza.

Cough with tearing pains in the larynx, worse from drawing in cold air but also can be worse in warm air or a warm room: worse in the evening.

Spasmodic cough resembling croup or whooping cough; hoarse, harsh, ringing, spasmodic cough excited by constant tickling in the larynx. Cough that produces a raw, splitting sensation in the larynx that is so acute and severe that patients make every effort not to cough.

Cold may also go down onto the chest with lots of secretions, coughing and rattling of mucus.

REMEDY SOURCE

Allium cepa is made fom the common onion. Onions have always been important in medicine and recognized for their usefulness in colds and infections. They were highly thought of by Hippocrates.

THE ALLIUM CEPA PERSONALITY

As it is primarily an acute cold remedy, there is no extensive psychological picture for Allium cepa. It is mostly used in a short-term situation, so there has been no need to observe long-term psychological symptoms to add to the remedy picture. There may be an uncharacteristic urge to eat raw onions.

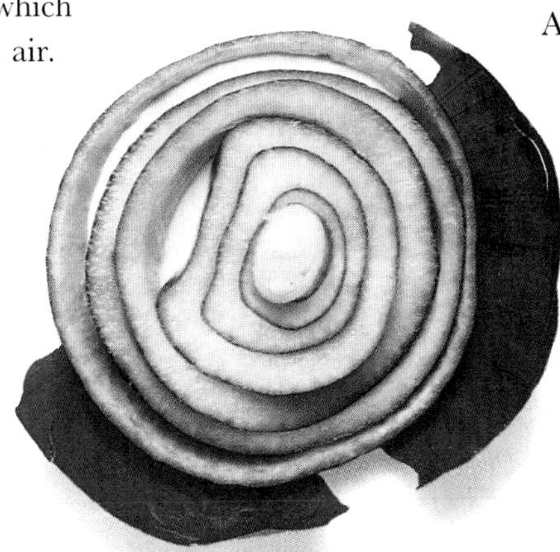

Red onion, the source for* Allium cepa. *Onions were well known as a folk remedy for everything from blood-cleansing to bee-stings, and so were an ideal candidate for homeopathic proving.

Antimonium crudum

- **Irritable, fretful**
- **Gloomy, sentimental, romantic**
- **Stomach disorders with all complaints**
- **Hot; worse for radiated heat**
- **Sensitive to cold**
- **Greedy, overeats, desires sour food**
- **White coated tongue**
- **Skin rough, horny, cracked**
- **Feet very sensitive**

INTRODUCTION

Known as 'the pig's remedy,' Antimonium crudum *is often associated with a greedy appetite and the stomach is the focus of all problems; whatever the symptoms, there will be some form of digestive upset as well. This remedy proves particularly useful in infants and old people.* Ant. crud. *and* Ant. c. *are the abbreviations for this remedy.*

THE MAIN SYMPTOM PICTURE

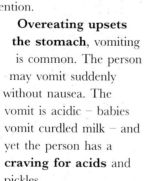

An Antimonium crudum child may show **irritability and fretfulness** similar to Chamomilla but while a Chamomilla baby can be demanding and wants to be carried around, the Antimonium crudum child does not want too much attention.

Overeating upsets the stomach, vomiting is common. The person may vomit suddenly without nausea. The vomit is acidic – babies vomit curdled milk – and yet the person has a **craving for acids** and pickles.

The Antimonium crudum **tongue** is distinctive: it has a **thick white coating**.

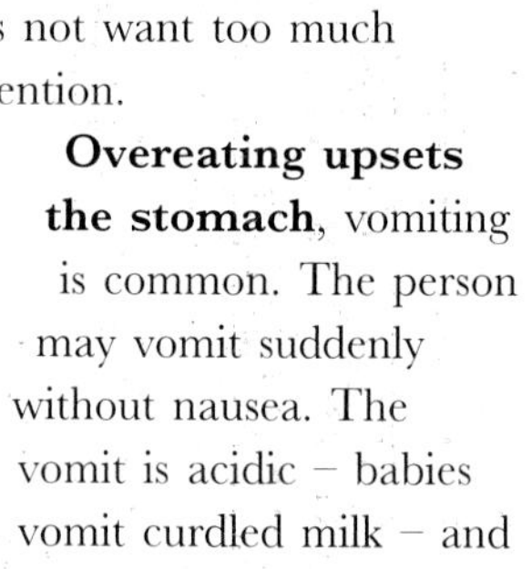

***Black sulphide of antimony, the source for* Antimonium crudum. *It was first proved by Hartlaub and Trinks and later by Hahnemann who published the results in his* Chronic Diseases.**

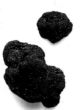

In long-term cases, the person may be obese, although by contrast Antimonium crudum may occasionally show emaciation and a loathing of food.

Antimonium crudum also comes up in acute situations such as measles, gastric flu and sunstroke. Patients are **worse for the sun and heat** generally, especially **radiated heat**. For example, in whooping cough, a coughing fit may be brought on by sitting in front of the fire. Although they feel hot, patients are **sensitive to cold** and are worse in cold **damp** weather. Antimonium crudum is well known for fitting the symptom picture of someone who is ill after falling into cold water during hot weather. They cannot adjust to sudden change of temperature and the stomach is affected.

Discharges have a lumpiness to them, such as the vomit of half-digested food, or lumpy diarrhea. The **skin** also has a lumpy quality and is **rough, horny**, crusty, and cracked. The nostrils, corners of the mouth and soles of the feet are particular areas which become cracked and sore. The **feet can be very sensitive**, not just from corns, cracks and horny nails, but also with complaints such as gout, sciatica, rheumatic pains, and inflamed tendons – all with some element of digestive disturbance at the same time.

REMEDY SOURCE

Antimonium crudum is prepared from black sulphide of antimony which occurs naturally as an ore.

THE ANTIMONIUM CRUDUM PERSONALITY

The peevish irritability of Antimonium crudum is gloomy and sulky, and there is a sentimentality to their gloominess. A typical subject would be a lovesick young person reading bad poetry in the moonlight. Adults feel very depressed, in the extreme suicidal, and they want to be left alone. They tend to eat beyond their capacity because however much they eat, their hunger is not appeased.

A CORN CURE

Used in low potencies, *Antimonium crudum* can be taken for long periods as a remedy for chronic calluses and corns on the feet.

Antimonium tartaricum

- **Chest complaints and gastric bowel disorders**
- **Face pale and sickly**
- **Feeble state, weakness, great drowsiness often**
- **Accumulation of mucus in the air passages**
- **Rattling breathing with the inability to raise phlegm**
- **Stomach troubles from sour food or drink**
- **Intense nausea**
- **Thirstless**
- **Worse lying down, warmth**
- **Better for vomiting**
- **Anxious and despairing**

INTRODUCTION

This remedy is most often needed in chest complaints and gastric or bowel disorders. The face may be pale and sickly with dark rings round the eyes and may be covered in cold sweat. A state of relaxation and weakness with little fever, a lack of reactive power, feebleness, great drowsiness which comes on often. Ant. tart. *and* Ant.t. *are the abbreviations for this remedy.*

THE MAIN SYMPTOM PICTURE

Every spell of cold, wet weather brings on coarse rattlings in the chest, a great **accumulation of mucus in the air passages**, or constant colds one after another. Patients lack the vitality to throw these conditions off; the chest steadily fills up with mucus; **rattling breathing with the inability to raise phlegm**. May be sinking rapidly into this unreactive state; suffocating on white mucus; lack the power to clear it but would be better if they could.

They **must sit up** in bed, breathing is **worse lying down**. Sometimes better for being fanned. They are **worse for warmth or too much clothing**, it makes them feel they are suffocating.

Mucous membranes covered in a thick white mucous discharge.

This weak, depleted state **does not come on early in an illness**. It comes with prostration, after several days and is most often found in patients of **low vitality, who are constitutionally weak or run down,** who are subject to catarrhal illnesses; most often needed in the elderly and in young infants.

REMEDY SOURCE

Antimonium tartaricum is made from tartar emetic, otherwise known as antimony potassium tartrate. It is extremely poisonous and a powerful emetic. It was used to treat the tropical disease *kala-azar* before less invasive forms of antimony were available.

Patients may loathe food; even plain water is vomited.

Thirstless and usually irritated if drink is offered; the child only grunts. May have intense desire for sour drink. Sometimes there is a desire for cold things, acids or acid fruits which cause vomiting. **Stomach troubles from sour food or drink** is another situation which may call for this remedy. Aversion to milk which is vomited. Vomiting, **intense nausea**, **prostration with coldness**, **cold sweat and drowsiness**, **sleepiness**. There may be giddiness between bouts of drowsiness. Vomiting ameliorates the nausea (unlike Ipecacuanha).

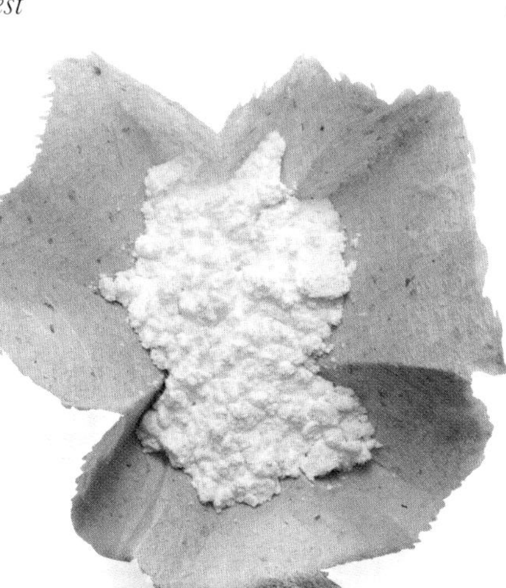

Tartar emetic, the source for **Antimonium tartaricum.** *Hahnemann proved this remedy, but there is no formal cataloging of its effects.*

THE ANTIMONIUM TARTARICUM PERSONALITY

This person does not want to be meddled or interfered with in this state; everything is a burden and they do not want to be disturbed. Irritability, anxiety and despair dominate. The sick child does not want to be touched or looked at; they want to be let alone. Babies may whine and moan pitifully, and become very irritable when disturbed. They may cling and want to be carried everywhere.

Apis mellifica

- **Complaints come on quite rapidly**
- **Worse for heat or warm room**
- **Better for cold**
- **Pains sting and burn**
- **Marked rapid swelling**
- **Thirstlessness**
- **Face flushed, red**
- **Tightness throughout the abdomen, fear that something will burst**
- **Scanty urine**
- **Rashes feel rough**
- **Skin sensitive to touch**
- **Fidgety**
- **Contradictory moods**

INTRODUCTION

Apis mellifica *may be needed after a fright, rage, anger, jealousy or hearing bad news. It may follow the disappearance or non-appearance of a rash, for instance if the rash of measles fails to develop fully or begins and then disappears.* Apis *is the abbreviation for this remedy.*

THE MAIN SYMPTOM PICTURE

Complaints come on quite rapidly in Apis as in Belladonna.

Patients are worse for **heat or in a warm room**. This is very marked, affects both the local conditions, such as pains and inflammations, and also the patient him- or herself; **better for cold** in any form, air or applications, etc.

Complaints may start on the right and go to the left. **Pains** characteristically **sting and burn** and are **better for cold**; however many other types of pain can occur.

REMEDY SOURCE

Apis mellifica is made from the honey bee. The entire insect, including its venom, is used to make remedy.

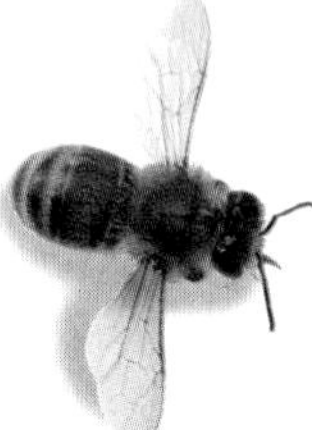

***The honey bee, source for the* Apis mellifica *remedy. Bee venom and tincture from the entire insect were proved by the* Central New York State Homeopathic Society.**

Swelling is also marked; rapid swelling may come and go rapidly. Mucous membranes swollen as if filled with water. Edematous eyes, eyelids, face or limbs.

Thirstlessness is also usual.

In delirium patients may fall into a stupor and even unconsciousness with twitchings, sometimes of one side only; the head rolls; pupils may be contracted or dilated; eyes red; **face flushed, red**. Patient lies as if benumbed and may become deathly pale if the room is overheated; they kick off the bed covers if they are able to.

Skin may be alternately hot and dry or perspiring.

A high-pitched shriek or cry in a tossing or stuporous child.

Many eye complaints with burning tears, swelling and redness. Discharges sting and burn, and are worse for heat and better for cold.

Suffocation from the radiated heat of a fire in a chill or fever.

Nausea, vomiting or retching, with great anxiety.

Tightness throughout the abdomen making it impossible to cough or strain for **fear that something will burst** or will tear loose. Patients are likely to bend forward and flex the limbs in order to gain relief from the tightness. Abdomen sore to touch.

Often there is **scanty urine**. There may be much urging to urinate, with smarting, stinging, and burning along the urinary tract. *Apis* is often needed in conditions where the skin is affected. **Rashes** feel thick, often **rough**; skin is **sensitive to touch**, tender. Urticaria. Also may be worse after sleep or touch.

THE APIS PERSONALITY

The Apis mental state is typified by fidgeting, restlessness and unpredictability, inappropriate emotional responses. The person may want company but reject affection, seethe with jealousy, burst into unprovoked tears. Fear of physical dissolution and even death is characteristic.

Argentum nitricum

- **Irritable, excitable, fearful, impulsive, and trembling**
- **Vertigo**
- **Fear brought on by anticipation**
- **Compressive head pains**
- **Catarrhal eye problems**
- **Violent pains with the sensation of a splinter**
- **Sore throat**
- **Ulceration with yellow pus**
- **Digestive problems with noisy flatulence and violent diarrhea**
- **Better for cold air, cold bath, cold drinks**

INTRODUCTION

Argentum nitricum *is a valued remedy for nervous persons, or for anyone suffering exam nerves or stage fright. It is also useful for people who do a lot of active brainwork – writers, artists, academics.* Argentum, Arg. nit. *and* Arg. n. *are the abbreviations for this remedy.*

THE MAIN SYMPTOM PICTURE

Compressive head pains, headaches which get worse with emotional or mental excitement; head feels large and may be better for being tightly bandaged.

If there are **eye problems**, there may be **purulent discharge** and swollen lids.

Pains are deep, sticking, **splinter-like pains**, sharp and shooting; they are better for cold, worse for heat. **Sore throats** present with sharp, sticking pain on swallowing and produce hoarseness; worse for heat, **better for cold drinks**. The throat is raw. The larynx is clogged with thick coryza.

If there is **ulceration**, there is much **golden**, **bloody pus**. Ulcers are red, raw and deep with hard edges.

There are many **digestive problems** associated with this remedy, often brought on by emotional disturbance or after eating sugar, which is craved but which disagrees. **Diarrhea**, often in **anticipation** of an undertaking or exam, may be noisy, violent and green, resembling flakes of spinach. There is great distention of the abdomen with **loud, bursting explosive flatulence**; person feels distended to bursting. All complaints are worse for heat and the patient feels suffocated in a warm room, or in a crowd.

REMEDY SOURCE

Argentum nitricum is made from silver nitrate ($AgNO_3$) known as lunar caustic to medieval alchemists.

THE ARGENTUM PERSONALITY

Argentum people are impulsive yet anxious, apprehensive, driven, restless and afraid of failure. The central idea is a mental weakness accompanied by an emotional state of excitability and irritability. This restless apprehension may manifest itself as claustrophobia, fear of crowds, or very commonly vertigo, and the compulsion to jump off a bridge or the fear of high buildings falling down on one. Irrational behaviour is possible.

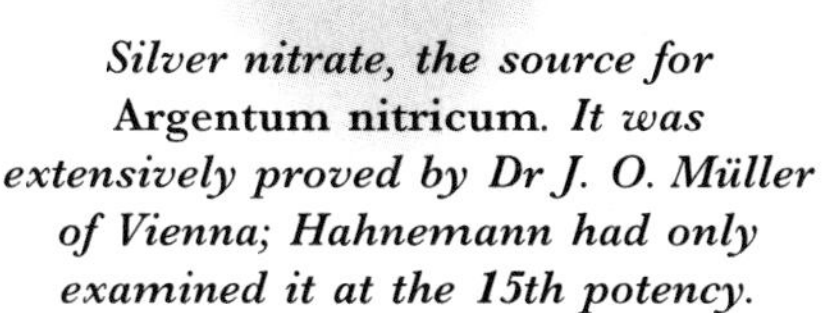

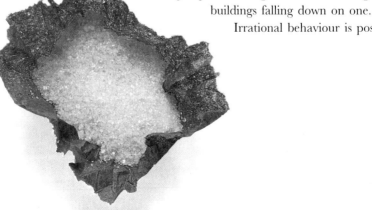

Silver nitrate, the source for **Argentum nitricum**. *It was extensively proved by Dr J. O. Müller of Vienna; Hahnemann had only examined it at the 15th potency.*

Arnica montana

- **First aid remedy**
- **Soreness of the body, as if bruised**
- **Prostration, weakness, weariness**
- **Averse to being talked to or even approached**
- **Hot and red head and face, cold extremities**
- **Persistent tiredness**
- **Worse in damp weather**
- **Better for lying down with head low**

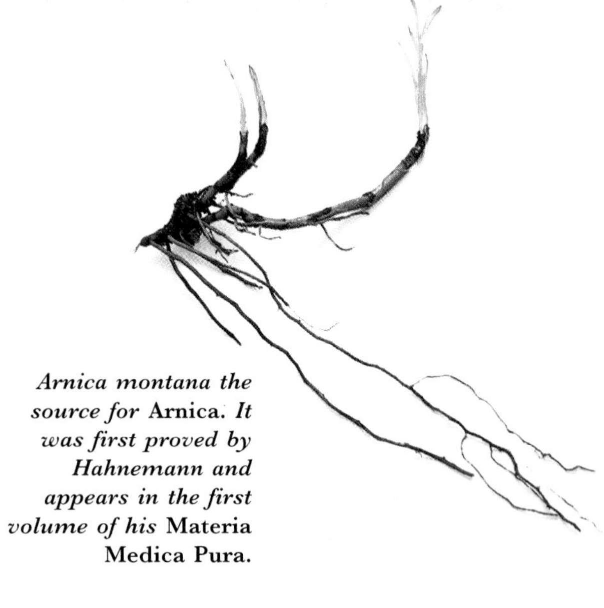

***Arnica montana* the source for Arnica. *It was first proved by Hahnemann and appears in the first volume of his* Materia Medica Pura.**

INTRODUCTION

The very sore body, as if bruised, marks out Arnica. The patient lies still, just turning a little from time to time because soreness makes the bed feel too hard. Arnica *is the prime remedy for bruises and the effects of trauma.* Arnica *and* Arn. *are the abbreviations for this remedy.*

REMEDY SOURCE

Arnica is made from *Arnica montana*, also known as Leopard's bane, fall herb and *Panacea lapsorum*. It grows high up in the Andes mountains and was often used as an infusion by South American indians to combat injuries sustained during climbing. The whole plant is used to make the remedy.

THE MAIN SYMPTOM PICTURE

In fevers, Arnica patients may be **greatly prostrated, weak and weary**, stuporous, almost unconscious, but they can be roused and will correctly answer your questions before lapsing back into the prostrate state. Because of their mental state, they may claim that they are not sick when clearly they are.

A patient may have a **hot and red head and face, cold extremities** and body. There is great thirst during the chill.

Patients bleed and bruise easily too; catarrhal complaints may be accompanied by inflamed mucous membranes which bleed easily.

In scarlet fever the Arnica state may come up when the patient is dusky, mottled and covered in red spots but the eruption does not come out (as in Antimonium tartaricum).

Joints may be swollen and sore.

Offensiveness of eructations, taste, flatus and stool – smells like rotten eggs (Baptisia tinctoria is even worse).

For someone who is sore as if bruised, with a sore throat, consider Phytolacca decandra, which also has a hot, red face and cold limbs and body.

There may even be stupor with involuntary discharge of feces and urine.

Many small boils may appear, one after another; they are painful and sore.

THE ARNICA PERSONALITY

People in an Arnica state want to be left alone; fear being touched because of the bodily soreness. **Averse to being talked to or even approached**; morose; obstinate; irritable; sad; fearful; stupid; horror of instant death; nightmares, night horrors.

FIRST AID REMEDY

Arnica is essential in the homeopathic first aid kit (see pages 240 to 245). It is helpful for every kind of wound or injury as it helps to stop bleeding, to heal the wound and to counteract shock and emotional trauma. As a cream, it is used externally on unbroken wounds, being particularly effective for bruising.

Arsenicum album

- **Anxiety**
- **Restlessness**
- **Weakness out of proportion to the illness**
- **Thirst for ice-cold water, little and often, just sips**
- **Burning pains better for heat**
- **Chilly**
- **Worse for cold**
- **Worse before and just after midnight**
- **Vomits everything**
- **Burns up and down**
- **Diarrhea with exhaustion and restlessness**

INTRODUCTION

Anxiety, restlessness, weakness out of proportion to the illness, burning pains which are better for heat, foul odors, chilly, worse before and just after midnight – these are characteristic of this remedy. Arsenicum *and* Ars. *are the abbreviations for this remedy.*

THE MAIN SYMPTOM PICTURE

Worse for cold air or applications; usually chilly and better for warm wraps, except for head complaints which are congestive and better in cool, fresh air. Often the skin is pale, cold and clammy.

Worse for movement, prostrated.

Anxiety is commonly intermingled with fear and takes the form of **restlessness**; it is a mental anxiety and uneasiness that makes the patient toss and turn, get up and walk about, move from place to place, one position to another, but they become so weak that eventually, in very serious diseases, they become prostrate. Commonly, too weak to move about but cannot keep still.

Thirst for ice-cold water, little and often just sips is another characteristic. They must drink because they are so dry, yet cold water disagrees with their stomach so they only take it in sips. In stomach complaints, they prefer warm things. In fevers there may be thirst for hot drinks during the chill, for sips during the heat, and a copious thirst during the sweat. The sweat usually ameliorates the condition.

Characteristically one finds **chills with a sensation of ice water running in the blood vessels**, which leads to an intensely hot fever with a sensation of boiling in the blood vessels, then comes prostration with marked chilliness. **Burning pains better for heat** are very characteristic of this remedy as is the **weakness out of proportion to the illness**.

Congestive, pulsating, burning in the head which is better for cold. All other burning pains elsewhere are better for heat.

Discharges are acrid and cause burning; better for heat.

A dry hacking cough and later a large quantity of thin watery or frothy mucus is spat out. Burning in the chest. Difficulty with breathing, wheezy; person must sit up to breathe and is much worse for any exertion.

Patient **vomits everything** with the prostration and anxiety; has a dry mouth, burning pains better for heat, better for warm water or milk; **pain burns up and down**. Gastritis. A very sensitive stomach, better for heat. Diarrhea and vomiting simultaneously, worse after eating or drinking. **Diarrhea with exhaustion and restlessness**, better for heat; foul smell. Rectum and anus burn and become raw.

Chilly, always taking colds; colds cause catarrh and sneezing, from every change in the weather. Catarrhs travel down to the larynx, with hoarseness, to the trachea, with burning worse for coughing, and to the chest, with constriction and a cough.

REMEDY SOURCE

Arsenicum album is made from arsenious oxide, familiar to the great poisoners in history and murderous protagonists in crime novels. In small, carefully prescribed doses, white arsenic promotes glossy hair, strong teeth and nails but taken unsupervised and carelessly, it is lethal.

THE ARSENICUM ALBUM PERSONALITY

People who need *Arsenicum Album* are restless and anxious, hopeless and despairing; fussy, faddy, fastidious and oversensitive. They fear night, being alone, things 'going wrong' or hurting someone.

***Arsenious oxide, the source for* Arsenicum album. *It was first proved by Hahnemann and appears in the second volume of his* Materia Medica Pura.**

Baptisia tinctoria

- **Toxic, septic conditions**
- **Intense aching and tenderness**
- **Rapid prostration to a serious state**
- **Discharges dark, foul**
- **Confusion, difficult concentration**

INTRODUCTION

The Baptisia symptoms may look similar to Gelsemium but the patient sinks rapidly into a serious state. They are restless but lack the energy to move around or even change position. The body aches and the bed feels hard as if lying on a board. Baptisia *and* Bapt. *are the abbreviations for this remedy.*

THE MAIN SYMPTOM PICTURE

Great prostration of the body is coupled with a restless, bewildered rambling of the mind. Patients are **confused** and find it **difficult to concentrate**, even falling asleep in the middle of talking. They may fall into a delirious muttering.

A patient needing *Baptisia* is likely to be very ill and in need of professional medical care.

Their face has a heavy, drugged look, dusky-colored and puffy or swollen. Eyelids feel heavy and eyes may be half-closed with a heavy pain in the head.

Lips look blue or are cracked and bleeding. **Mouth and breath are foul**, as is the tongue which has a dirty yellow-brown coating, often just in a central stripe. **Painful ulcers** appear in the mouth and throat. **Ear infections** can rapidly become serious and are more likely to appear on the right side.

Patients may have breathing difficulties with a great desire for air. They can wake up fighting for air or be afraid to go to sleep in case they suffocate.

They are very thirsty but need to take frequent short drinks as large quantities, or any food, may cause nausea or sudden vomiting. Despite this great thirst they may pass little urine.

This remedy was traditionally used in typhoid. Today Baptisia states may be found in septicemia, miscarriage, gastric flu, severe infection and other such states.

REMEDY SOURCE

Baptisia is produced from *Baptisia tinctoria*, the wild indigo, also known as horse-fly weed, indigo weed and rattlebush. It is native to North America, and was once used as the basis for indigo dye.

THE BAPTISIA PERSONALITY

As it is primarily an acute remedy for the desperately sick, and therefore of limited range, there is no extensive psychological picture for Baptisia tinctoria. There will be great restlessness, incoherent thoughts and the person may feel as if their body parts have become separated and scattered about. There may also be a fear of food and being poisoned.

Wild indigo, the source for* Baptisia tinctoria. *It received a small proving, involving only seven volunteers, and the results appeared in* The North American Journal of Homeopathy *(1857 and 1859)

Baryta carbonica

- **Slow immature child**
- **Early senility**
- **Shy, insecure, clings to the familiar**
- **Chilly, worse for cold and sun**
- **Complaints come on slowly**
- **Underdeveloped physically**
- **Swollen glands**
- **Sore throat**
- **Aversion to sweets**
- **Anorexia**

INTRODUCTION

This is a useful remedy for children, or sometimes for adults who give the impression of being in their second childhood. There is an immaturity about these children, perhaps they are failing to develop at a rate that might be expected, especially when illness retards their development. Baryta carb. *and* Bar. c. *are the abbreviations for this remedy.*

THE MAIN SYMPTOM PICTURE

A child lacks spark and brilliance – the opposite of precocious – and is **timid and shy**. Baryta children hide when a stranger is around, or cling to their mothers. Any change of routine or unexpected event upsets them.

The child is late in walking, late in talking, falls behind at school. He or she can be late reaching puberty, and even when grown up, cling to childish thoughts and ways, remaining **immature** and shy.

The picture may be seen in acute states, for example when a child has been ill. When a healthy child recovers from an acute illness such as measles or chicken pox this often heralds a sudden spurt of growth or development – for example the child suddenly grasps how to walk or how to read when they had been struggling with this skill before the illness. In the Baryta carb. child, this energy surge does not occur; instead they become withdrawn and seem to have slipped backwards.

In older people, insecurity and anxiety can manifest as obsessive behavior; in particular, they can become preoccupied with some aspect of their appearance. Premature aging and **early senility** respond well to *Baryta carb.* when the picture fits.

Patients are **chilly and sensitive to cold**, but **worse for being in the sun**. Typically symptoms come on several days after the person has been exposed to the cold. **Complaints** in general **come on gradually**.

The **under-development** is seen on the **physical** as well as the mental and behavioral levels. One part of the body may fail to develop, particularly the testicles. Emaciation, poor hearing, tooth decay and dim vision are all possible expressions of this trend.

REMEDY SOURCE

Baryta carbonica is made from barium carbonate ($BaCO_3$), a soluble salt of barium, a poisonous alkaline earth.

Glands swell and harden, and the Baryta carb. picture is one to consider in glandular fever. There is a great tendency for sore throats and enlarged tonsils.

Although patients may desire sweets there is more likely to be an **aversion to sweet** things and fruit; they may also refuse hot meals, preferring cold food. Generally they feel worse for eating, and *Baryta carb.* may be useful in anorexia, particularly **anorexia nervosa** in a teenage person who is having trouble accepting puberty.

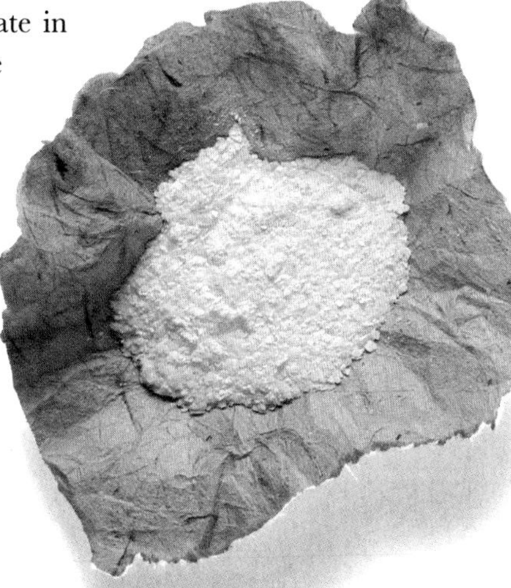

***Barium, the source for* Baryta carbonica. *It was proved by Hahnemann and appears in the first edition of his* Chronic Diseases.**

THE BARYTA CARBONICA PERSONALITY

Mental dullness, inattention, amnesia and fear of trifling things characterize Baryta carbonica. There may be a fear that people are jeering, and a sensation of cobwebs festooning the face, which no amount of brushing will dislodge.

Belladonna

- **Complaints come on suddenly and with great violence**
- **Violent heat**
- **Redness – bright, shiny red skin**
- **Intense burning in the inflamed parts**
- **Swelling**
- **Very sensitive to pains which come and go suddenly**
- **Congestion with throbbing all over**
- **Hot head and cold extremities**
- **Great dryness of mucous membranes**
- **Dry skin but often sweats on covered parts**
- **Twitching and jerking, starts and jumps in fevers**
- **Worse for motion**
- **Worse at 3pm and at night**

INTRODUCTION

Like Aconite, Belladonna *is suited to plethoric, vigorous, healthy constitutions, robust children and babies where the complaints come on suddenly and with great violence, then subside just as suddenly. It is not to be used in prolonged, continuous or recurrent states or in complaints which come on gradually.* Bell. *is the abbreviation for this remedy.*

THE MAIN SYMPTOM PICTURE

Extremely liable to take cold; sensitive to a draft, especially on the head, as Hepar sulph. and Silica.

Violent heat, so intense that it lingers on the hand after touching the patient's skin. All sorts of inflammations and fevers.

Redness: **bright, shiny red skin** especially of face, mucous membranes etc. Later it may become a little dusky and mottled.

Burning: **intense burning** in the inflamed parts. The throat burns like fire; the skin burns in scarlet fever and inflammations.

Swelling: inflamed parts swell rapidly, are very sensitive to touch with the sensation as if they would burst, with pressing, stinging, burning pains.

Great sensitivity to pains, which **come and go suddenly**. Much suffering; **worse for motion**, jarring, cold, touch, pressure, light. Patients want to be warmly wrapped, unlike Apis.

Congestion with throbbing all over and burning; blood vessels throb and pulsate as do local inflammations; hammering pains in the head if person moves. The more congestion there is, the more excitability. In fever, they become **delirious**, see horrible faces, animals, etc.; a wild state, even, which is sometimes better for eating some light food. Vertigo.

REMEDY SOURCE

Belladonna is made from *Atropa belladonna,* deadly nightshade. The whole plant is used to make the remedy.

Congestive headache worse for stooping, lying down; wants to wrap head up in scarf, blanket etc.

Hot head and cold extremities; rush of blood to the head. Eyes red and bloodshot.

Burning dryness and sense of constriction in the throat. **Great dryness of mucous membranes** with copious thirst, or person may be thirstless; often craves lemons or lemonade in fevers. **Dry skin, but often sweats on covered parts**.

Tongue may have red edges and white central coating. Offensive, putrid taste.

Twitching and jerking, **starts and jumps** – more common in fevers; even may be convulsions. Restless sleep, full of dreams of violence, nightmares, moaning and groaning.

Dryness produces tickling, leading to a dry, barking cough; violent cough, and may produce a little blood-stained mucus. Once mucus is raised there is relief for a while and then cough repeats. Chest very sore and tight, children may cry before they cough. Tickling and burning in the larynx with violent paroxysms of coughing. Headache as if head would burst with the cough.

Most complaints are better for keeping still; frequently **worse at 3pm and at night**.

THE BELLADONNA PERSONALITY

The Belladonna mental picture is one of violent intensity, the brain in turmoil. Lively and charming when well, Belladonna becomes violent when ill.

Deadly nightshade, the source for **Belladonna.** ***It was first proved by Hahnemann and appears in the last edition of the first volume of his*** **Materia Medica Pura.**

Bellis perennis

- **Injury or trauma to deep-seated tissue**
- **After abdominal surgery**
- **Great soreness and bruised sensation**
- **Waking at 3am**
- **Worse for getting wet**
- **Recent and remote effects of injury**

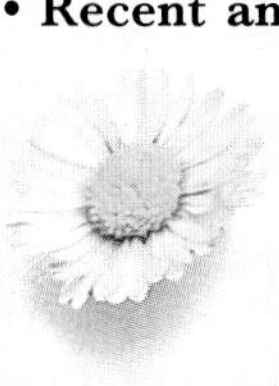

- **Tired and wants to lie down**
- **Feeling downtrodden**

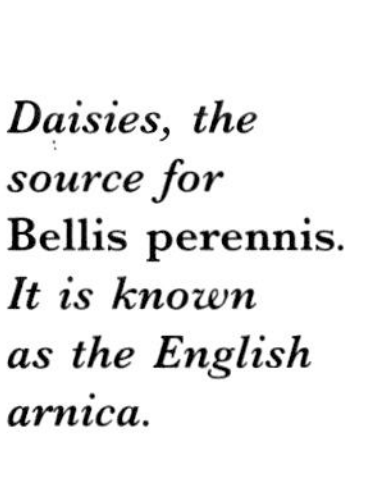

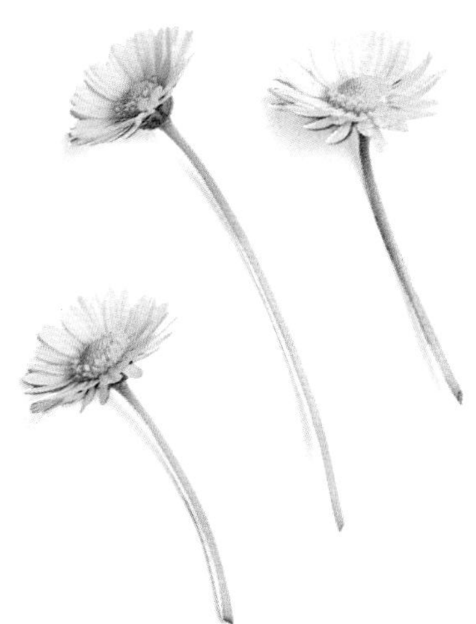

Daisies, the source for **Bellis perennis**. *It is known as the English arnica.*

INTRODUCTION

Bellis, *the daisy, is also known as woundwort or English arnica. Its uses are similar to those of* Arnica, *but for wounds which are deeper within the body, such as abdominal or pelvic surgery.* Bellis *and* Bell. p. *are the abbreviations for this remedy.*

THE MAIN SYMPTOM PICTURE

REMEDY SOURCE

This remedy is made from *Bellis perennis*, the common daisy. The whole plant is used to make the remedy. Daisies are also used in herbalism for coughs and catarrh problems, arthritis, rheumatism and diarrhea.

There is a general **bruised sore feeling**. Pains are worse for heat and better for cold. *Bellis* is useful for pains and swelling that occur from **injury or trauma to deep-seated tissue** rather than surfaces of the body. As well as **surgery** and **deep damage from accident** or illness, particular uses are for a blow to the breast, and for stomach pains after taking an icy drink when overheated.

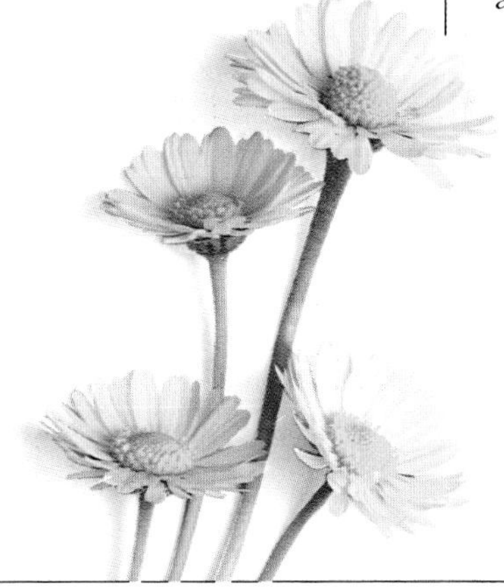

Like *Arnica*, *Bellis* can be used for either **recent or remote effects of injury or trauma**. As a general rule, long-established, deep-seated problems need treatment with higher potencies, so advice from an experienced homeopath should be sought.

Patients are generally **worse for getting wet**, and *Bellis* is a good remedy for sprains and bruises from overwork. For these reasons, *Bellis* has gained a reputation as a useful remedy for gardeners. It is also often of great help to the elderly where the picture fits.

Patients may wake early, or **wake at 3am** and be unable to go back to sleep. If this symptom occurs it is advisable not to take the remedy at bed time.

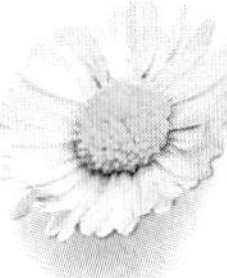

THE BELLIS PERSONALITY

The Bellis personality usually shows few mental symptoms, but like Arnica they may say they are well when they are very ill. Longer established cases of aches and pains may develop a sense of feeling downtrodden – like a daisy in the grass trodden on by everyone's feet. They are tired and want to lie down.

Bryonia alba

- **Complaints come on slowly, are continuous or remittent**
- **Much worse for motion**
- **Worse for heat and stuffy rooms**
- **Better for pressure**
- **Extreme irritability**
- **A sluggish state of mind**
- **Headache accompanies almost all other illnesses**
- **Stitching pains, lies on the painful side**
- **Chest painful and held when coughing**
- **Dryness of mucous membranes**
- **Great thirst for large quantities of cold water**

***White bryony, the source for* Bryonia alba. *It was an early proving by Hahnemann and appears in the second volume of his* Materia Medica Pura.**

INTRODUCTION

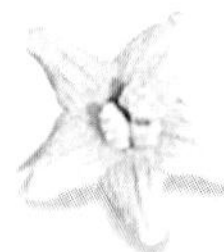

Bryonia *is a very important homeopathic remedy and the source has a long history as a medicinal remedy. It has been used in vertigo, melancholia, gout, hysteria, jaundice, mania, delirium, deafness, pleuritis, sciatica, uterine complaints, and asthma, to name only a few. It was one of the earliest remedies to be proved by Hahnemann and is selected for complaints of the lung and the digestive system, and arthritic conditions.* Bryonia *and* Bry. *are the abbreviations for this remedy.*

THE MAIN SYMPTOM PICTURE

Complaints begin a day or more after taking cold, especially if overheated or if the sweat is suppressed by cold air or water, or from exposure to dry, cold winds. They may also follow some mortification or hurt feelings.

Complaints often commence in the morning and may follow several days of preparation – feeling languid, tired, stupid in the head – and may increase gradually into violence. **Complaints come on slowly, are continuous or remittent**.

Much worse for motion. They desire to keep perfectly still; the more and the longer they move, the more they suffer. Better for **pressure**, and holding the affected parts parts still.

Extreme irritability; do not want to talk or be disturbed and may later fall into a state of stupor, even bordering on unconsciousness. **A sluggish state of mind**, not excitable; when roused from stupor they may be confused, want to go home etc., a low type of delirium, **not** the flashing wild excitement of Belladonna. Delirium may start at 9pm and last all night like the fever. Chill at 9pm too. (This is a common time of aggravation for Bryonia complaints).

Patients may be indecisive and not know what they want. Sometimes their anxiety and an uneasy feeling compel them to move, like Arsenicum, and even though it makes the pains worse, they cannot keep still; or the pains can be so violent that they also have to move but it still makes the pains worse.

Worse for heat, better for cold. In themselves and their congestive complaints, they are worse for heat and better for cold (like Apis, Pulsatilla etc.). Some rheumatic complaints are better for heat though.

Headache may be on its own or **the forerunner of other complaints; it accompanies almost all other illnesses**. There may be

REMEDY SOURCE

Bryonia comes from white bryony, a member of the gourd family; there are two species, *Bryonia diocia* and *Bryonia alba.* Hahnemann used *Bryonia alba* to make his provings, but both plants are suitable. The rootstock is used to make the remedy. It is very poisonous. The French call it the devil's turnip.

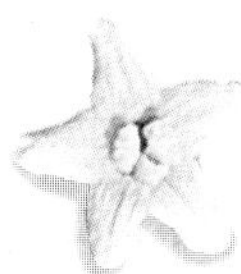

mental dullness and confusion with a bursting headache; usually better for tight pressure. Headache with nausea, with faintness.

Splitting, violent, congestive headache, a pressure pain; headache as if the skull would split. Worse for motion, even the winking of an eye; exertion is impossible, they keep perfectly quiet and still, in the dark because symptoms are made worse by light. Worse for **heat and stuffy rooms**, stooping, sitting up after lying down, coughing. Often look rather besotted with a congested mottled and purple face; a bloated face but no edema.

Stitching pains (like Kali carb.) **but better if patient lies on the painful side** (unlike Belladonna or Kali carb.); they lie still and are better for pressure. They hold their heads tight when coughing because of the splitting headache.

Many complaints start in the nose with sneezing, coryza with red eyes, and headache. They may progress to the throat, larynx and down onto the chest. Burning and tickling of the chest. Patients feel sore, lame and bruised all over (Arnica more so). The **chest** may be **painful and they hold it when coughing** and lie on the painful side to keep it still and put pressure on it. A chill with much pain in the chest, a short, hard, racking, dry cough with scanty or rusty-colored sputum. They take short rapid breaths because of the pain if they breathe deeply; pleurisy. Affinity for the right side with pain and pneumonia. A violent cough racks the body, sometimes with a headache and copious mucus. Cough worse after eating, movement, going from cold to warm air.

Dryness of mucous membranes, from lips to anus. Lips very dry, children tend to pick them; mouth dry.

Great thirst for large quantities of cold water at long intervals.

Toothache better for cold and pressure. There may be loss of or an alteration of taste, with a dry brown tongue and even, rarely, thirstlessness. Dry, sore throat with the thirst but cold drinks may bring on the cough and pains. In stomach complaints, warm drinks ameliorate.

Thickly coated white tongue. Sore throats with blistering, flaking ulceration.

Patients may crave what their stomach is averse to; indecisive. Sitting up may cause nausea and faintness. **Disordered digestion with the sensation of a stone or weight in the stomach** (like Nux vomica, Pulsatilla). Bitter taste in the mouth (like Pulsatilla; Nux vomica is sour). Nausea and vomiting worse for motion. Complaints follow errors in the diet, especially at the beginning of a warm spell after cold weather. **Constipation with dry, hard stools is most characteristic** but there may also be diarrhea which is worse in the morning, for movement and from overeating.

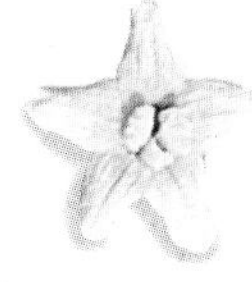

All complaints are usually better for sweat. Generally worse after eating, and at 9pm. Pains, except in the abdomen, are better for pressure.

THE BRYONIA PERSONALITY

The Bryonia personality is typified by the accountant, insurance salesman, or bank manager. Calculating, prudent, methodical, preoccupied with security, convinced that his method is best, but anxious and worried about poverty and his inability to control the future. This fearfulness may disable him, making it difficult to move or speak.

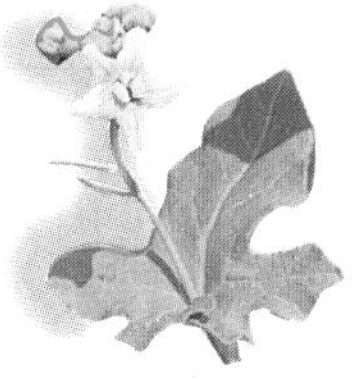

The flowers of white bryony, a climbing hedgerow plant which blossoms in early summer.

Calcarea carbonica

- **Complaints may follow exposure to cold water**
- **Full of congestions**
- **A chilly patient; sensitive to cold air**
- **Coldness with sweats**
- **Sweats in patches**
- **Relaxed tissues and blood vessels**
- **Weakness**
- **Glands, especially lymph nodes, hard, inflamed and sore**
- **Sourness**
- **Sweats about the head on the least exertion**

INTRODUCTION

Calcarea carbonica *is a very important remedy in homeopathy. It is primarily prescribed to rebalance calcium levels or correct malfunction in calcium metabolism. Calcium is vital to the efficient function of the body; it combines with proteins to form essential compounds. If calcium is not well absorbed, or if there is excess or deficiency, many disorders can occur.* Calc. *and* Calc. carb. *are the abbreviations for this remedy.*

THE MAIN SYMPTOM PICTURE

The Calcium carbonica subject may be **full of congestions**. Cold feet and hot head.

A chilly patient; sensitive to cold air, raw winds, a draft, a storm. Takes cold easily. Coldness of parts especially lower legs and feet. Worse in cold air, after ascending or exertion.

Coldness with sweats. Sweats in patches, in various places; head, forehead, back of neck, front of chest, feet. If patient gets into a sweat and stops still too long, the sweat will stop suddenly and a chill or a headache comes on.

Relaxed tissues and blood vessels – varicose veins, piles etc. with possible burning in varicose veins.

Weakness, worse after exertion, out of breath. Fever or headache from exertion.

Glands, especially lymph nodes, become **hard, inflamed and sore**. Abscesses in deep tissues.

Sourness; sour vomiting, diarrhea, smell of the body, breath etc. Tendency to looseness of the bowels, worse in the afternoon.

Tired and exhausted mentally and physically; break down in a sweat and become excited and irritable.

Headaches are stupefying, benumbing and bring on confusion of the mind. Headache from suppressed coryza. Pulsating headache if severe.

The more marked the congestion of the internal parts, the colder the surface becomes.

Thick yellow discharge from ears **or nose** after cold weather.

Sore throats in those that take cold frequently, one straight after another; chronic sore throats with constant dry, choking feeling and pain on swallowing. There may be painless hoarseness, which may be worse in the morning.

Colds all settle on the chest; very tired; expectoration of thick, yellow mucus, may be sour and offensive. Cough is better in cold, wet, wind.

Rheumatic joints, stiffness on rising from a seat.

***The European edible oyster, the source for* Calcarea carbonica.**

REMEDY SOURCE

This important remedy is also known as *Calcarea ostrearum*. It derives from the natural secretions of the European edible oyster, *Ostrea edulis*. It is made from the layer of fine crystals of calcium carbonate found in the middle layer of the oyster's shell.

FIRST PROVING

Calcarea carbonica was first proved by Samuel Hahnemann and appeared in the first edition of his book *Chronic Diseases* published in 1828.

THE CALCAREA CARBONICA PERSONALITY

The psychological picture of Calcarea carbonica shows a tetchy, stubborn, indecisive individual who finds mental effort extremely taxing and decision-making almost impossible. Despair and generalized fearfulness hamper any progress and the subject may feel stagnant and immobilized. In response, he or she may withdraw from the world and appear indifferent, or become supersensitive.

Calc. fluorica

- **Dilated veins**
- **Enlarged, hard glands**
- **Poor teeth**
- **Swelling around joints**
- **Gastritis with green discharges**

INTRODUCTION

This is one of the tissue salts, with an affinity for connective tissue, so it is useful for such disorders as dilated veins and enlarged glands. Calc. fluor. *and* Calc. f *are the abbreviations for this remedy.*

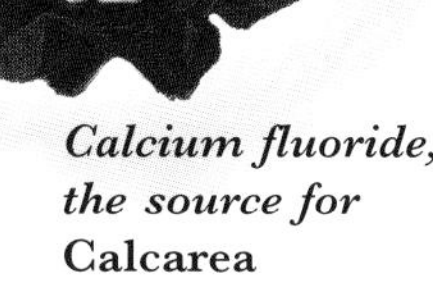

***Calcium fluoride, the source for* Calcarea fluorica.**

THE MAIN SYMPTOM PICTURE

EMEDY SOURCE

lcarea fluorica made from fluorspar, lcium fluoride. It is tissue salt occurring in bones, teeth and skin.

There is a general sluggishness and weakness. The body becomes flabby where there has been a long term Calc. Fluor. state.

Calc. Fluor. is used for **swelling around the joints** and tendons and general stiffness, weakness and lack of tone in these areas, perhaps after injury. Also **enlarged, hard glands**, varicose veins, bleeding piles and hard lumps in the breast or testicle.

Poor tooth enamel links this remedy with the benefits of fluoride for teeth. This remedy may help a teething baby, particularly if the teeth are late.

Calc. fluor. also has a use in **gastric disturbances** where there is vomiting and /or watery diarrhea which may be **grass green** in colour. Also useful when acute indigestion is the result of overexertion, particularly mental effort.

Where heart disease is due to weakness in the blood vessels, *Calc. fluor.* may be a useful support.

THE CALCAREA FLUORICA PERSONALITY

Calcarea fluorica is a tissue salt that works directly at the cellular level of body repair and therefore does not have a precise psychological picture. However, there may be an obsession with incipient financial ruin (however unlikely) and trivia.

Calc. phosphorica

- **Often needed by growing children**
- **Headaches in school-age children**
- **Growing pains**
- **Neck pains**
- **Complaints from grief and bad news**
- **Useful in puberty**
- **Aids bone growth**

INTRODUCTION

This remedy matches very well the problems of adolescence and children during growth spurts, although old people may also need it. Calc. phos. *and* Calc. p. *are the abbreviations for this remedy.*

THE MAIN SYMPTOM PICTURE

REMEDY SOURCE

The remedy is prepared from phosphate of lime made by adding dilute phosphoric acid to lime water.

During the growing period, many children need this remedy. Where a child is failing to thrive, slow in learning to walk, with weak legs and slow and painful dentition, **growing pains, headaches from studying**, this remedy may be considered. For complaints during teething, delayed dentition or soft teeth that decay easily; watery green diarrhea may feature during teething. The remedy **helps bone repair** if a fracture is slow to heal; it is also useful for infants who are intolerant of milk.

After a growth spurt, children may have pain and are drained of energy. **Useful in puberty**. Smoked meats may be craved. **Painful neck from drafts**, neck appears weak; head may bob about. There may be a sensation of numbness and crawling on the skin. **Ailments from grief** and unrequited love.

***Calcium phosphate, the source for* Calcarea phosphorica.**

THE CALCAREA PHOSPHORICA PERSONALITY

The main theme is discontent and restlessness; people who need this remedy do not know what they want, are often indifferent emotionally and lack stamina. Mental exertion is a strain.

Calendula officinalis

- **First aid remedy**
- **Cuts and open wounds**
- **After childbirth**
- **Much bleeding after tooth extraction**
- **Excessive pain out of proportion to injury**

INTRODUCTION

Calendula *is a very useful first aid remedy. Homeopaths recommend it as a basic ingredient in a home first aid kit; it is primarily used on cuts, grazes, shallow wounds and scalds.* Calendula *cream or lotion is normally available over the counter and does not need to be specifically prescribed by a homeopathic practitioner.* Calendula *and* Calen. *are the abbreviations for this remedy.*

THE MAIN SYMPTOM PICTURE

Calendula has an affinity with soft tissue conditions. Excessive pain is most characteristic. It helps clot formation and keeps a wound clean.

Most frequently used as a first aid remedy for **cuts**, scalds, minor burns and **open wounds**. Most often used in the form of a cream, lotion or a tincture, diluted with boiled water. Follows *Arnica* well. Use *Arnica* for the trauma of the accident and follow with *Calendula* to promote and speed healing of the cut. In deep cuts ensure the wound is clean before using *Calendula*, to prevent the cut healing over too rapidly and trapping dirt, germs or a foreign body inside.

Do not use *Calendula* for puncture wounds or very deep cuts, as it will promote rapid healing and may seal the infection inside the wound.

It is indicated when great pain is associated with the injury; the pain seems to be excessive for the degree of damage.

It is also useful **after childbirth.** Drops of *Calendula* lotion may be added to a warm bath or applied direct with a warm, damp sponge.

It is also useful **after tooth extraction** where there is much bleeding. *Calendula* lotion should be diluted with cold boiled water to make a mouthwash. This can be used as long as bleeding persists (although you should seek professional advice if bleeding gets worse or has not stopped completely after 12 hours). Alternatively, the remedy can be taken as a tablet.

REMEDY SOURCE

Calendula is made from the common or pot marigold, *Calendula officinalis.* Extracts from this unassuming plant have great healing properties, being anti-inflammatory and anti-microbial. Marigold is also important in herbal medicine, where it is used for skin problems and to treat internal and external fungal infections.

THE CALENDULA PERSONALITY

As it is primarily a first aid remedy used in response to minor accidents, there is no extensive, detailed psychological picture for Calendula. Anyone who suffers minor wounds will find *Calendula* helpful and healing. It is mostly used in acute short-term situations that are rapidly resolved, so there has been no need to observe long-term psychological symptoms to add to the remedy picture. Calendula subjects may be irritable or frightened, but mental symptoms may not show in an acute situation.

MARIGOLDS

Marigolds are named for Mary, the mother of Jesus. The pot marigold, a native of southern Europe, is a bushy hardy annual which grows to a height of 60cm (24in). It has long, narrow, light green leaves and bright orange or yellow daisy-like flowers; the leaves and stems give off a strong, pungent scent. Marigolds grow easily from seed and thrive well even in poor soil and bad conditions. Flowers are produced from late spring onwards. Marigolds can also be grown under glass for winter flowers.

Marigold, the source for* Calendula officinalis. *The whole plant is used to make the remedy.

Camphora officinarum

- **Colds**
- **Fevers**
- **Convulsions**
- **Collapse and state of shock**
- **Inflammation of bladder**
- **Cramps**

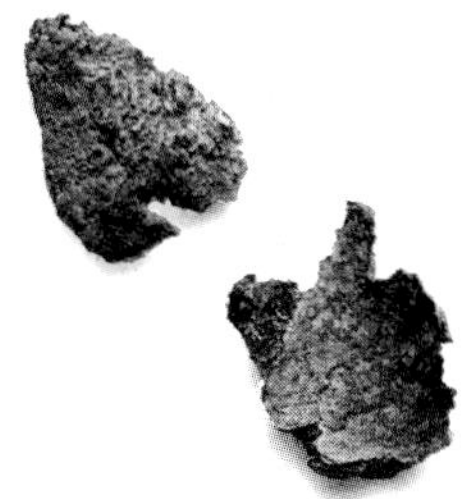

INTRODUCTION

Coldness, cramps and convulsions with awful anguish characterize this remedy. There is the unusual state of a person who is icy cold to touch but cannot bear to be covered. Persons who need Camphor *may go from extremes of mental excitement and violence to states of physical prostration and exhaustion.* Camphor *and* Camph. *are the abbreviations for this remedy.*

THE MAIN SYMPTOM PICTURE

This remedy is useful at the first stages of a **cold** when chilliness is intense, there is sneezing and the person feels better for uncovering.

The Camphor fever presents as a shaking chill with cold skin, better for uncovering. The patient wants cold air and open windows, then suddenly experiences a flash of heat and wants to be covered and warmed with hot water bottles, then becomes icy cold again and wants to be uncovered. There may be sudden, serious inflammatory **fevers** with rapid alternation of heat and cold, followed by rapid prostration. **Convulsions** may follow.

In extreme cases, the patient **collapses**, the body surface is cold with pale face and blue lips, but he or she cannot bear to be covered and is better for uncovering. There may be a burning in the stomach and a burning thirst. Sudden attacks of vomiting, diarrhea with rice-water stools. Nose cold, tongue blue, skin and breath cold; better for uncovering.

There may be **inflammation of the bladder**. Person feels excitable, mind frenzied, very cold but wants cold air, open windows and uncovering. As for fevers, he or she may have a flash of heat and want to be warmed, but then coldness returns and the covers are off again. Burning pains in the bladder and powerful spasms of bladder; may be retention of urine.

Cramps may be accompanied by a state of coldness, jerking of muscles, trembling. Cramps in calves. Numbness, tingling and coldness; cracking of joints, icy-cold feet and aching as if sprained.

Better for drinking cold water, for discharges and for thinking of pain; worse for cold drafts, after shock and for night suppression (not emptying bladder in night).

REMEDY SOURCE

Camphor is made from the wood of the mature camphor tree, a member of the laurel family. Camphor has always been valued for its medicinal properties. A piece of camphor bark worn around the neck was once thought to protect against infection.

THE CAMPHOR PERSONALITY

Persons in need of this remedy are characterized by cold. They are anxious, fearful of people in the dark; they feel isolated and forsaken – left out in the cold – and may have a tremendous rage at others. They feel rejected, hurt and unable to be comforted or warmed. They often feel better if they think about their pain.

***Camphor bark, the source for* Camphora officinarum.**

Cantharis

- **Cystitis with great pain**
- **Violent inflammation**
- **Burning pains**
- **Restlessness, excitement, mania**
- **Great thirst but aversion to water**
- **Burns and skin eruptions that look like burns**
- **Scanty urine**
- **Stabbing headache**
- **Cannot bear bright light**
- **Insect bites**
- **Angry and excitable**

INTRODUCTION

Made from a source commonly known as Spanish fly, a traditional aphrodisiac, this remedy can exhibit sexual frenzy in extreme cases.

It has an affinity with the urinary system. Its common use is for cystitis, particularly severe cases with strong symptoms. Canth. *is the abbreviation for this remedy.*

THE MAIN SYMPTOM PICTURE

Inflammation of the urinary tract **is sudden and intense**. The **pain is burning** and patients are afraid to pass urine because of the severe pain. The pain has been described as like 'drops of molten lead' in the urethra.

Urgency and frequency in passing urine are common, but urine is often scanty or retained, only a small amount is passed each time.

They are **angry and excitable**, **manic** in extreme cases. There is a great **restlessness** but they feel better for rest and warmth.

The remedy has an association with hydrophobia. The patient is **worse for drinking** and even from seeing or hearing water. They cannot bear the thought of water even though they have a burning thirst. This symptom may present as difficulty in swallowing liquids.

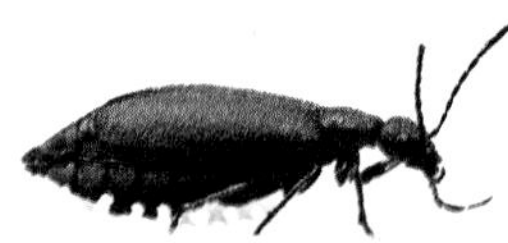

The Spanish fly, or blister beetle, the source for **Cantharis.** *It was proved by Hahnemann and appears in his* **Lesser Writings.**

They also cannot bear bright dazzling lights, particularly when the eyes are inflamed and burning. Headaches have a violent stabbing pain.

Cantharis is also useful in cases of burns. The **skin may have suffered burns**, including sunburn, or develop blisters or **eruptions that look like burns**. Also for insect bites where the Cantharis picture of great pain and excitability fits.

Cantharis patients may deteriorate rapidly to serious conditions. Skin symptoms can lead on to gangrene, serious cases of cystitis may lead to kidney and urethral damage. Unless symptoms disappear or improve greatly within a reasonable time, professional treatment should be sought.

THE CANTHARIS PERSONALITY

The person who needs *Cantharis* will be confused, with a head full of weird notions; they may be maniacal, in a raging fury or in a sexual frenzy. They may suddenly lose consciousness. There may be great thirst but they are unable to swallow easily; there may be no appetite and a marked aversion to food.

REMEDY SOURCE

Cantharis is made from the blister beetle, or Spanish fly *Lytta vesicatoria*, which has a reputation as an aphrodisiac. The insect lives on olive trees and honeysuckle all over southern Europe and western Asia. The whole insect, dried and powdered, is used to make the remedy.

Carbo vegetabilis

- **Coldness**
- **Sluggish circulation**
- **Bloating and belching**
- **Desire to gulp air**
- **Violent cough**

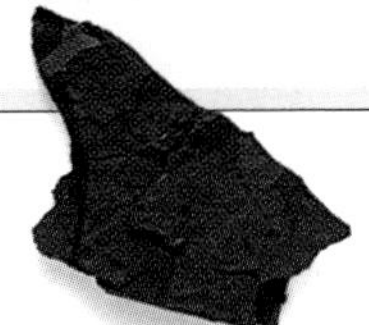

INTRODUCTION

Carbo vegetabilis *is commonly used for digestive problems. There is much wind, especially in the higher part of the stomach and frequent belching, which brings relief.*

The remedy is often appropriate where the digestion is weak and the general constitution is not healthy. After overindulgence in rich food the Carbo veg. picture may be seen. Typically this patient lives on junk foods and does not eat many nourishing, digestible foods. They crave salt, sweets, and coffee and may desire alcohol even though it disagrees with them. Fatty foods and, in particular, milk causes flatulence. Carbo veg. *and* Carb. v. *are the abbreviations for this remedy.*

REMEDY SOURCE

Carbo vegetabilis is made from black charcoal. Hahnemann used birch wood, but modern homeopathic remedies derive from beech-wood charcoal.

THE MAIN REMEDY PICTURE

The **stomach feels bloated**, as if it is pressing up on the diaphragm. Hiccups and even fainting may occur. This picture is frequently seen in pregnancy in an otherwise healthy woman where the baby presses upwards on the stomach.

It is often suited to elderly people, where the constitution is broken down, weak and sluggish. But a similar Carbo vegetabilis picture may come on suddenly in a healthy person who suffers a severe shock or accident.

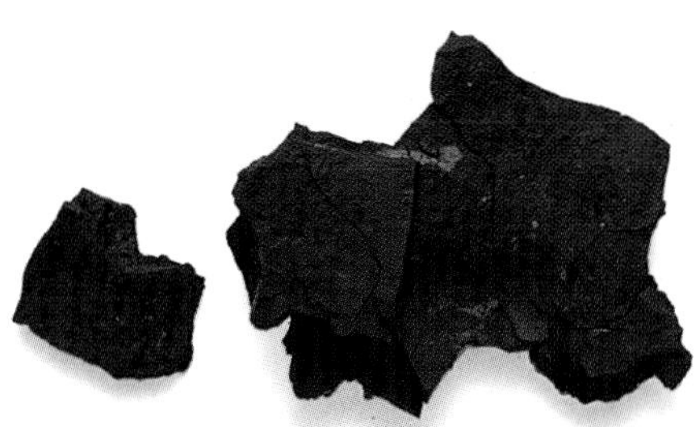

Charcoal, the source for **Carbo vegetabilis.** *A proving appears in the sixth volume of Hahnemann's* **Materia Medica Pura.**

Carbo vegetabilis also has an affinity for the chest, with effects usually felt in the lower chest. Colds go down to the chest and there is **violent** and paroxysmal **coughing**.

There is a sense of suffocation and a **great desire for air**. Patients **like to be fanned**. Carbo vegetabilis may be a useful remedy in whooping cough where the picture fits.

The circulation is generally sluggish. Patients are chilly, limbs are cold and blue and the sweat and even the breath feels cold. Skin quality may be poor, but this may not be seen in minor or acute cases.

THE CARBO VEGETABILIS PERSONALITY

The Carbo vegetabilis person is tired of life; desponding, despairing, listless, torpid, lazy, disinterested in everything, but will have swift mood swings to excitability and irritation. There may be fear of the dark, of closing the eyes, and of seeing ghosts. Mental processes are clouded, short-term memory is sluggish, and there may be tears and suicidal inclinations.

Causticum

- **The Causticum cough**
- **Burning thirst but aversion to drinking**
- **Drowsiness by day, insomnia by night**
- **Restless legs at night**
- **Sudden emotional stress**
- **Long-standing worry**
- **Creaking joints, especially knees**
- **Better for warm moist weather**

INTRODUCTION

This remedy is used for problems with the neuromuscular system (weakness, stiffness, cramps, convulsions, neuralgia) and for pains in the joints and tendons. It is also indicated as the carer's remedy, helpful to people who are looking after a convalescent or chronically ill relative and who may have to spend long weary nights 'on duty'. Caust. *is the abbreviation for this remedy.*

THE CAUSTICUM COUGH

This remedy has a well-known picture called the **Causticum Cough**:

Rawness and tickling in the throat with a dry cough. Burning in the throat not better for swallowing. Dry, raw, hoarse, even complete loss of voice; hoarseness worse mornings.

Hard, dry cough racks the whole chest. Tracheal irritation – a raw streak down the center of the upper chest.

Chest seems to be full of mucus; if only patients could cough a little deeper, they feel they would be able to shift it and get it up. Struggle and cough until exhausted or until they find that a little cold drink will relieve.

Cough worse when breathing out.

Leak of urine may occur with each cough. Soreness in the chest with the cough.

Inability to expectorate and obliged to swallow any sputum that is raised; it may taste greasy.

Dry cough with pain in the hip, involuntary urination.

THE MAIN SYMPTOM PICTURE

Patient is chilly but does not like extremes of heat or cold. Appetite banished at the sight of food; desire for spicy things and cold fizzy drinks, **although not always able to drink**.

Condition may result from exposure to cold, dry wind, lack of sleep, chronic illness or the legacy of a previous illness.

Symptoms come on slowly and the person gets weaker and must lie down.

Pains are tearing or drawing, and painful areas tender to touch; worse for cold, windy weather and thinking about them; better for rain. Local paralysis may occur. Symptoms may recur at full moon.

Headaches may cause nausea; there may be a tight scalp or a feeling of space between brain and skull. Better for warmth.

Ear ache accompanied by tinnitus and deafness.

Toothache made worse by cold air; a tendency to bite cheek or tongue while chewing. Griping, cutting colic better for lying down or for bending over double.

Involuntary leaking of urine may occur during coughing, sneezing or emotional excitement; frequency of urine, passed in large quantities.

Drawing and tearing pains in limbs; **joints** stiff and **creaking**; overuse of muscles may produce temporary partial paralysis; there may be acne on cheeks and forehead or behind the ears. Warts on hands and face. Soreness from old scars.

Complaints worse in dry, windy weather, after exposure to drafts, getting wet, movement, at night and early evening. **Better for warm moist weather** and being warm in bed.

REMEDY SOURC

This remedy is made from a mixture of slake lime (calcium hydroxide $Ca(OH)_2$) and potassium bisulphate $K_2(SO)_3$, following Hahnemann's carefully researched method.

THE CAUSTICUM PERSONALITY

People who need *Causticum* are usually worn out mentally and physically, and are weepy, anxious, hypersensitive and very easily emotionally upset. They are prey to fretful fears, and may be tetchy and hypercritical. Empathy with other people's suffering is a marked feature.

Slaked lime and potassium bisulphate, the source for **Causticum.** ***A proving appears in the second volume of the second edition of Hahnemann's*** **Materia Medica Pura.**

Chamomilla

- **Great sensitivity, especially to pain**
- **Great irritability and oversensitiveness**
- **Angry, snarling crying; piteous moaning**
- **Teething**

Wild chamomile, the source for **Chamomilla.** *A proving appears in the second edition of the third volume of Hahnemann's* **Materia Medica Pura.**

INTRODUCTION

Chamomilla *is an important remedy for nervous or psychological afflictions, and is indicated when pains seem to be disproportionate to their obvious cause. It is a good remedy for people with a low tolerance of pain and no mental strategies to deal with their afflictions. It is particularly useful for newborn babies and teething problems.* Cham. *is the abbreviation for this remedy.*

THE MAIN SYMPTOM PICTURE

Great sensitivity especially to pain, also to impressions, surroundings and persons. **Great irritability and oversensitiveness**. Cross, ugly, spiteful and snappish. This state may arise from anger, a temper, being contradicted, feeling mortified or from physical pain itself.

Angry, **snarling crying**, piteous moaning. These states are often found in the child and it is this emotional picture that will usually indicate the remedy. Patients may be driven to a frenzy by the pains, with a total loss of consideration for others; they may be quarrelsome, argumentative and rude. Children are often snappish and cannot be touched; they want to do as they please yet do not know what pleases them! An irritable, peevish state that can occur with inflammation anywhere. They may whine and cry; sputter about everything; not know what they want and never be satisfied, capriciously rejecting the things they have just asked for and display **temper**. Sometimes better for passive motion; they want to be carried the whole time but even then, they may not be quietened for long and will demand to be carried by someone else.

With ear ache children may screech out, cannot keep still with the pain and may be violently excited by it. Ear ache may be very sensitive to the cold. **Very sensitive to pain** which makes them mad, cannot bear the pain, sweat with the pains. Sometimes there is numbness with the pains.

Thirsty, for cold water usually. High fever with sweating especially on the head, one cheek red and one pale.

Very useful in **teething,** especially if the child is in an oversensitive, capricious state where nothing pleases and the teething is worse for heat and at night, and better for cold applications; also for teething accompanied by green, foul diarrhea smelling of rotten eggs; colicky pain and bloating.

Most complaints come on in the evening or night and usually subside by midnight. May be worse at 9am. Often worse for heat but not better for cold in general (unlike Pulsatilla and Apis). In fact cold may bring on most troubles.

REMEDY SOURCE

Chamomilla is made from *Matricaria chamomilla*, the German chamomile or wild chamomile, a member of the daisy family.

THE CHAMOMILLA PERSONALITY

The person who needs *Chamomilla* – most often a child – is restless, irritable and hypersensitive, unable to bear being touched, or even spoken to or looked at. Any pain is described as unbearable. Nothing can please or comfort this state; people are easily offended and may become moody and resentful and refuse to speak to anyone.

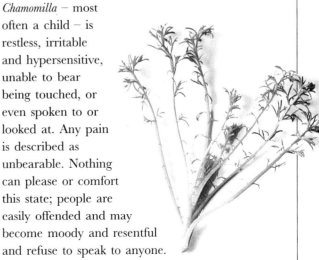

Cimicifuga racemosa

- **Great pain**
- **Hypersensitive state of mind and body**
- **Black depression**
- **Post-natal and menopausal depression**
- **Painful rheumatism and back and joint complaints**
- **Shock-like pains**
- **Slow childbirth**
- **Heavy painful periods**

INTRODUCTION

This remedy has an affinity with the nervous system and the pelvic region and reproductive organs. It is useful when symptoms veer from mental to physical and back again, and mental symptoms improve when physical complaints get worse. Symptoms appear mostly on the left side.

The nerves are particularly affected, so the Cimicifuga patient is in a sensitive state, pains are very bad and they feel very chilly. Cimicifuga *and* Cimic. *are the abbreviations for this remedy.*

THE MAIN SYMPTOM PICTURE

Arthritis, **rheumatism**, lumbago and such disorders of the joints are accompanied by **great pain**. Rheumatism may alternate with mental states – when the depression lifts the **joint pains** are more severe.

All sorts of **back pains** occur, stiff neck, aching shoulders, pain between the ribs and down the back of the thighs. In headaches the pain may shoot down the spine and relief is gained from bending the head back and applying pressure to the back of the neck; cool open air is also beneficial.

Angina may respond well if it has the characteristic strong, **shock-like** pains and the Cimic. picture of depression and hypersensitivity.

All sorts of **disorders of the uterus and ovaries** occur with the Cimicifuga picture, including prolapse and **heavy**, **painful periods**. The remedy also has uses in **childbirth** and cases of early miscarriage, always where there is much pain and sensitivity.

REMEDY SOURCE

Cimicifuga is made from *Cimicifuga racemosa,* also known as *Actaea racemosa,* a perennial herb native to North America. Its local names include black cohosh, bugbane and black snake root. The remedy is prepared from the dried roots. Native Americans used the plant for rheumatism, snakebite and gynecological complaints.

THE CIMICIFUGA PERSONALITY

The Cimicifuga patient is emotionally hypersensitive and will snap irritably and appear restless and highly strung. He or she talks a lot, speaking rapidly in a high-pitched voice and switching constantly from one subject to another. In severe cases, hysteria and even hallucinations may occur.

Patients are in a state of depression as if they were living under a black cloud. The state emerges during pregnancy, post-natally, or at the menopause, or possibly as the result of some accident or trauma.

***Black snake root, the source for* Cimicifuga racemosa. *It was proved in America, and results appear in the third volume of the* North American Journal of Homeopathy.**

Cinchona officinalis

- **Oversensitive senses**
- **Pains feel worse for light touch, better for hard pressure**
- **Ailments often caused by loss of vital fluids**
- **Complaints return at a regular time of day or year**
- **Fevers**
- **Headaches**
- **Bloated abdomen**

***Leaves from the quinaquina tree,. the quills of which form the modern source for* Cinchona officinalis. *It was proved by Hahnemann himself in his very first homeopathic proving and the results of his observations underpin the theory of homeopathy. An account of the proving appears in the last edition of the third volume of Hahnemann's* Materia Medica Pura.**

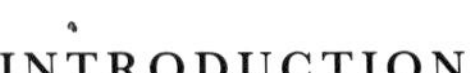

INTRODUCTION

This remedy is also known as China, *which is also its abbreviation. In the seventeenth century, bark from* Cinchona officinalis *was introduced into Europe by Jesuits who had found it in South America. It was known as Jesuit Powder, Peruvian bark, or simply 'the bark' and found to cure 'the ague'. This is the remedy that Hahnemann tried on himself, the inspiration for homeopathy itself.*

THE MAIN SYMPTOM PICTURE

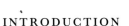

Extreme sensitivity to touch; hypersensitive tissues. Also great sensitivity to all external impressions such as motion, noise, cold air, drafts, smoking. People become easily excited, nervous and full of worries.

Weakness and **debilitation from loss of vital fluids** such as hemorrhage, diarrhea, excessive lactation, suppurating wounds. Patient is weak, oversensitive, nervous, may have twitching limbs, liable to feel faint and sleepless.

Complaints often return every other day or **regularly** in season **at the same time**.

Headaches feel as if skull will burst, the head throbs, it is worse for being in the sun, sitting or lying down; the patient feels that he or she must walk. Pain is worse in the temples and spreads from occiput (the back of the head) over the whole head and the scalp is very sensitive.

Fevers. Continued debility after flu; often very chilly; chill, heat, and sweat in stages. Chill, then thirst, then heat, then thirst. Red hot face, cold hands, drenching sweat at night; tropical fevers, intermittent fevers. Chill starts in breast.

Abdomen is bloated and distended to bursting point with constant loud belching which does not relieve. The patient may have sore bowels, loud eructations, and feel immobilized; they may have copious painless diarrhea, worse at night or after fish, fruit or wine. Often hiccups and nausea, and vomiting with bitter eructations; worse at night and after eating. **Better for hard pressure on the abdomen**, bending double and lying down.

THE CHINA PERSONALITY

People who need *China* are often living on the edge of their nervous capacity. They have strong imaginative powers and love to daydream about positive, wonderful things. They do not like superficial exchanges with others and are irritable, chilly, excitable, and easily offended. They can be contemptuous and can hurt others' feelings while being oversensitive themselves.

REMEDY SOURCE

China derives from *Cinchona officinalis*, the quinaquina tree, native to the eastern slopes of the Andes. The tree is also the source of the allopathic drug quinine.

Cocculus indicus

- **Travel sickness**
- **Anxiety, preoccupation**
- **Aversion to food**
- **Nausea, vomiting**
- **Dizziness**
- **Bad effects of sleep loss**
- **Sweaty hands**

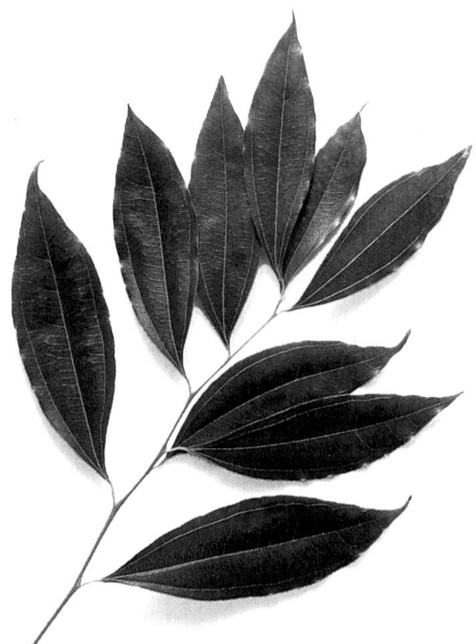

***Indian cockle, the source for* Cocculus indicus. *It was proved by Hahnemann and appears in the third volume of his* Materia Medica Pura.**

INTRODUCTION

Cocculus indicus *is the primary homeopathic remedy for travel sickness.*

Apart from travel sickness, the other occasion on which the Cocculus picture arises is after a period of lack of sleep. All the physical and mental symptoms can be seen with a marked irritability. Cocculus *and* Cocc. *are the abbreviations for this remedy.*

THE MAIN SYMPTOM PICTURE

Headaches are accompanied by **vertigo**, nausea, numbness, staggering when walking; complaints are made worse by getting up, in motion or looking at moving objects, after sleep, eating and drinking; better for lying down. Neck muscles feel too weak to hold head up. **Eyes feel bruised**; vision blurred with spots before the eyes.

THE TRAVEL SICKNESS REMEDY

The best known use for *Cocculus* is in the prevention and cure of travel sickness in both children and adults.

If taken before a journey begins, it may prevent any symptoms occurring, while a dose at the end of the journey can rapidly dispel the bad effects of travelling.

Patients may be apprehensive concerning travel, particularly those who panic when faced with air travel. The after-effects of this fear leave them weak and shaking. They seem preoccupied with their own inner thoughts and fears and may lose track of time while in this absorbed state.

There is giddiness and nausea with palpitations and constriction of the chest, a dry throat, sweaty palms, a flushed face and frequent urge to urinate. The mouth is wet with saliva and has a metallic or bitter taste. Vomiting is likely, even at the mere sight or smell of food.

The sense of smell is acute; there is a dry throat, slurred speech; stitch pain and tightness in the chest.

Nausea and vomiting precipitated by food or the thought of food; much saliva before vomiting. Pains in liver and abdomen; flatulent colic late at night, feeling of 'something alive' in stomach. Possible constipation; diarrhea following drinking water; frequent urge to urinate.

Stiff, heavy limbs, very painful to move; tendency to shake; numb hands with stinging fingertips. There may be an itchy rash especially in the evening.

REMEDY SOURCE

Cocculus comes from the fruits of *Anamirta cocculus*, a native of India and Sri Lanka. It is also known as the Indian cockle, Levant nut, or fish berry. The fruits contain a potent stupefying drug; thrown into the water they release enough of it to stun fish. The drug was also the basis of a kind of 'Mickey Finn', tipped into the beer of drunken sailors who had just been paid, to make them easy to rob.

THE COCCULUS PERSONALITY

The person who needs *Cocculus* appears dull and stupid, unable to finish a sentence or a train of thought; alternatively they may be chatty, joking and wanting to sing. They are melancholy and easily provoked into anger or react badly to insults. May be worried about others and neglectful of self. The Cocculus state may be brought about by anger or sadness, but is most often a response to travel motion.

Coffea cruda

- **Excitable and oversensitive**
- **Mentally overstimulated**
- **Senses acute**
- **Restless, sleepless**
- **Trembling limbs**
- **Toothache**

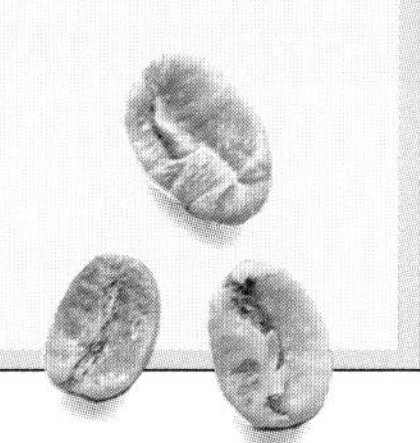

INTRODUCTION

Many healthy people have 'proved' coffee by drinking too much, too strong and developing the typical picture of the Coffea *remedy. When a similar picture arises from some disease – perhaps toothache or pre-menstrual tension – where no coffee has been drunk but the patient responds well to potentized* Coffea, *we have a good demonstration of how homeopathy works.* Coffea *and* Coff. *are the abbreviations for this remedy.*

THE MAIN SYMPTOM PICTURE

The nerves are **oversensitive** and **overexcitable**. Both the **mind** and body are restless and **overactive**. Symptoms may be the result of some trauma such as a fright, great fatigue or an unhappy love affair.

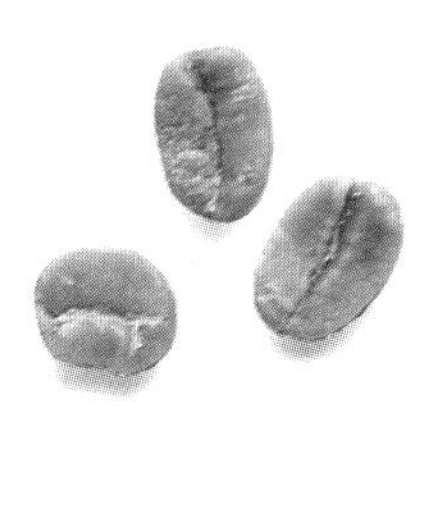

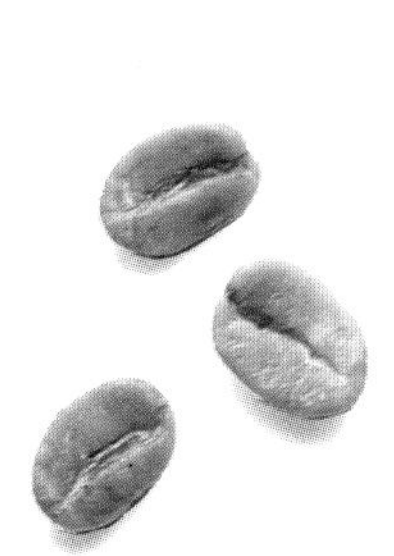

Laughter and tears come easily and follow each other in quick succession. The brain is buzzing and patients often find **sleep impossible** because of mental activity.

All **senses are more acute** – noise, smells, touch can become unbearable.

Toothache occurs either alone or accompanying other conditions, such as a menstrual period.

Hands tremble and **limbs twitch**. The skin is sensitive and itching. Generally, the patient feels driven to desperation by the symptoms.

This remedy is useful for acute pre-menstrual symptoms where the picture fits. Persistent PMS or difficult periods require deeper, long term constitutional treatment.

REMEDY SOURCE

Coffea is made from the raw berries of the coffee tree.

THE COFFEA PERSONALITY

The Coffea cruda personality is hallmarked by classic symptoms brought on by too much caffeine in the bloodstream. The mind is hyperactive, bursting with ideas, the memory becomes phenomenal, reams of poetry, or statistics, may be declaimed. There is an equally speedy descent into gloom and despondency and a tendency to work so hard that 'burn-out' is inevitable.

Coffee berries, the source for* Coffea cruda. *It was proved by Hahnemann himself and four other people.

Colocynthis

- **Complaints from anger and indignation**
- **Violent cramping abdominal pains**
- **Paroxysmal**
- **Severe face pain**
- **Vertigo**
- **Sciatica**
- **Neuralgic eye pains**

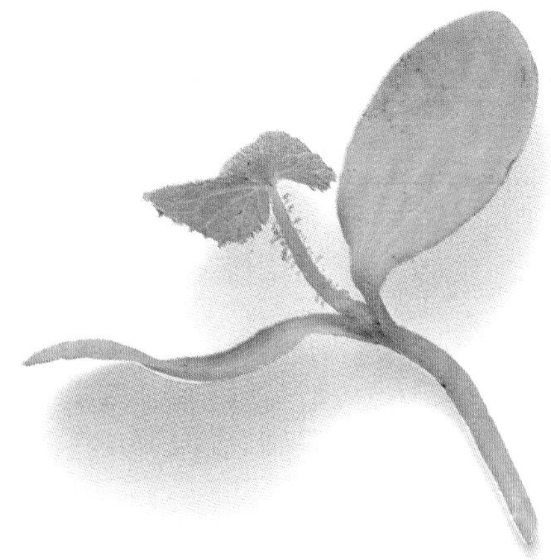

***Leaves from the plant of the bitter cucumber, the gourd of which is the source for* Colocynthis. *A proving appears in the sixth volume of Hahnemann's* Materia Medica Pura.**

INTRODUCTION

Colocynthis *was well known as a purgative by Arab and Greek physicians. In the homeopathic repertoire it is an important remedy for severe cramping colic.* Coloc. *is the abbreviation for this remedy.*

THE MAIN SYMPTOM PICTURE

Pains are severe, paroxysmal, tearing and neuralgic, and occur in the face, abdomen and along the nerve tracks. Sudden **violent cramping pains in the abdomen**, sensation as though intestines are being crushed between two stones. Cutting, clutching, tearing neuralgic pains which come on in waves and grow in intensity and are so severe the person twists and turns and screams with pain. Patients may be so distressed they are compelled to bend double and apply hard pressure; they bend over backs of chairs or lean heavily on round bedpost heads to gain relief. They are better for bending double, pressing hard on the abdomen, and heat.

REMEDY SOURCE

Colocynthis comes from a gourd, *Cucumis colocynthis*, known as the bitter cucumber or bitter apple. It grows around the Eastern Mediterranean. The fruit is bitter and poisonous.

Nausea appears only when pain becomes intense and patients eventually vomit. Awful **spasms** are experienced while passing jelly-like stool; excessive urging to stool; flatulence makes symptoms better.

Tongue is coated and person is weak and very restless with pain. Infant screams with colic pain and is relieved by lying on abdomen.

Severe neuralgia **face pain**, feels like hot wire, spreads over face in waves usually on the left side; feels better for pressure, heat and anger.

Vertigo experienced when moving head quickly, particularly to the left. **Sciatica** experienced as cramping pain in hip as though screwed in a vice. Better for pressure, lying on the affected side; better for heat, worse for motion.

Severe burning, cutting and sticking pains in eyes, better for pressure; sensation of eye falling out of socket when bending over.

Headaches give tearing pain in scalp, severe gnawing pain in head, person cries out. Worse for moving eyes and anger or emotion, better for pressure and heat.

THE COLOCYNTHIS PERSONALITY

People who need this remedy are often haughty and easily offended. They become morose, easily angered and indignant and their complaints often follow anger and indignation. They are restless and extremely anxious and weak with pains; everyone irritates them and they want to be alone.

Conium maculatum

- **Coldness**
- **Paralysis**
- **Hardening**
- **Sensation of a lump**
- **Progressive illness**
- **Better for heat and sunshine**
- **Suited to the elderly**

INTRODUCTION

Conium maculatum *is a remedy particularly suited to the elderly. It is usually indicated after another remedy has been prescribed to deal with acute problems.* Conium *and* Con. *are the abbreviations for this remedy.*

THE MAIN PICTURE SYMPTOM

The picture of a patient in need of *Conium* shows the same feeling of **coldness and slow paralysis** that Socrates is said to have suffered as he died. It is often needed in serious illness, such as cancer, which has gradually overtaken the system. It suits slow, **progressive disorders**, particularly of the nerves – for example, multiple sclerosis.

Patients may show an aversion to company but at the same time a fear of being alone – perhaps shutting themselves alone in a room after ensuring there are other people in the house.

A MELANCHOLY REMEDY

'No, no, go not to Lethe, neither twist
Wolf's Bane, tight rooted, for its poisonous wine
Nor suffer thy pale forehead to be kiss'd
By nightshade, ruby grape of Proserpine.
Make not your rosary of yew-berries...
...For shade to shade will come too drowsily
And drown the wakeful anguish of the soul.'

Keats' 'Ode on Melancholy' romanticizes slow, creeping death from poisonous plants. He might well have included Conium maculatum *amongst these. Hemlock, as it is commonly known, is the plant whose juice the Greek philosopher Socrates is said to have drunk.*

They are very chilly and much worse for being exposed to the cold, they **need warmth,** and love to soak up the sun.

The **hardening process** affects all levels and may often show itself as hardened glands or as tumors after injury. Cataracts and lumps in the breast or testicles are found in Conium and when these problems are combined with a general slowness and debility, this is often a **useful remedy for the elderly**.

Sometimes no actual lump is present but the person has the **sensation of a lump**; for example, has a sore throat which feels as if there is a lump in it.

In stomach problems such as ulcers or stomach cancer, the pain may feel better if the person sits or lies with the knees pulled into the chest. Eating also relieves the pain but only for a couple of hours. There may be a craving for coffee, salt, and sour things, but milk, and sometimes bread, disagree and even small amounts of alcohol cause complete prostration.

Constipation and difficulty passing urine are due to general paralysis and hardening of the parts, as for example in prostate problems where the urine can only dribble weakly.

REMEDY SOURCE

Conium maculatum is made from hemlock - common hemlock, spotted hemlock, poison hemlock or herb Bennett, the plant used as an executioner by the Greek and Roman judiciary. It bears a striking resemblance to sweet cicely (*Myrrhis odorata*), but should never be eaten in mistake for it, as the results will almost certainly be fatal. The remedy is prepared from the whole plant in flower.

THE CONIUM MACULATUM PERSONALITY

The mind is slow and tired – there is emotional apathy where 'the wakeful anguish of the soul' has certainly been drowned.

It can be difficult to hold thoughts together, so subjects become attached to certain ideas, with a stubbornness which makes them irritable and quarrelsome if contradicted.

***Hemlock, the source for* Conium maculatum. *A proving appears in the fourth volume of Hahnemann's* Materia Medica Pura.**

Cuprum metallicum

- **Spasms and cramps**
- **Better for touch of hands**
- **Tense and nervous**
- **Worse for suppressed discharges**
- **Menopausal problems**
- **Worse for hot weather and sun**
- **Vertigo**
- **Cramping stomach pains**

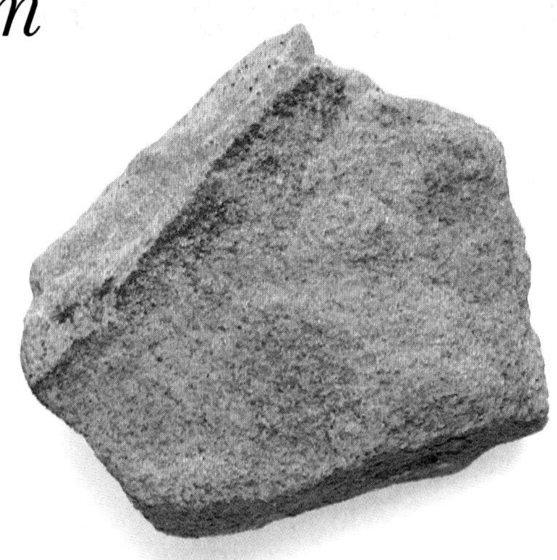

INTRODUCTION

Cuprum metallicum *is characterized by extreme contrasts: violent symptoms followed by exhaustion; ravenous hunger followed by anorexia, deep sleep disturbed by frenetic twitching and jerking.*

The spasms and violent cramps mean that Cuprum *has a useful place in the treatment and control of epilepsy. Convulsions appear to move in an upward direction, sometimes beginning in the toes or fingers.* Cuprum, Cuprum met. *and* Cupr. *are the abbreviations for this remedy.*

THE MAIN SYMPTOM PICTURE

Other forms of Cuprum **cramps** include angina pectoris, after-pains following childbirth, and knotting and jerking of the limbs. **Having someone put their hands over the affected part** can relax and relieve the painful **spasms**. Anything that induces a state of relaxation is beneficial.

Mental and emotional symptoms also show someone who **is tense, nervous** and generally strung-up. This could show itself by the person being very talkative, or taciturn, experiencing fits of rage or alternating between hysterical weeping and unprompted laughter.

Cuprum may be of help pre-menstrually if the picture fits. This remedy has the characteristic that symptoms are **worse if a discharge is suppressed**, so PMS may be worse if a period is late; may be useful at the time of the **menopause** when a period does not appear.

Vertigo and headaches, cramping pains in the stomach, and spots that do not develop are typical symptoms. Patients are generally **worse in hot weather and especially if out in the sun**.

REMEDY SOURCE

Cuprum metallicum is made from dry powdered copper. Copper as a trace element is essential to the healthy maintenance of the body.

THE CUPRUM METALLICUM PERSONALITY

The person who needs this remedy is a bundle of contradictory moods: silently sullen then chatty, malicious and spoilt, tricky, changeable and tending to get angry very quickly; patients may want to run away. They may be in a maniacal frenzy or a catatonic trance, or may alternate between these states.

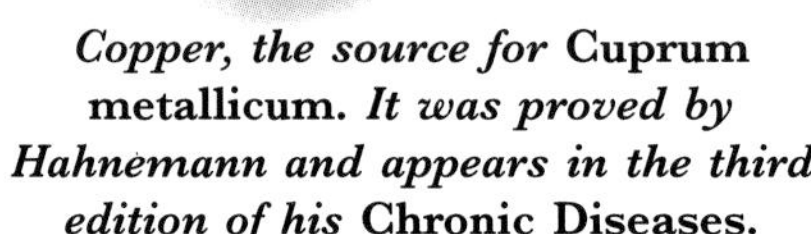

***Copper, the source for* Cuprum metallicum. *It was proved by Hahnemann and appears in the third edition of his* Chronic Diseases.**

Dioscorea villosa

- **Severe abdominal colic**
- **Flatulence**
- **Gall bladder colic**
- **Pains shift suddenly**
- **Better for stretching out**
- **Renal colic**
- **Period pains**

INTRODUCTION

This remedy is used for many kinds of pain and colic. It is especially useful for severe, unbearable, sharp, cutting, twisting, griping pains that dart about and extend to distant parts of the body. Pains are sudden and uncontrollable and may stop and start in different places. They are better for stretching out and worse for doubling up – completely opposite to the Colocynthis colic *picture.* Dioscorea *and* Dios. *are the abbreviations for this remedy.*

THE MAIN SYMPTOM PICTURE

Abdominal colic presents severe griping, cutting pains in and around the umbilicus. Violent twisting colic occurs in paroxysms or as if the intestines had been grasped and twisted. Pains may shift suddenly to a different site – often fingers and toes. Pains can radiate from the abdomen to back, chest and arms. There is much rumbling and **flatulence** and hurried desire for stool, which does not relieve colic. Patients feel worse for tea and doubling up, better for stretching out, bending backwards, and walking in open air. They may have early morning yellow diarrhea which drives them from bed.

Gall bladder colic is accompanied by cutting, sharp pain radiating from gall bladder to chest, back and arms; pain shifts location. **Better for** belching, **stretching out**, bending back; worse for doubling up.

Renal colic with pains in back, shooting down into legs. Patient is flatulent, with cold clammy sweat; better for standing upright.

Period pains which are cutting and griping radiate from the uterus and alternate with cramps in the fingers and toes. The woman may have vivid dreams; pain may be better for bending backwards and stretching, worse for doubling up.

***Leaves from the wild yam, the source for* Dioscorea villosa.**

THE DIOSCOREA PERSONALITY

People who need this remedy are easily made nervous and troubled. They may call things by the wrong names. They often have feeble digestive powers.

REMEDY SOURCE

Dioscorea is prepared from *Dioscorea villosa*, the wild yam, a tropical plant native to West Africa. This plant was the source material for the first oral contraceptives.

Drosera rotundifolia

- **Worse lying down and after midnight**
- **A dry cough with tickling**
- **Coughs that are spasmodic**
- **Stitching pains in the chest**
- **Better for motion**

INTRODUCTION

This remedy has an affinity with the respiratory system and long bones, and is indicated where there are tubercular complaints. It is an important remedy for whooping cough, and for other spasmodic, constrictive, exhausting coughs. Drosera *and* Dros. *are the abbreviations for this remedy.*

THE MAIN SYMPTOM PICTURE

The patient feels worse lying down and after midnight, and when drinking and eating; may have pains in teeth after drinking hot liquids.

Pains in the chest which are better for pressure.

A tickling cough comes every few hours with increasing intensity. It may lead to vomiting or hemorrhage. A tickling or crawling in the larynx provokes the cough and wakes the patient.

Constriction is felt in the throat, larynx or chest with the spasmodic cough; the patient can hardly get any breath; a suffocation with the spasm in the chest and larynx and constant violent paroxysms of coughing; this is **worse lying down**. Constriction prevents swallowing. Clutching, cramping, burning is felt in the larynx.

REMEDY SOURCE

Drosera is made from *Drosera rotundifolia*, a bog-loving insectivorous plant. Local names include youth wort, red rot, round-leaved sundew and devil's ear. The remedy is prepared from the whole fresh plant. The plant is used by herbalists for bronchitis and whooping cough.

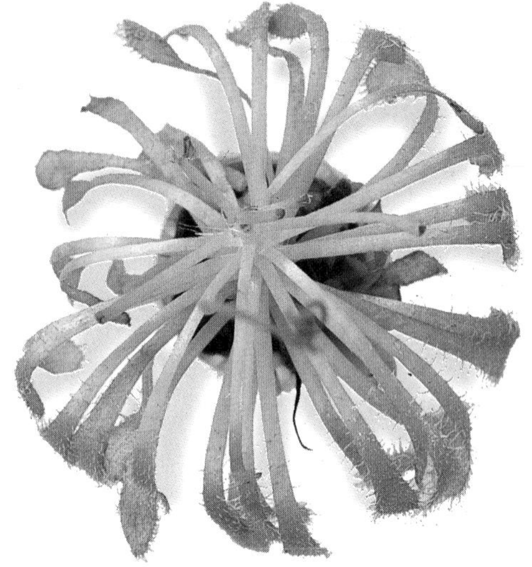

***Round-leaved sundew, the source for* Drosera rotundifolia. *It was proved by Hahnemann and appears in the fourth volume of his* Materia Medica Pura.**

The patient has a deep-sounding, hoarse cough; mucus is tenacious or dry.

Coughing spasm occurs every 2–3 hours, and is **worse lying down** at night until 3am.

Stitching pains in the chest are worse for coughing and better for pressure; the patient holds the chest as in Bryonia. Pain in top of abdomen, better for holding it while coughing.

Chill and fever are worse after midnight; patient has cold, copious sweat, hot head and cold extremities, and no thirst.

Patients may have shivering at rest, **better for motion**.

They feel generally better in the open air.

THE DROSERA PERSONALITY

People in need of *Drosera* may be strong and silent but fussy about small matters. They may be afraid of being alone and yet feel persecuted by others. Night is dreaded. The patient may be very cold, even in bed, and shivers a lot. Snoring may interrupt sleep. There is a distaste for acidic food and pork.

Dulcamara

- **Affinity for catarrhal states of mucous membrane**
- **Onset with every change of the weather, especially from warm to cold**
- **Perspiration that is checked**
- **Catarrh from taking cold**
- **Worse from cold, wet weather**

INTRODUCTION

Dulcamara *has a strong affinity for catarrhal states of the mucous membranes.*

Symptoms tend to alternate, often with asthmatic condition followed by skin rash or joint pains and then asthmatic problems once again. Symptoms tend to be on the left side. Pains are relieved by movement. Dulc. *is the abbreviation for this remedy.*

THE MAIN SYMPTOM PICTURE

REMEDY SOURCE

Dulcamara is prepared from *Solanum dulcamara*, the woody nightshade, a relative of *Belladonna*. It is also known as amaradulcis, or bittersweet. The remedy is made from green shoots and leaves, but not the berries, which are poisonous.

Onset is often caused by **every change of the weather, especially from warm to cold**; **from perspiration that is checked** especially if hot; **from taking cold**; from **cold, wet weather**.

Patients are worse in cold, damp weather, worse in the autumn, in the evening and at night, at rest. They are better for dry, calm weather, for motion, for rising from a seat, for warmth.

Diarrhea may come on when there are hot days and cold nights; the nature of the stools may keep on changing (as in Pulsatilla). Infant diarrhea may be like this. There are yellow or yellowy-green, slimy and undigested stools. Frequently there is a mass of slimy substance. Diarrheas come on after taking cold.

There may be back and neck pains and stiffness from cold and damp.

Fevers may come on from going into cold air while hot; patients may have trembling, aching bones and muscles; or be in a dazed state; they cannot remember things.

Sore catarrhal eyes result from taking cold.

There is a tendency for mucous membranes to ulcerate and for the ulcers to spread.

Sore throat occurs every time patients breathe cold air when overheated, especially if it is cold, damp air.

An urge to urinate may come if the patient becomes chilled.

There may be dry, teasing winter coughs; a dry, rough and hoarse or a loose cough with copious mucus. The patient feels worse lying down, or in a warm room, and better in the open air.

Cold sores may appear on the lips or genitalia.

A HERBAL CONNECTION

Solanum dulcamara also has an important place in the herbalists' repertoire, where it is generally called bittersweet. The stems and leaves are used to make ointments to treat psoriasis, eczema and ulcers. It is also taken as a tincture and an infusion for diarrhea and rheumatic problems.

THE DULCAMARA PERSONALITY

The mental state of the Dulcamara type is restless and confused, with a compulsion to keep on the move. Impatient desire for something is followed by indifference when the object is achieved. Dulcamara patients may be hungry but not want food.

Drowsiness prevails in the daytime but sleep is disturbed at night by restlessness.

***The woody nightshade, the source for* Dulcamara. *It was proved by Hahnemann and appears in his* Materia Medica Pura.**

Eupatorium perfoliatum

- **Aching in bones, which feel as if they would break**
- **Winter colds with much sneezing, coryza and headache which feels as if head would burst**
- **Chill at 7–9am, intense aching in bones before the chill**
- **Worse for motion**

INTRODUCTION

An aching in the bones as if they would break is the main feature of this remedy and accompanies all of its complaints. Otherwise, Eupatorium is very similar to Bryonia. Eupatorium *and* Eup. per. *are the abbreviations for this remedy.*

THE MAIN SYMPTOM PICTURE

Winter colds with much sneezing, coryza and bursting headache which **is worse for motion**, in a person who is chilly and wants to be warmly wrapped and has much aching in the bones. There can be fever or thirst and patients are generally worse for motion. After a few days, fever may go onto their chest or settle in the liver to cause a bilious fever or even jaundice.

An attack may begin with the sensation as if the back were breaking, with great shivering all over, a congestive headache and flushed face. There is high fever; bilious vomiting and aching bones. There may be stomach pains after eating. Patients want to keep still but the pains can be so severe that they must move, so sometimes they appear restless.

The chest may be sore, with a dry, racking, teasing, hacking cough which is worse for motion; it is similar to Bryonia and Phosphorus. There is hoarseness in the morning, with a sore, aching chest.

Patients are very sensitive to cold air, as much as in Nux vomica which also has aching bones and desire to be covered and in a hot room. Nux vomica has dreadful irritability of temper whereas Eupatorium tends towards overwhelming sadness.

There may be chill at 7–9am, and intense aching in bones before the chill. There is often a thirst, but during the chill cold water often makes this worse. There is vomiting of bile between the chill and the heat. Patients burn all over with the heat and feel hotter than their temperature would justify. There is usually little sweat. A violent headache may be present during the chill and it can be worse for sweat. Fever every third day.

REMEDY SOURCE

This remedy is made from *Eupatorium perfoliatum,* a member of the hemp agrimony family. It is also used in herbal medicine for digestive problems, cystitis and sore throats.

THE EUPATORIUM PERFOLIATUM PERSONALITY

The psychological picture of Eupatorium perfoliatum type is one of great sadness, restless anxiety and listlessness. People needing this remedy often sit in a characteristic way, with their hands resting flat on their knees and their shoulders raised, in an attempt to support the chest during labored breathing.

***Hemp agrimony, the source for* Eupatorium perfoliatum.**

Euphrasia officinalis

- **In fevers the chills predominate**
- **Catarrh; catarrhal headaches**
- **Profuse, watery, excoriating discharge from the eyes with a bland, runny discharge from the nose**
- **Marked affinity for the eyes**
- **Worse in daytime**
- **Better lying down**
- **No cough at night**

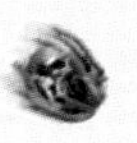

INTRODUCTION

This is a remedy suitable for catarrhal complaints but it also has a marked affinity for the eyes. Euphrasia *and* Euph. *are the abbreviations for this remedy.*

THE MAIN SYMPTOM PICTURE

A chilly person who cannot get warm. In fevers the **chills predominate,** with the fever mostly in the day; the patient is red faced with cold hands. Often perspiration is confined to the upper body.

Catarrhal headaches; often has a headache with eye complaints or coryza, a bursting, bruised headache with dazzling from bright lights or headache in the evening.

Catarrh may be with or without fever.

There is a tendency to accumulate sticky mucus on the cornea, removed by blinking.

Profuse, watery, excoriating discharge from the eyes, with a bland, runny discharge from the nose are very strong symptoms for this remedy.

Dry, burning, biting pressure in the **eyes**, as if from dust, with itching. Swollen mucous membranes, red and enlarged blood vessels; inflammation of all the tissues of the eye; contracted pupils. There may be a purulent discharge too. Patient has many tears in cold air and windy weather. The lids may be very sensitive and swollen; the margins itch and burn. Blepharitis. A fine rash about the eyes; pain in the eyes is worse for open air and light; lots of tears.

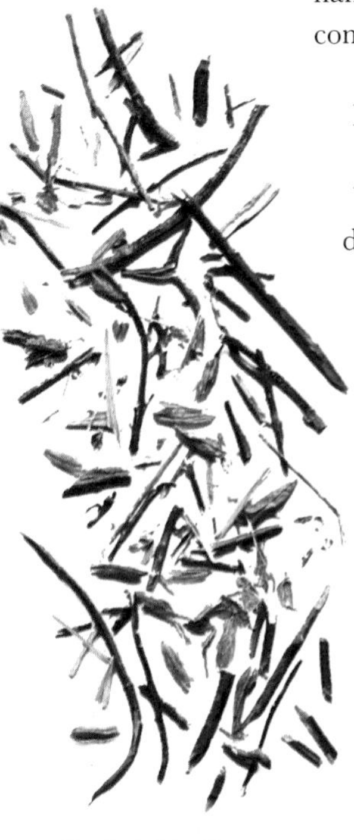

Eyebright, the source for **Euphrasia officinalis.** *The illustration shows the dried plant.*

Sneezing and fluent, bland coryza; the mucous membranes of the nose may be swollen and after a day or two the coryza may extend to the larynx with a hard cough.

Coryza is worse lying down at night and worse in the open air and windy weather.

Cough is worse in the daytime and is better lying down. It sometimes comes on in the open air. There may be hoarseness in the morning; irritation in the larynx with compulsion to cough, followed by pressure beneath the sternum. Abundant secretions in the larynx causing a loose cough with rattling in the chest; copious expectoration with or after the coryza. Difficulty breathing may be better lying down at night and worse in the morning, when there may be copious, and usually easy, expectoration. **No cough at night**, as in Bryonia. Usually loose, but sometimes can be a dry cough.

REMEDY SOURCE

This remedy is made from *Euphrasia officinalis*, better known as eyebright. It is also a popular remedy in herbalism, where it is best known as a cure for eye problems such as conjunctivitis and blepharitis.

THE EUPHRASIA PERSONALITY

As it is primarily an acute remedy for eye problems, there is no extensive psychological picture for *Euphrasia officinalis*. It is mostly used in a short-term situation, so there has been no need to observe long-term psychological symptoms to add to the remedy picture. It is more effective to look for the accompanying mental state and find a remedy to match that.

The growing plant, eyebright, also a herbal remedy for eye problems.

Ferrum phosphoricum

- **Complaints often come on from overexertion**
- **The early stages of many illnesses**
- **Great weakness and the desire to lie down**
- **Hemorrhagic complaints**
- **Nosebleeds**
- **Worse in the open air**
- **Better for gentle motion**

INTRODUCTION

The onset with Ferrum phosphoricum is not quite as rapid or violent as with Belladonna or Aconite but it is not quite as torpid and slow as with Gelsemium. Complaints often come on from overexertion. Ferrum *and* Ferr. p. *are the abbreviations for this remedy.*

THE MAIN SYMPTOM PICTURE

Great weakness with the desire to lie down is a strong feature, as are **hemorrhagic complaints**; problems involving some sort of bleeding. There may be fainting spells but the patient is more alert than in Belladonna. There are congestions and a vascular fullness, pulsations and rushes of blood. Flushes of the face and a flushed face – a false kind of plethora that is often confined to well-defined circular patches on the cheeks. The appearance of the patient may not be one of illness because of these pink cheeks.

There may be nervousness at night, and trembling limbs, though not as anxious as Aconite. Sometimes patients are loquacious and mirthful when ill. Often the mind is confused when trying to think; they have difficulty concentrating and can become forgetful, dull and indifferent as they tire; better for cold washing of the face.

Patients are sensitive to the open air and worse from it; always taking cold.

Soreness throughout the body is worse for jar and walking. Many complaints are worse from lying in bed and from rest and are better for slowly moving about, but the great lassitude compels patients to lie down. Subjects are restless at night with the fever, forever tossing about.

There may be numbness of affected parts, stitching, tearing pains and patients may be oversensitive to pain.

Ear infections with a purulent discharge, itching and noises in the ears or Eustachian catarrh may occur.

Coryza may be acrid and purulent or a bloody discharge. **Nosebleeds** may come with the coryza, with fear or with a headache, when the head is congested and hot.

Dry lips with a flushed face. Dry cough which is worse for cold, eating and deep breathing, with a mucous coryza or dryness. Sore chest or stitching pain with the cough or deep breathing. There is mucus of all sorts.

Backache, a stiff neck, wry neck.

Chills in the afternoon and at night, a shaking chill. Fever has a dry heat with thirst, flushes of heat and perspiration.

There may be cold extremities or heat all over.

Patients may desire sour things but are worse for eating or drinking them.

Worse in the open air; for physical exertion, after eating; cold drinks; sour food; standing; patients are better for gentle motion, as Pulsatilla.

REMEDY SOURCE

Ferrum phosphoricum is made from iron, a very important trace element in the body.

Iron phosphate ($Fe_3(PO_4)_2$), the source for* Ferrum phosphoricum. *This is one of the twelve tissue, or mineral, salts identified by Dr Wilhelm Schuessler (1821-98).

THE FERRUM PHOSPHORICUM PERSONALITY

As it is a tissue salt, *Ferrum phosphoricum* works directly on the body at a cellular level and so there are few outstanding mental symptoms in the overall picture. Any symptoms that may show are usually a result of fluctuating oxygen levels in the blood.

Gelsemium sempervirens

- **Complaints may follow fear, shock, embarrassment or fright**
- **Insidious onset**
- **Slow, congestive complaints and headache**
- **Congestion of the head**
- **Face flushed, dusky**
- **Mottled skin**
- **Cold extremities**
- **Disturbed sensations**
- **Paralytic state of sphincters**
- **Ptosis**

INTRODUCTION

The complaints of Gelsemium may follow fear, shock, embarrassment or fright. There is an insidious onset of complaints, several days after exposure or shock, etc. Colds and fevers are of a low grade, not violent. Slow, congestive complaints and headaches. Congestion of the head is most marked. It is suited to the warmer climates and milder winters. Gelsemium. *and* Gels. are *the abbreviations for this remedy.*

False jasmine, the source for* Gelsemium sempervirens. *It was first introduced into the homeopathic canon by Dr Hale in 1862.

THE MAIN SYMPTOM PICTURE

Congestive headaches, with most violent pain in the occiput; sometimes hammering, pulsating pain. So violent sometimes that patients cannot stand up, but lie perfectly exhausted. Often better for lying still, bolstered up by pillows. Better for pressure and for alcohol, which stimulates the person; worse for mental exertion, smoking, lying with the head low, heat of the sun. **Face is flushed, dusky**, mind dazed, eyes glassy, pupils often dilated, cold extremities; there is **mottled skin**, scanty urine, cramps in fingers, toes and back.

Dizziness with blurred or double vision.

Cold extremities, with hot head and back; face purple during congestion, high fever. Great coldness and chills run up and down the back; pains can go up the back too. Chattering teeth and shaking, even without a sense of coldness. High fever in the afternoons may progress to a continued fever with **little thirst** and marked head complaints, a dazed mind, etc. Patients are as still as in Bryonia but it is because they are so weary, not from the pain, and the head is more congested than in Bryonia. Profuse, exhaustive sweats; patient too weak to move.

Coryza with sneezing and a watery discharge, and cold extremities. It goes down to the throat with redness and swelling, enlarged tonsils, hot head, congested face, heavy limbs. Onset is gradual.

There may be tearing pains in nerves, sciatica, numbness, **disturbed sensations**. Disturbance of vision before attacks; double, dim, misty vision or nystagmus.

Palpitations with fever. A sense of weakness or 'goneness' in the heart region extends to the stomach, creating a sensation of hunger. The heart's pulse is feeble, soft and irregular (unlike Aconite or Belladonna).

Paralytic states of sphincters – involuntary stool and urination. Weakness of extremities or just awkward and clumsy. **Ptosis.**

Diarrhea from sudden excitement or emotion, bad news, fright, or anticipation of some ordeal.

THE GELSEMIUM PERSONALITY

A feeling of great weight and tiredness runs all through the remedy; patients feel so weary and heavy that they must lie down and lie still, trembling if they attempt to move. In fevers, children may have a fear of falling and hold on tight. They are in a state of nervous excitement when awake, though they lie thinking of nothing in particular because their minds will not work in an orderly way. They may be dazed and talk as if delirious, forgetful; worse for mental exertions and averse to speaking or even having company present; too tired to communicate and not wanting to make the effort.

REMEDY SOURCE

Gelsemium is made from Carolina jasmine (*Gelsemium sempervirens* or *Gelsemium nitidum*); it is also known as yellow jasmine and false jasmine and is a native of North America. The remedy is made from the fresh roots and bark of the plant's rhizome.

Glonoin

- **Violent symptoms**
- **Disordered circulation**
- **Headaches and migraines**
- **Worse for heat, artificial light**

INTRODUCTION

It comes as no surprise that symptoms in the Glonoin picture are characteristically quick and violent, bursting and expansive, as this is potentized nitro-glycerine. It is truly an explosive remedy.

Nitro-glycerine is used in allopathic medicine for heart complaints, and in homeopathy it has an affinity for blood and the circulation. Throbbings, palpitations, pulsations and cardiac pain are all violent. Glon. *is the abbreviation or this remedy.*

THE MAIN SYMPTOM PICTURE

Glonoin can be very useful in severe **headaches and migraine** where the picture fits. There is a sensation of over-fullness in the blood vessels, nausea and vomiting are likely and the head feels hot. Any kind of **heat makes the patient worse,** particularly hot sun, while open air and cold applications feel beneficial. They may hold the head, but any kind of pressure, even wearing a hat, can become unbearable.

REMEDY SOURCE

Glonoin is prepared from nitro-glycerine, a highly unstable chemical compound ($C_3H_5(ONO_2)_3$). It is a thick oil made by treating glycerine with nitric and sulphuric acid, and is the explosive component of dynamite.

The eyes are affected and feel hot and dry, with a wild or protruding look. Vision is impaired with visual disturbances, **aggravated by artificial light**.

Patients feel better after a good long sleep, but may feel giddy and heady on waking.

The Glonoin picture may be seen before or during a period, or at the menopause where hot flushes sweep up the body.

THE GLONOIN PERSONALITY

As it is primarily an acute remedy for sunstroke, there is no extensive psychological picture for Glonoin. It is mostly used in a short-term situation, so there has been no need to observe long-term psychological symptoms to add to the remedy picture. However, pain may be felt as so unbearable that the sufferer wants to jump out of the window.

THE TYPESETTER'S REMEDY

Glonoin was a useful remedy for the blinding headaches suffered by Victorian typesetters and printers who had to work under the fierce heat of incandescent gas lamps. Glonoin patients cannot bear heat on top of or on the back of their heads.

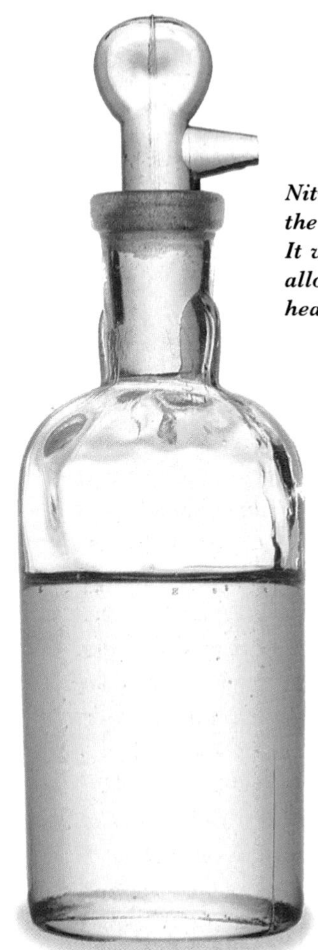

Nitro-glycerine, the source for* Glonoin. *It was also used as an allopathic drug for heart disease.

Hepar sulphuris calcareum

- **Chilly, irritable and hypersensitive**
- **Onset from exposure to dry, cold winds**
- **The least uncovering of a hand or foot causes chilliness**
- **Oversensitivity to impressions, touch, surroundings, cold and pain**
- **Quarrelsome, nothing pleases, everything disturbs**
- **Catarrhal states**
- **Sweating all night without relief**
- **Worse for cold**
- **Better for heat and wet weather**

INTRODUCTION

This remedy has a strong affinity with the nervous system, the respiratory system, the skin and the mucous membranes of the mouth and throat. Hep., Hepar, *and* Hepar sulph. *are the abbreviations for this remedy.*

THE MAIN SYMPTOM PICTURE

Caused by **exposure to dry, cold winds** or after the premature disappearance of a rash.

All the complaints are **worse for cold**. Patients want the room to be warm and to be well covered. The **least uncovering of a hand or foot causes chilliness** or cough.

Oversensitive to impressions, touch, surroundings, cold and pain. Intense suffering, even apparently without sufficient cause. Pains are severe, sharp and sticking; very sensitive inflammations and ulcerations; splinter pains in the throat worse from swallowing. There may even be fainting with the pains.

Tendency to suppuration – glands, ulcers, boils, injuries.

Catarrhal states; coryza with much sneezing and obstruction on going into a cold wind. Initially watery, later thick, yellow and offensive smelling – often like decomposed cheese. All discharges can smell of rotten cheese, or may smell sour.

Copious catarrhs of the throat and pharynx; splinter pains; patient is extremely sensitive to touch; pain on swallowing.

Loss of voice and dry, hoarse bark, especially in the mornings and the evenings, **worse for cold** and dry winds, worse for uncovering.

This is a great remedy for croup for sensitive children who have been exposed to cold air or dry, cold winds and have come down with croup the following morning ; worse morning and evening. It may follow *Aconite* if an attack returns the next morning. The more rattling there is in the chest, the more it is like Hepar. There may be a loose cough in the day and a dry, paroxysmal cough in the evening and night.

The catarrhal state may be lower down in the trachea, which becomes extremely sore from much coughing for days and weeks. Again this is worse morning and evening – a rattling, wheezing, barking cough in an oversensitive, chilly patient. The patient may cough and sweat; much sweating throughout the night, which does not relieve.

Sweating all night without relief is found in many complaints. Sweats easily.

Ear infections with a bloody, purulent, cheesy smelling discharge and sticking pains. Offensive, thick eye discharges too.

They may hate fat and love vinegar, pickles and other sour things, spices, strong tasting foods.

Better for heat and wet weather, damp.

Worse for lying on the painful side, touch, pressure, motion, exertion, tight clothing.

Flowers of Sulphur, one of the source ingredients for* Hepar sulphuris calcareum.** ***A proving appears in the fourth volume of Hahnemann's **Materia Medica Pura.**

THE HEPAR PERSONALITY

Hepar subjects are delicate, oversensitive people who become extremely irritable. Angry, abusive and impulsive, they are quarrelsome, nothing pleases, and everything disturbs. They desire a constant change of people, surroundings or things.

REMEDY SOURCE

Hepar sulphuris calcareum is made from Liver of Sulphur, a form of calcium sulphide (sulphurated potash). Hahnemann directed the source to be made from equal parts powdered oyster shells and Flowers of Sulphur.

Hyoscyamus niger

- **Confusion, passive stupor**
- **Sudden short outburst**
- **Twitchings and tremblings**
- **High fever**
- **Starts up during sleep**
- **Worse when covered**
- **Better for warmth**
- **Cough is better for sitting up**
- **Eyes sensitive to light**

INTRODUCTION

Hyoscyamus *belongs to the same botanical family as* Belladonna, *so there are certain similarities between the homeopathic pictures of these two remedies. Both show disturbances of the brain and there is high fever in both. Hyoscyamus, however, is generally more passive in its reactions; the patient may be too weak to respond in the active way of Belladonna, so this remedy is therefore often useful in the elderly.* Hyoscyamus *and* Hyosc. *are the abbreviations for this remedy.*

THE MAIN SYMPTOM PICTURE

There is **confusion** and even delirium but it is mumbling and bumbling, with a detachment from the real world. Any violent outbursts soon die down and patients sink back into a **passive stupor**.

On the physical level, there is not enough energy to express symptoms fully.

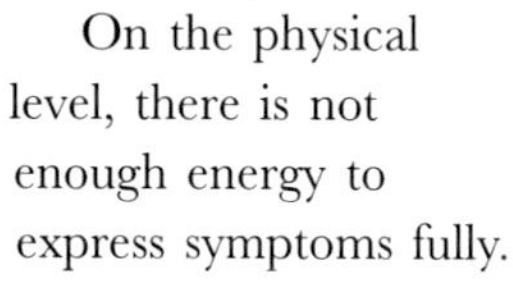

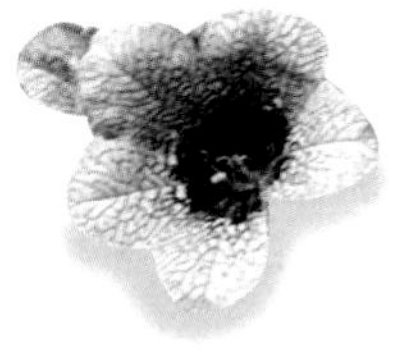

Where an illness has been strongly suppressed, this picture may break through. For example, someone who has been 'dosing himself up' with medicine to keep going may eventually break down and develop a *Hyosc.* flu.

Twitchings and tremblings occur. **When asleep they may suddenly sit up** in bed and then lie down again, or they may sob and cry out in their sleep. They cannot bear the touch of clothes on the skin and **do not like to be covered over**, even though they are **better for warmth**. The **eyes are sensitive to light** and disturbance of vision may continue after other symptoms subside. The **cough is dry** and **worse when lying down** – immediately the patient sits up, it stops.

REMEDY SOURCE

This remedy is made from *Hyoscyamus niger*, black henbane also known as hairy henbane, stinking Roger or hog's bean. It thrives in garbage heaps and badly kept cemeteries and is extremely poisonous. The remedy is made from the whole plant.

THE HYOSCYAMUS PERSONALITY

There is a general sense of lack of self-expression, which may show itself as muttering to imaginary people, suspicion or obsession. Hallucination and delusions of all kinds may occur. There is an urge to count things – this is the patient who lies in bed counting the flowers on the wallpaper.

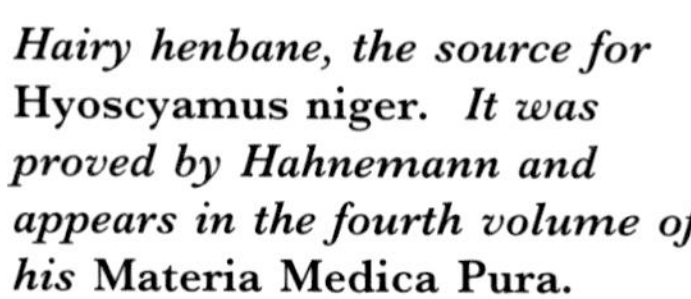

***Hairy henbane, the source for* Hyoscyamus niger. *It was proved by Hahnemann and appears in the fourth volume of his* Materia Medica Pura.**

Hypericum perforatum

- **First aid remedy**
- **Injuries to parts rich in nerves**
- **Pain shoots along nerve path**
- **Gaping wounds**
- **Pain worse for motion and pressure**
- **Spinal injuries**

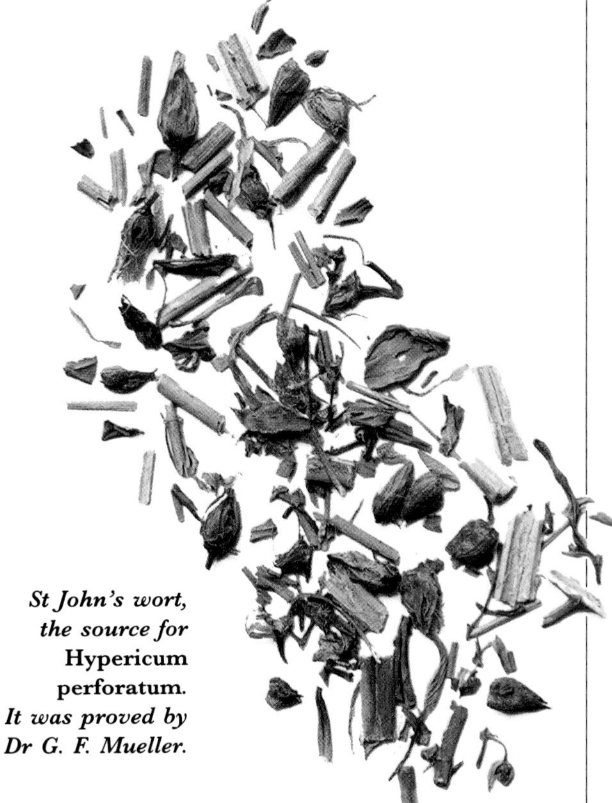

St John's wort, the source for* Hypericum perforatum. *It was proved by Dr G. F. Mueller.

INTRODUCTION

Hypericum *has an affinity with the nervous system, especially the sheaths of the nerves and the meninges of the brain. It is particularly recommended for wounds involving nerves, and can be used after* Ledum *for puncture wounds caused by animal bites. It is also indicated for injuries to the head (concussion), spine or coccyx.* Hypericum *and* Hyper. *are the abbreviations for this remedy.*

THE MAIN SYMPTOM PICTURE

Hypericum is used mainly as a **first aid remedy** where there is **damage to parts of the body rich in nerves**, such as fingers, nails, lips.

In particular *Hypericum* is for **injuries to the spine** such as a blow to the top of the head or coccyx that jars the spinal column. Also useful after a lumbar puncture or spinal injection.

This remedy is usually associated with great pain. Typically the **pain shoots along the path of the nerve**, for example from an injured hand or foot, up the arm or leg. The painful part feels much **worse if it is moved or touched**, for example toothache is better if the patient keeps still and lies on the painful side.

Patients are nervous and cry out with pain. *Hypericum* deals with the shock of injury, but where there has been trauma such as in an accident or tooth extraction, *Arnica* can be given first.

Hypericum is useful for **gaping wounds** where the nerves are damaged and there is much pain. Compare with *Calendula,* which is better suited to superficial cuts.

Also suitable for old scars which are still painful.

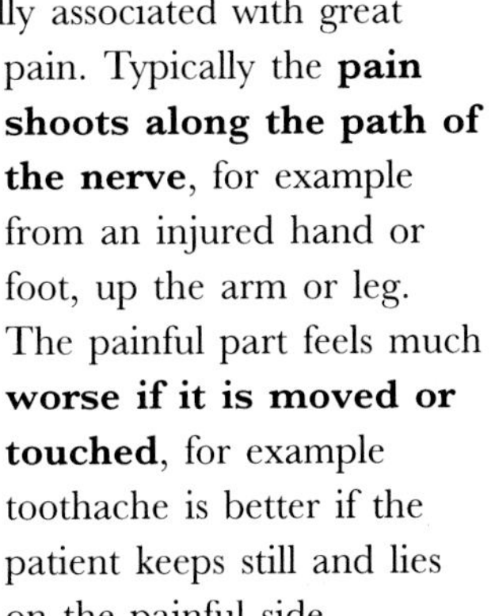

REMEDY SOURCE

Hypericum is made from *Hypericum perforatum,* St John's wort, which has been an important remedy for herbalists and conventional medicine as well as in homeopathy. Herbalists used it to heal wounds. The remedy is made from the whole fresh plant.

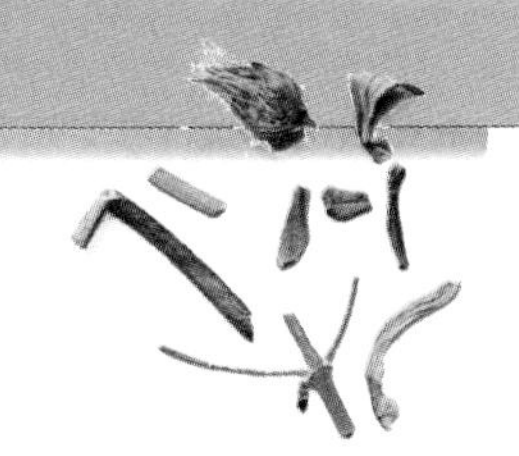

THE HYPERICUM PERSONALITY

As this is mainly a first aid remedy, the mental picture is usually characterized as severe depression following injury involving the nerves. Memory may be impaired.

A SAINT'S REMEDY

St John's wort is named for John the Baptist. The black 'perforation' marks on the leaves were considered to be a symbol of St John's beheading at the behest of Salome, Herod's daughter. Medieval herbalists construed the marks as stab wounds and so used the herb as a cure for cuts.

Ignatia amara

- **Sensation of a lump**
- **Cough and sore throat**
- **Loss of appetite or overeating**
- **Sleeplessness**
- **Grief, bereavement, broken love affair**
- **Much sighing**

INTRODUCTION

In Ignatia, look for some recent grief or emotional upset. The remedy has a strong mental and emotional picture and may bring comfort and relief to someone who is unhappy, even if he or she shows no obvious physical symptoms. Ignatia *and* Ign. *are the abbreviations for this remedy.*

THE MAIN SYMPTOM PICTURE

The throat is often affected. There is a **sensation of a lump** in the throat and the pain is lessened when swallowing solid food. There is a sense of constriction in the throat after an emotional shock. One **cough** causes patients to keep on coughing. This can feel like choking and they need to take a deep breath.

In ear complaints there may be deafness or noises in the ear and patients may prefer to be in a noisy place or to play music, as this seems to help their hearing problems.

If there is an **appetite it is probably insatiable**. They crave raw food and indigestible things, preferring cold food to a hot meal, but not wanting to eat fruit. *Ignatia* is often useful in **eating disorders such as anorexia and bulimia,** where there is a strong emotional element. In cases of long-term eating disorders it is essential to seek professional help, counselling and dietary advice as well as constitutional homeopathic treatment.

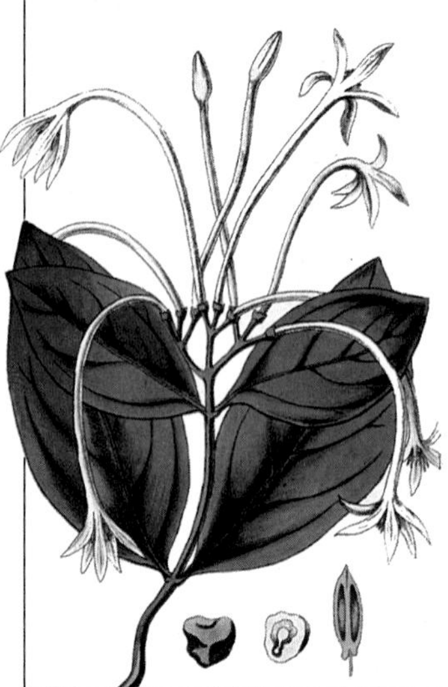

***St Ignatius' bean, the source for* Ignatia amara. *It was first proved by Hahnemann and appears in the third edition of the second volume of his* Materia Medica Pura.**

If patients are feverish they will not be thirsty, but thirst reappears if they are chilly. Digestive symptoms include hiccups, flatulence and painful piles which feel better when walking about.

The heart is a focus for symptoms at all levels. Emotional heartache may be coupled with, or replaced by, anxiety and palpitations. Yawning and sighing show the desire to draw deep breaths into this region.

The *Ignatia* remedy is closely related to *Natrum mur.* and it may sometimes be difficult to choose between them. Ignatia people generally respond to grief in an emotional way; Natrum mur. people are more likely to hide their emotional grief and produce physical symptoms. *Ignatia* generally suits recent grief and *Natrum mur.* more long-term distress.

REMEDY SOURCE

Ignatia amara is made from the fruits of *Strychnos ignatia,* also known as St Ignatius' bean. The remedy is made from the heavy, pebble-like seeds embedded in the bitter pulp of the fruit.

Sleep may be impossible or very light so the slightest thing causing waking. Bad dreams and sleepwalking may occur as a result of emotional stress.

THE IGNATIA PERSONALITY

Ignatia people may sigh a lot and want to be alone to brood and cry. They may start to weep if asked what is the matter, and can have bouts of hysterical sobbing.

They can also laugh hysterically. In fact, they show many contradictory symptoms at all levels. Symptoms can also change rapidly (in a similar way to Pulsatilla); for example, they may refuse food, or may overeat in their misery; they may be very sensitive to pain or appear not to be troubled by something that looks painful.

They are nervous and apprehensive. A bright child suddenly bursts into tears because he is worried about an exam; a person who has been upset by a friend sulks and flies into a temper.

They often develop nervous headaches with the sensation of a nail being driven into the skull. They can also suffer from nervous paralysis, spasms and twitching.

Ipecacuanha

- **Rapid onset over a few hours**
- **Prostration comes in spells**
- **Nausea and vomiting accompany all complaints**
- **Vomiting does not relieve the nausea**
- **Bronchitis of children with coarse rattling, coughing, gagging and a sense of suffocation**
- **Great desire for fresh air**

INTRODUCTION

Nausea and vomiting run right through this remedy, especially if the vomiting does not relieve the nausea. Often an acute complaint begins with nausea and vomiting, with a clean tongue. The stomach and bowels feel relaxed, as if hanging down. Ip. *is the abbreviation for this remedy.*

THE MAIN SYMPTOM PICTURE

Onset is rapid. Prostration comes in spells, unlike Arsenicum, where it is continuous.

Complaints may come on from suppressed emotions or vexations. Nausea may come from eating rich foods, as in Pulsatilla, and after dietary indulgences.

Violent chills may occur, with the face flushed bright red or bluish-red.

Colds settle in the nose, which may stuff up at night with much sneezing and blowing out of mucus and often blood; nosebleeds with every cold. Colds descend and produce hoarseness, then rawness of the trachea, then to the chest with suffocation and a great accumulation of mucus, but there is an expulsive power to the cough (unlike in Antimonium tartaricum).

Dry, teasing, hacking cough with a sense of suffocation. Patients choke and gag and get red in the face. Bloody sputum. Whooping cough may be like this, or even asthma.

Bronchitis of children with **coarse rattling, coughing, gagging and a sense of suffocation**, weight and anxiety in the chest, after a rapid onset. They look dreadfully sick, drawn and pale; again, the condition has come on rapidly. Mucus in the chest will not come up; rattling and wheezing.

Wheeziness is worse in damp weather, better for sitting up and fresh air. Often patients **desire fresh air very much**. Cough with inclination to vomit, without nausea; the nausea is usually intense, though.

Generally thirstless except in the fever, which is prolonged and with nausea.

Headache as if bruised all through the bones of the head and down into the root of the tongue, with nausea. Nausea may precede the headache.

Dysentery like diarrhea with awful tenesmus; the patient may pass a little blood or green slime. Constant nausea; vomits bile; vomits everything taken in, with great prostration and great pallor. Copious diarrhea, often of green slime or mucus. Much crying and straining at stool in the infant. Colic with nausea and green stools; fermented, foamy stools.

Worse for damp, overeating.

Better for open air, rest.

REMEDY SOURCE

Ipecacuanha is made from *Cephaelis ipecacuanha*, a perennial plant native to Brazil. The remedy is made from the dried root. *Ipecacuanha* was used as an anti-dysentery drug in Brazil and France in the seventeenth century, and later became popular for a variety of ailments. Mixed with opium and potassium sulphate, it was sold as the wide-spectrum panacea known as Dover's Powder.

THE IPECACUANHA PERSONALITY

The person who needs *Ipecacuanha* is malcontent, impatient and full of nebulous, unsatisfied desires; tends to be sulky, out of temper and scornful of others. He or she feels nauseated by everything.

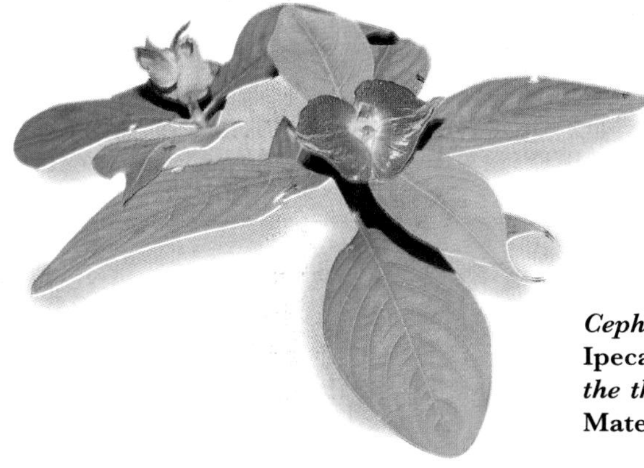

***Cephaelis, the source for* Ipecacuanha. *A proving appears in the third volume of Hahnemann's* Materia Medica Pura.**

Iris versicolor

- **Burning pains**
- **Profuse urination**
- **Profuse watery vomit and diarrhea**
- **Worse for heat and during hot weather**
- **Occurs at regular intervals**
- **Migraine**

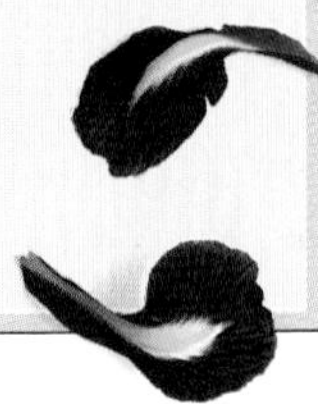

INTRODUCTION

Iris *is a useful remedy where there are strong burning pains with rapid and profuse elimination. It is appropriate where there are strongly marked symptoms, and in such cases professional advice may be necessary.* Iris *and* Iris.v. *are the abbreviations for this remedy.*

THE MAIN SYMPTOM PICTURE

In stomach disorders the whole digestive tract feels as if it is burning. There is constant nausea; vomiting is sudden with **large quantities of acrid watery vomit. Diarrhea is also watery and burning**; in cystitis there is burning along the whole of the urethra after urination.

REMEDY SOURCE

Iris is prepared from *Iris versicolor.*

These gastric states can occur with a headache, as in migraine, and may come on with a marked **periodicity**, meaning that they occur at regular intervals, weekly or monthly. For example, this person may be well all week but suffer **migraine** with burning gastric symptoms every Sunday.

Symptoms may come on, or get worse, around 2am, and are **worse for heat or during hot weather**.

THE IRIS PERSONALITY

The mental state may not be significant, but Iris subjects are likely to feel dull and low in spirits.

Iris, the source for* Iris versicolor. *There are remedies made from several different members of the Iris family, but this is the most often used.

Jaborandi

- **Eye complaints with profuse tears**
- **Much salivation**
- **Profuse sweat**
- **Dry skin**
- **Useful for mumps**
- **Possible pre-menstrual remedy**

INTRODUCTION

Jaborandi *is a remedy that is particularly useful in glandular complaints, but it does not have a very wide application. The source,* Pilocarpus jaborandi, *is used to make the allopathic drug pilocarpine.* Jab. *is the abbreviation for this remedy.*

THE MAIN SYMPTOM PICTURE

The glands are strongly stimulated in this remedy and it has a particular affinity for the eyes. Twitching, smarting and all sorts of **visual disturbances** occur, all accompanied by a **profuse flow of tears**.

REMEDY SOURCE

Jaborandi is prepared from *Pilocarpus jaborandi*, a woody shrub native to Brazil.

The mouth produces **much saliva**, even when the throat feels dry. Similarly there is a **lot of sweating**, even though the **skin is dry** and sometimes red. Coughing produces much thin mucus.

The Jaborandi state is one that can occur pre-menstrually and may be accompanied by hot flushes.

As a glandular remedy, it may be useful in **mumps** if the picture fits.

THE JABORANDI PERSONALITY

The mental state is one of nervous excitement, but not talkative. Provings of *Jaborandi* give the mental symptom 'has a fixed idea she will murder all her family with a hatchet'. This symptom is not likely to occur – if it does, seek urgent professional assistance!

Kali bichromicum

- **Catarrhal remedy**
- **Copious, ropy, mucus discharges from mucous membranes anywhere**
- **Wandering pains and very severe pains in small spots**
- **Always suffering with nasal catarrh**
- **Better for warmth**
- **Worse in the morning**

INTRODUCTION

This remedy has an affinity with skin and mucous membrane. Thick ropy mucus is characteristic. There may also be alternation of symptoms, with catarrhal symptoms clearing up when diarrhea appears, for instance. Kali bich. *and* Kali bi. *are the abbreviations for this remedy.*

REMEDY SOURCE

Kali bichromicum is prepared from bichromate of potash which derives from chromium iron ore.

THE MAIN SYMPTOM PICTURE

There may be **copious, ropy, mucus discharges from mucous membranes anywhere**; great long string of mucus; jelly-like mucus.

The catarrhal symptoms may alternate with joint symptoms and rheumatic pains in the winter. In the summer, diarrhea alternates with rheumatic complaints.

Wandering pains (as in Pulsatilla) **and very severe pains in small spots**, such as can be covered by a thumb tip, are characteristic. Sharp, stitching pains too. Pains often appear and disappear rapidly (as in Belladonna).

A chilly person, everywhere, especially in the back of the neck. Pains and cough are made better by warmth or warm bed.

Always suffering with a nasal catarrh; pressing pain in the root of the nose with a chronic catarrh and if exposed to the cold the discharge dries up and a headache begins (as in Kali carbonicum), often starting with dim vision. The pains may be pulsating, shooting, burning, better for warmth and pressure. One-sided pains or even just in spots. Often retching and vomiting occur with the headache and sometimes vertigo; worse in the morning, at night, for motion, and stooping.

Very red, inflamed throat with swollen tonsils, swollen neck and even suppuration; with this the pain extends to the ears. There may be a dry burning sensation; a dry mouth, ropy mucus, mouth ulcers. The uvula can be edematous. Intense pain in the root of the tongue on protrusion may be present or the sensation of a hair on the tongue. Yellow coating at the base of the tongue or a dry, smooth, glazed, cracked tongue.

Copious, thick, ropy mucus from the larynx; hoarseness, rough voice, dry cough. Cough worse for breathing, worse in damp, cold weather and may be better in a warm bed at night. Stitching pain with the cough. Much wheezing and tightness in the centre of the chest. There is a characteristic pain from the sternum to the back with the catarrh and the cough. A tickling, dry, hard cough; great soreness in the chest on coughing or deep breathing. Hard coughing on waking, better lying down, warm bed, worse for cold air, undressing, deep breathing. Ropy, yellow or green mucus with rattling in the chest.

Digestion is suspended and food lies like a load in the stomach; fullness and distress come on immediately after eating. Much fetid eructation. Averse to meat but may desire beer, which produces vomiting and diarrhea.

Worse at 2–3am, in the morning, for motion.

Ulcers of mucous membranes can be deep, as if punched out.

THE KALI BICHROMICUM PERSONALITY

The person needing *Kali bichromicum* is listless and low; there may be distrust of strangers, or even misanthropy. Memory is poor and there is aversion to mental and physical effort. There may be an intolerance of carbohydrate foods.

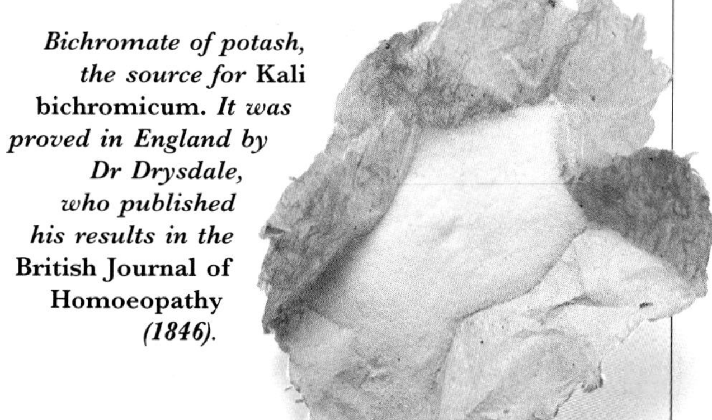

Bichromate of potash, the source for* Kali bichromicum. *It was proved in England by Dr Drysdale, who published his results in the* British Journal of Homoeopathy *(1846).

Kali carbonicum

- **Sensitive to every draft or air movement**
- **Stitching pains**
- **Pains that fly around**
- **Worse from 3–5am**
- **Dry, hacking, barking cough in cold air**
- **Swelling between eyelids and eyebrows**

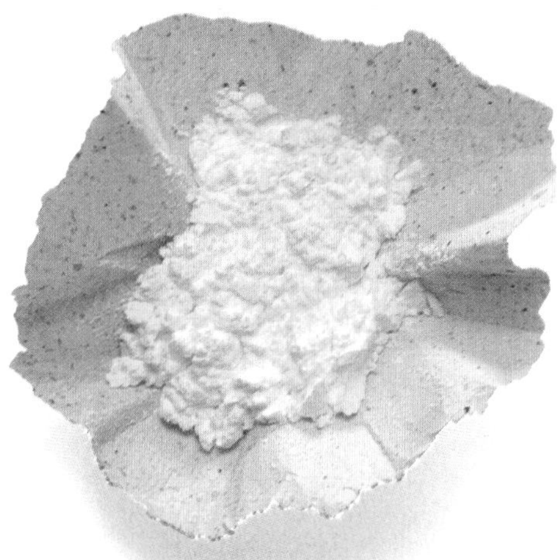

***Potash, the source for* Kali carbonicum. *It was proved by Hahnemann and appears in the first edition of his* Chronic Diseases.**

INTRODUCTION

This remedy is indicated when the delicate potassium/sodium balance of the body is upset. Potassium is essential for the transmission of impulses in the central nervous system, and malfunction is experienced as the stabbing pains which characterize the remedy. Kali carb. *and* Kali c. *are the abbreviations for this remedy.*

THE MAIN SYMPTOM PICTURE

REMEDY SOURCE

Kali carbonicum is made from potash (K_2O), the carbonate of potassium. Potassium is an important tissue salt in the cell structure of the body.

These people are worse in wet weather and worse in cold weather. They tend to be sensitive to every change in the atmosphere; they cannot get the temperature exactly right. **Sensitive to every draft or air movement.**

Sensitive to cold, always shivering. Their nerves may be painful when cold and if the affected part is kept warm the pain goes to some other place that is uncovered. **Stitching pains**, burning, tearing pains. **Pains that fly around**, wander from place to place.

Worse from 3–5am.

Catarrhal, congestive headaches from cold air, which clears the nose and brings on a headache (as in Kali bich.). In a warm room, the nose discharges and fills up, which ameliorates the headache; a thick, fluent, yellow discharge.

Colds tend to locate in the chest.

Dry cough day and night with vomiting of food and some phlegm, worse after eating and drinking, worse evenings.

Chronic bronchitis. Dryness, a **dry**, **hacking**, **barking cough in cold air**, which is when they feel most uncomfortable; copious expectoration of mucus in the warm which produces a general amelioration. Expectoration may be very offensive, tenacious, lumpy, blood-streaked or like thick, yellow or yellow/green pus, often with a pungent, cheesy taste. Mostly patients have a dry hacking cough with morning expectoration, increasing to a most violent, gagging cough with vomiting and sensation as if their head would burst or fly to pieces. The face begins to swell and the eyes to protrude with the cough and then comes **edema between the eyelids and the eyebrows**, even to the extent of a little water bag forming.

Wheeziness worse from 3–5am, better leaning forward or rocking, as in Arsenicum; with rattling in the chest, rattling cough and stitches in the chest with respiration, as in Bryonia, or between breaths. Sputum of small round lumps.

Pain in the lower right chest through to the back (as in Mercurius), worse lying on the painful side (opposite to Bryonia).

Great flatulence, everything eaten turns to gas.

THE KALI CARBONICUM PERSONALITY

The mental picture of Kali carbonicum is one of exhausted, touchy irritability. Kali carbonicum people want company but tend not to get on with anybody. They are very sensitive to noise and complain about everything. They are usually fearful of the future, of death, or even of ghosts.

Kali muriaticum

- **Thick white discharges**
- **Ulcerated throat**
- **Blocked sinuses**
- **Blister-like eruptions**
- **Worse for eating**
- **Dark menstrual flow**
- **Constipation**
- **This remedy is a tissue salt**

INTRODUCTION

This remedy is one of the tissue salts and works well in low potency in acute situations. It is particularly useful for ear ache with blocked Eustachian tubes and for indigestion and diarrhea from a surfeit of rich, fatty foods. It also works well in the secondary stages of any inflammatory complaint. Kali mur. *and* Kali m. *are the abbreviations for this remedy.*

REMEDY SOURCE

Kali muriaticum is made from potassium chloride (KCl). It is one of the 12 tissue, or mineral, salts identified by Dr Wilhelm Schuessler (1821-98).

THE MAIN SYMPTOM PICTURE

Secretions are thicker than the watery Natrum mur. kind, and are milky or greyish white and sticky, sometimes lumpy. In colds and flu the ears, nose and **sinus** areas feel swollen and **blocked up** with a thick catarrh. This seems to be worse in bed at night.

The **throat is sore and ulcerated** and the tonsils swollen; there may be ulcers in the mouth. *Kali mur.* is also useful in conditions such as chicken pox when the spots have come out and **blister-like** eruptions can be seen on the skin.

They are better for cold drinks but may have **no appetite for food** as eating brings on indigestion or nausea.

They are worse for open air, drafts and damp, but no better when lying in a warm bed.

Kali mur. is useful during a **period** where the **flow is dark** and clotted. Other symptoms may be a bloated abdomen, **constipation** and painful breasts. A **thick, milky-white discharge** between periods may also respond well to *Kali mur.*

THE KALI MUR. PERSONALITY

As a tissue salt, *Kali muriaticum* is a remedy that works directly on the cellular level of the body. Therefore, there is no outstanding psychological profile and it would be more effective to take careful notes of the mental state and look for a remedy to match it.

A COMBINATION CURE

The 12 tissue salts are used in various combinations to treat specific problems. *Kali muriaticum* forms part of six such combinations. For example, combination remedy D (with *Kali muriaticum*, *Kali sulphuricum*, *Calcarea sulphurica* and *Silica*) is useful for minor skin eruptions, and combination remedy S (with *Kali muriaticum*, *Natrum phosphoricum* and *Natrum sulphuricum*) is good for 'holiday tummy' (queasiness and stomach upsets).

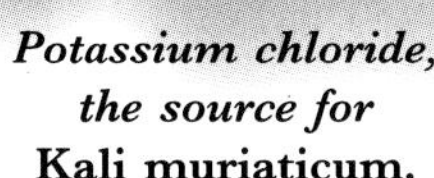

Potassium chloride, the source for **Kali muriaticum.**

Kali phosphoricum

- **Septic conditions**
- **Insomnia**
- **Tiredness**
- **Nervous excitement**
- **Dry nose and mouth with offensive discharge**
- **Worse for exertion, better for rest**
- **This remedy is a tissue salt**

INTRODUCTION

Kali phosphoricum *is a tissue salt and works well in low potency.* Kali phosphoricum *has the nervous excitability of Phosphoros but is used where there are septic conditions in the body and the discharges are yellowish and putrid. The remedy is useful even when there are no physical symptoms but the brain seems under- or overactive.* Kali phos. *and* Kali p. *are the abbreviations for this remedy.*

THE MAIN SYMPTOM PICTURE

Patients are extremely **tired** and feel weak and depressed, especially if they are worn out by work and stress. Sleep is difficult – *Kali phos.* is a great remedy for **insomnia**. Post-natal depression often fits this picture.

They may be sleepless from worry or after a shock or bad news that creates a state of hurry and restlessness. The remedy is also useful for hyperactive children and children who suffer nightmares and sleepwalking due to their **nervous excitability**. Pain in the nerves (neuralgia, toothache) may also be helped.

REMEDY SOURCE

Kali phosphoricum is made from potassium phosphate (K_2PHO_4). It is one of the 12 tissue, or mineral, salts identified by Dr Wilhelm Schuessler (1821-98).

Although headaches are better for fresh air, they are generally worse for going out in the cold and the person wants to lie down in the dark.

A **dry itchy nose with unpleasant discharge** occurs in a cold and also in hay fever. The **mouth is** similarly **dry but offensive**. *Kali phos.* eases nervous asthma where the picture fits and may be useful for acute attacks in combination with a deeper constitutional remedy, particularly *Pulsatilla* or *Carcinosin* (a nosode made from cancerous tissue).

Patients may have a great desire for really cold drinks and sweet things; children may demand ice lollies but refuse all other kinds of food (the Phosphorous child prefers ice cream).

Generally they are **worse for all kinds of exertion**, stress and anxiety and are **better for warmth** and **rest**.

THE KALI PHOSPHORICUM PERSONALITY

As a tissue salt, *Kali phosphoricum* is a remedy that works directly on the cellular level of the body. Therefore, there is no outstanding psychological profile, although the phosphorus element may be characterized by sleeplessness, nerviness and weariness of the brain.

STUDY AID

Taken in combination with *Calcarea phosphorica* and *Natrum phosphoricum* (made from sodium phosphate), *Kali phosphoricum* is an excellent remedy for soothing exam nerves and calming anxious students who study too hard.

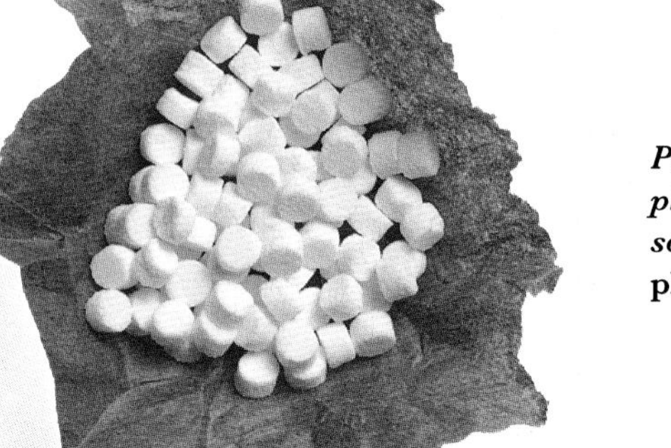

***Potassium phosphate, the source for* Kali phosphoricum.**

Kreosotum

- **Rapid decay of teeth with putrid odour**
- **Diarrhea, vomiting, teething**
- **Menstrual problems**
- **Nocturnal enuresis in children**
- **Profuse bleeding from small wounds**
- **Offensive, excoriating discharge**

INTRODUCTION

Kreosotum *is often used for states of putridity. Its main characteristics are excoriating discharges, pulsations all over the body, profuse bleeding from all over the body and bad teeth and gums.* Kreos. *is the abbreviation for this remedy.*

THE MAIN SYMPTOM PICTURE

In children, gums are very painful and swollen lips are red and bleeding. Corners of mouth tend to be raw and sore. In addition, child often has loose, acrid diarrhea and the crease between the buttocks is red and excoriated.

REMEDY SOURCE

Kreosotum derives from phenols produced from beechwood tar.

In adults, after eating there is a burning pain in the stomach, a sense of fullness and nausea which ends up in **vomiting,** with soreness and acrid fluid. Worse for cold things; better for warm food and drinks.

Early **decay of teeth** with spongy, bleeding gums and a putrid flow from the mouth. Teeth may be black and crumbly or have black spots; they may come through discoloured and decayed.

Kreosotum is indicated frequently for **problems around the menstrual period**, worse for lying, and during urination, better for sitting or walking. The woman feels great weakness and may have yellowish skin. When she starts her menstrual flow, she complains of swelling and rawness of genitals, flow is copious or clotted, often black, and may be fetid and excoriate genitals and thighs; she may have intense itching of the vagina. Often the woman is excited, restless, with a headache constant buzzing and roaring in her ears and has difficulty hearing. Menstrual flow may stop and

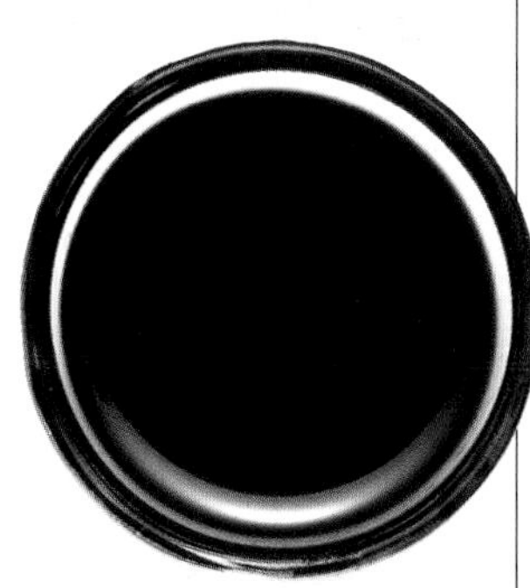

Beechwood tar, the source for* Kreosotum. *It was proved by Dr Wahle of Rome.

start and be lumpy and profuse. Frequently indicated for gushing leucorrhea which is offensive, corrosive and very itchy; may look like bloody water and stains linen yellow. It has a peculiar odor of green corn.

Bedwetting in the first part of the night; child dreams of urinating and cannot get out of bed quickly enough. Urine is very offensive.

Pin pricks bleed profusely, and the patient has copious nosebleeds. Dark, prolonged hemorrhage from nose, eyes, uterus, anus, chest. Wherever there is a mucous membrane there is rawness and excoriation.

Discharges from body **are offensive**, bloody, acrid and very putrid.

Better for warm food, warmth, motion and sitting.

A KREOSOTE MNEMONIC

This poem was devised to help homeopathic students commit *Kreosotum* to memory.

This is the Kreosotum *state*
Discharges hot, excoriate
From mucous membrane, wound or gum
Profuse and easy bleedings come
Sanguineous oozings, frightful stenches
Which Kreosotum *only quenches*
Leucorrhea acrid, putrid, stains
Like red hot coals her pelvic pains
Dentition painful, futile too
Teeth decay as soon as through
For cholera infantum note
With teething troubles – Kreosote

THE KREOSOTUM PERSONALITY

The person who needs *Kreosotum* is irritable, his wants are numerous and he is dissatisfied with everything. It is a state of irritability and chronic dissatisfaction. There is tearfulness with every emotion and throbbing all over the body. A Kreosotum child is very irritable, doesn't know what it wants, tends to scream the whole night long, must be nursed to sleep in parent's arms.

Lac caninum

- **Pains which change sides**
- **Sore throats**
- **Menstrual problems**
- **Mastitis**
- **Rheumatism**

INTRODUCTION

In ancient times, bitch's milk was used to cure problems with the uterus. It was revived as a homeopathic remedy in 1888. It is a very valuable remedy for sore throats, diphtheria, rheumatism and complaints around menses and lactation. It has a most interesting symptom of erratic pains which alternate sides – the symptoms move from right to left then back again, or the reverse. The person may desire salt. Lac. c. *is the abbreviation for this remedy.*

THE MAIN SYMPTOM PICTURE

Headaches. There is a sensation of floating in the air. **Pain appears on one side of the head then the other**. Occipital pain extending to forehead. Blurred vision and nausea and vomiting at the height of the attack. Worse for noise, better for quiet. Brain feels alternately contracted and relaxed.

REMEDY SOURCE

The remedy is derived from bitch's milk.

Sore throat. Swallowing is difficult and painful. Sore throat begins with a tickling sensation which causes a cough, then sensation of a lump on one side. Condition then ceases, only to commence again on opposite sides, then alternates. Sore throat begins and ends with menses. Often begins on left side of throat and extends to ears. Shining, glazed appearance of throat as if varnished. Tonsils inflamed, sore, red and shining. Diphtheric membrane is silvery white, like china. Worse for swallowing solids, touch and extension of throat; better for cold drinks.

Female complaints include severe pain in right ovary region which then changes to the left side and alternates. Better for menstrual flow; escape of gas from vagina, menses gushing, hot, early. **Mastitis and breast problems**. Breasts inflamed, painful; patient must hold them up going up and down stairs. Worse for jarring, better for menstrual flow. Mastitis worse for jarring and dries up milk.

Rheumatism with swelling of the lower extremities affecting the limbs alternately. Pain in limbs as if beaten. Stiffness and swelling of joints and sensitivity of fingers. Pains shift from one side to the other. Worse for motion and heat, and better for cold.

Menses better for open air, cold, cold drinks; worse for touch and jarring, pressure.

THE LAC CANINUM PERSONALITY

The mental state of a Lac Caninum patient is one of oversensitivity of all the senses. Low self-esteem, generalized fearfulness and anxieties arising from powerful imaginings and delusions. Despondent, absent-minded, restless, and nervous, with delusions that one is infested by snakes or vermin.

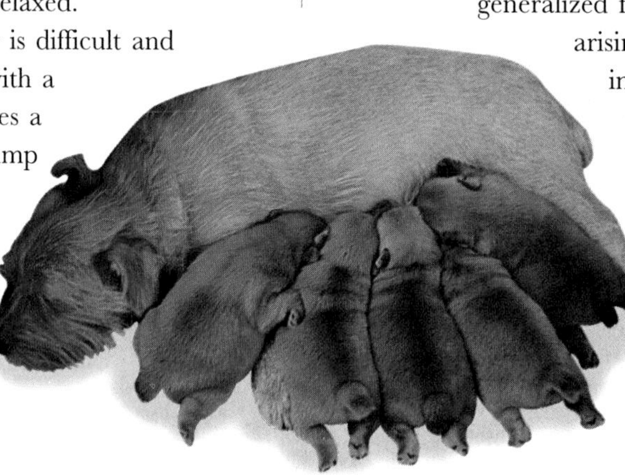

Bitch's milk provides the source for* Lac caninum. *The remedy was revived in New York and provings were cataloged in* Materia Medica of the Nosodes and Morbific Products, *1888.

Lachesis

- **Worse on waking**
- **Complaints get worse during sleep**
- **Worse in spring time, on going from cold to warm or on becoming warm**
- **Better for onset of a discharge**
- **Surging waves of pain**
- **Face is congested, mottled, purplish and engorged**
- **Complaints on the left side or go from left to right**
- **Neck is very sensitive to touch**

INTRODUCTION

Lachesis *has great affinity with the blood and the central nervous system. It is indicated for throat complaints and menopausal problems, and has been used to treat the physical effects of alcoholism. It is a very powerful remedy, useful in many complaints.* Lach. *is the abbreviation for this remedy.*

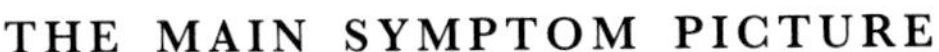

THE MAIN SYMPTOM PICTURE

The modalities are likely to lead to this remedy:

Complaints are **worse on waking**; they get worse during sleep.

Worse for light touch or pressure.

Worse in spring time, on going from cold to warm or on becoming warm. The patient cannot breathe in the heat.

Better for onset of a discharge, e.g. menses or a nasal catarrh.

Surging waves of pain and the face is **congested, mottled, purplish and engorged**. Puffed eyelids and face. The inflamed parts take on a bluish, purplish tint. The person hates constrictions about the neck or abdomen.

Complaints are characteristically on the **left side or go from left to right**.

Headache on waking, which began during sleep. Face very pale with the headache. Waves of pain, worse after moving. Bursting, pulsating headache, **pressure and burning on the vertex** and the senses are overwrought; worse for noise, cannot stand the touch of the clothes, especially about the neck. Dim vision and flickerings with the headache and a very pale face, maybe vertigo. Relief often comes with a discharge such as the menses or coryza.

The bushmaster snake, the source for* Lachesis. *It was first proved accidentally by Constantine Hering in 1837 during a bungled attempt to extract snake venom while conducting scientific research in the Amazonian jungle.

Dyspnea; patients wake from sleep with a sense of suffocation or choking which can come on during sleep, a sense of strangulation when lying, and especially when anything is around the neck; **neck is very sensitive to touch**. They wake with this sense of suffocation and must sit up and bend forward or else must rush to the open window; they feel they must take a deep breath.

The **cough is dry, suffocating,** as in Spongia, and tickling. There is little secretion and much sensitiveness, worse for pressure on larynx; larynx is painful to touch. Cough worse after sleep, as Spongia; coughs early in sleep at about 11pm.

Throat problems are worse for empty swallowing or swallowing liquids. Pains go to the ears and are worse for hot drinks (unlike Lycopodium). Painful hawking of mucus which starts on left and goes to right. Purplish hue to the inflammation. Throat and neck sensitive to the slightest touch.

REMEDY SOURCE

Lachesis is prepared from the venom of *Lachesis muta*, the deadly surucucu snake from South America, also known as the bushmaster. It is a pit viper, related to the rattle snake. The remedy is made from the venom.

THE LACHESIS PERSONALITY

The Lachesis mental picture is one of unattractive egocentricity – and disregard for others. These people have no empathy with others, are unstable, devious, selfish, jealous, and self-publicizing. They may be gloomy, taciturn or loquacious and are full of schemes to take over the world but tend to achieve nothing.

Ledum palustre

- **First aid remedy**
- **Puncture wounds**
- **Rheumatic joints**
- **Chilly but averse to warmth**
- **Thirst for cold water**
- **Bad dreams**

INTRODUCTION

Ledum *is often selected for respiratory and rheumatic complaints. Hahnemann maintained that the remedy 'is suitable for the most part only in chronic maladies in which there is a predominance of the coldness and deficiency of animal heat.'* Ledum *is a useful first aid remedy for puncture wounds, such as from a nail, thorn, bite or sting. The wound may not bleed much but becomes puffy and swollen.* Ledum *and* Led. *are the abbreviations for this remedy.*

THE MAIN SYMPTOM PICTURE

In accidents with trauma it may be appropriate to give *Arnica* first. If the wound is gaping or bleeding heavily, *Hypericum* or *Calendula* should be considered.

In **puncture wounds**, particularly from garden tools or dirty instruments, professional advice should be sought immediately to prevent risk of tetanus.

Injuries to the eyes, especially from a blow. The area is bloodshot and bruised and the eye may weep.

Ledum is also useful in **joint pains**, particularly in pains of the feet and ankles. Heels feel sore and soles are so painful it is difficult to walk; ankles are easily sprained.

There may be violent **thirst for cold water**.

Pains are **better for** cold and being bathed in cold water. Although the person is **chilly** and the body is cold to touch, any kind of **warmth aggravates the symptoms**, including a warm bed or warm room. May throw off bed covers or get out of bed in search of coolness. Restless sleep disturbed by **bad dreams**.

REMEDY SOURCE

Ledum is made from *Ledum palustre*, a small shrub also known as wild rosemary, marsh tea or Labrador tea, a native of northern Europe and Canada. The remedy is prepared from the whole fresh plant or dried twigs.

THE LEDUM PERSONALITY

The Ledum mental state is one of self-pitying discontent. It has been compared to the state exhibited by an alcoholic 'on the wagon'.

According to the homeopath Dr James Tyler Kent, *Ledum* 'counteracts the effects of whisky and takes away the desire for it.'

***Wild rosemary, the source for* Ledum palustre. *It was proved by Hahnemann and appears in the fourth volume of his* Materia Medica Pura.**

Lycopodium clavatum

- **Complaints are on right side, go from right to left or from above downwards**
- **Chilly patient, pains better for warmth**
- **Head complaints better for cold and worse in a warm room**
- **Often worse from 4–8pm**
- **Sore throats better for warm drinks**
- **Flatulence and belching**
- **Fullness after a very few mouthfuls**

INTRODUCTION

Lycopodium *is reputed 'to act on the entire organism'. It is a remedy often selected by homeopaths for chronic disease. People who need* Lycopodium *are often physically weak or weakened by chronic disease. There are many physical symptoms.* Lycopodium *and* Lyc. *are the abbreviations for this remedy.*

REMEDY SOURCE

Lycopodium is made from *Lycopodium clavatum,* also known as wolf's claws, club moss, lamb's tail or fox tail, a mossy plant native to mountain pastures and heaths. The remedy is made from the spores produced by the fruits of the plant.

THE MAIN SYMPTOM PICTURE

Complaints are on the **right side, go from right to left or from above downwards**.

A **chilly** patient with **pains better for warmth,** except the **head complaints** which are **better for cold and worse in a warm room**; **symptoms often worse between 4–8pm**.

There may be marked nervous excitement and possibly even prostration.

Headache is better for cool air and motion until the patient becomes warmed up, which then makes it worse; worse for lying down, warm wraps and noise. Throbbing, pressing, bursting headache.

Periodical headaches and headaches with stomach complaints. Often better for eating and comes on if a meal is missed; headache with hunger.

Headache from suppressed nasal discharge, when a chronic, thick, yellow discharge is replaced by an acute, watery coryza with sneezing, then comes a headache which subsides when the thick, yellow discharge returns.

Thick, yellow, offensive ear discharges with loss of hearing and dry cough. Ear infections with eczema around and behind the ears.

Colds may settle in the nose and usually go to the chest, with much whistling, wheezing and dyspnea, worse for exertion. There is a dry, teasing cough with throbbing, burning and tickling in the chest.

***Club moss, the source for* Lycopodium clavatum. *It was proved by Hahnemann and appears in the first edition of his* Chronic Diseases.**

Sore throats better for warm drinks, especially if they go from the right to the left side of the throat.

Patient has cold extremities and a hot, congested head; wants the head uncovered.

Great flatulence and belching are marked symptoms of this remedy. Everything eaten turns to wind and patients may feel **full and distended after only a very few mouthfuls,** with momentary relief from belching. Gnawing pains and burning with gastritis and ulcers. Better for warm drinks. Noisy rumbling, diarrhea of all kinds. Patients may have strong desire for sweets.

The urine may contain a substance that looks like red sand or gravel. A headache may come on after the gravel stops coming out in the urine. Patients may be irritable on waking.

THE LYCOPODIUM PERSONALITY

The Lycopodium subject is diffident, conscientious, meticulous but self-conscious, fearful of the future and of failing. They dislike public appearances and may take offence easily and harbor grudges. Unsustained outbursts of anger or temper tantrums are common, as are black moods of despondency.

Magnesia phosphorica

- **Severe cramping pains**
- **Abdominal cramps**
- **Infant colic**
- **Right-sided pains**
- **Menstrual cramps**
- **Writer's cramp**

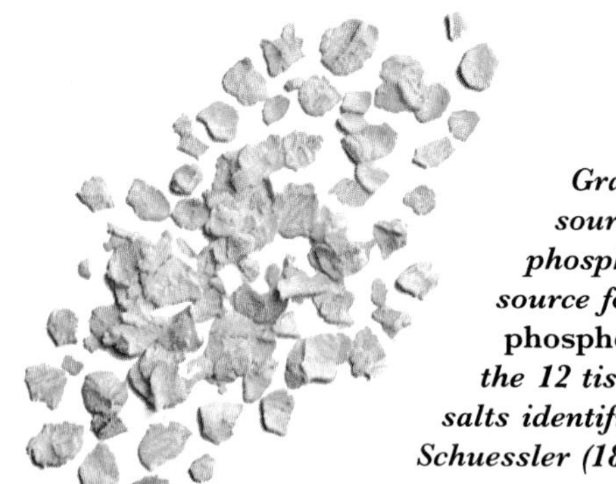

Grain cereals, a r[...] source of magnesiu[...] phosphate, itself the source for* Magnesia phosphorica. *It is one [...] the 12 tissue, or minera[...] salts identified by Dr Wilh[...] Schuessler (1821-98).

INTRODUCTION

Magnesia phosphorica *is a superb anti-spasmodic remedy with all pains relieved by heat. It is probably the remedy most frequently indicated for menstrual cramps.* Mag. phos. *and* Mag. p. *are the abbreviations for this remedy.*

THE MAIN SYMPTOM PICTURE

Cramping pains which can spread in all directions, so severe they cause doubling up. Relieved by heat (often a hot-water bottle firmly pressed into abdomen). Better for heat application and hard pressure. Back ache may accompany pains and the person has a clean tongue. Worse for uncovering and cold drafts.

Abdominal cramps, sharp, cutting, pinching, griping, intense cramps which radiate, and pain comes and goes, shooting and darting like lightning. Person groans with pain, accompanied by much flatulence; better for doubling up, heat and hot applications and hard pressure; worse for cold, drafts, and night.

Pains are right-sided and person has clean tongue. **Colicky pains** make baby draw up legs; better for warm hand pressing on abdomen; diarrhea accompanies and baby screams with pain.

The modalities of Mag. phos. are similar to those of Colocynthis, but Colocynthis pains are often due to anger and vexation and not so greatly relieved by heat. Pain as if band drawn tightly round abdomen.

Headaches, throbbing, with red face. Sudden pains that come and go; often begin in occiput and extend over head. Better for tight bandaging round head, warm room; worse for cold, drafts and at night.

Spasms about the eyes with squinting, especially on right side. Stiffness, numbness and awkwardness of nerves from prolonged exertions. This applies to the long use of hands and fingers such as writers experience, or harpists and pianists after hours of practice. Also carpenters' or **workers' cramps** from prolonged use of certain tools; repeated stress injury. Better for heat and pressure.

Toothache worse for cold drafts and touch; better for doubling up, warmth, warm applications, hard pressure.

REMEDY SOURCE

Magnesia phosphorica derives from phosphate of magnesium, a tissue salt present in various parts of the body. It is also found in grain cereals.

THE MAGNESIA PHOSPHORICA PERSONALITY

People who need this remedy are often sensitive and artistic, intellectuals who are nervous, intense and restless and suffer from cramps and colics. Often outgoing and impulsive, physically they are thin, weak and very sensitive, languid, forgetful, disinclined to mental effort, may stammer, complain of cold in spine. They crave sugar, but loathe coffee.

Mercurius

- **Sensitive to both heat and cold**
- **Offensive odor to breath, sweat, discharges, stools, etc.**
- **Glands affected; inflamed and swollen**
- **Ulcerations of mucous membranes**
- **A tendency to suppuration**
- **Catarrhs of mucous membranes**
- **Copious salivation; often with a metallic taste**

INTRODUCTION

Mercurius *is also known as* Mercurius vivus; *it is one variety on the Mercurius theme. For others, see* Mercurius cyanatus *on page 94. This remedy is called for when slight activity produces disproportionate exhaustion.* Mercurius, Merc. *and* Merc. v. *are the abbreviations for this remedy.*

THE MAIN SYMPTOM PICTURE

Sensitive to both heat and cold or open air.

Offensive odors to breath, sweat, discharges, stools, etc.

Worse at night; pains in joints or inflammations which get hard. Worse in the warmth of the bed.

Glands affected: inflamed and swollen.

Ulcerations of mucous membranes.

Tendency to suppuration: it comes on rapidly with burning and stinging (as in Apis).

Catarrhs of mucous membranes: discharges start thin and excoriating and later become more thick and bland.

Rheumatic complaints.

Complaints with sweating which is offensive, may be profuse but does not give relief, and may even make patient worse.

Copious salivation: often with a **metallic,** sweet or salty taste. Sometimes a sense of dryness with intense thirst. Trembling. Delirium in the acute illness. Many complaints are worse when patient lies on the right side.

REMEDY SOURCE

Originally the source for this remedy was the ammonium nitrate salt of mercury. Hahnemann considered that the procedure was too complicated, and substituted metallic mercury (Hg) as the source. In the fifteenth century, mercury-based medicine was used to treat syphilis.

Repeated swellings and abscess formation. Patients sweat all over, without being hot, and slowly emaciate. Abscess keeps on discharging, with no tendency to heal.

In a child: after scarlet fever or a suppressed ear discharge, with sweating of the head, dilated pupils, rolling of the head; worse at night. In such lingering febrile conditions, *Mercurius* may be needed.

In fevers, patients may feel a creeping chilliness in the evening which may increase as night progresses. They are very sensitive to drafts and have cold hands and feet. Their sweat is profuse and offensive, and often makes things worse.

In chronic catarrh, and with a thick discharge suppressed, possibly by a cold, a severe headache comes on in the forehead, face, ears. Much heat in the head with headaches; bursting, constricting pains.

Eye catarrh worse when sitting by the fire; every cold settles in the eyes in rheumatic patients. Colds may also go to the chest and linger.

Mercury, the source for **Mercurius.** *It was proved by Hahnemann and appears in the last edition of the first volume of his* **Materia Medica Pura.**

Ears and nose produce a horrible, sticking, green discharge. Ear infection with rupture and suppuration.

The **tongue may be swollen, flabby, spongy, taking the imprint of the teeth**, coated, foul with copious saliva. Nothing tastes right. Gums may be swollen, spongy and bleeding.

Sore throat may have a swollen, spongy appearance, with flat spreading ulcers. Sensation of great dryness. Difficulty in swallowing because of the pain and paralytic weakness. Quinsy.

Sour stomach with wind, regurgitation, reflux, nausea, food sitting like a load, the characteristic taste and salivation. Milk disagrees with them.

Tenesmus with diarrhea.

Affects the lower right chest with stitches through to the back (as in Kali carb.).

Almost everything will make them worse and virtually nothing will bring relief.

THE MERCURIUS PERSONALITY

The Mercurius subject is restless and anguished, feels guilty and tormented and frightened by trivial matters. Memory and willpower may be impaired; they may be indifferent, suicidal or even feel murderous for no reason.

Mercurius cyanatus

- **Throat infections**
- **Tonsils**
- **Talkative**
- **Weakness and prostration**
- **Worse at night**

INTRODUCTION

Mercurius cyanatus *has many similarities to the other* Mercurius *remedies.* Merc. cyan. *is the abbreviation for this remedy. Most commercial outlets stock only* Merc. solibilis *which is the most commonly occurring mercury picture. Other mercuries include* Merc. vivus *which is very close to* Merc. sol., Merc. corrosivus *(a powerful disinfectant),* Merc. dulcis *ear catarrh),* Merc. iodatus flavum *(glands and throat),* Merc. iodatus ruber *(lymphatic glands). These mercuries, along with* Merc. cyan., *usually have to be ordered from a pharmacy.*

THE MAIN SYMPTOM PICTURE

Merc. cyan. has the instability of mercury but is particularly useful in cases of toxemia and severe infections. It is best known for its use in diphtheria, and although this disease is rarely seen in the West these days, if a child has a bad reaction to a diphtheria innoculation, the Merc. cyan. picture could come up.

PROOF IN THE POISON

In February 1899, Dr Henry C. Barrett of New York, who was being systematically poisoned by bicyanide of mercury, was diagnosed as suffering from diphtheria, giving an inadvertent proving of the remedy. He recovered.

Because this remedy has an affinity for the mouth and throat area, it is useful for **sore throats** and **tonsillitis**. Despite pain in the throat, patients are likely to be **talkative** with an excitable anger.

The main feature is great **weakness and prostration**. Like all *Merc.* remedies, everything seems to make them feel worse – heat, cold, rest, motion, etc. – and nothing really ameliorates the symptoms.

Symptoms are **worse at night**, particularly headaches, which can be very severe. There is much saliva in the mouth, especially at night, and it may dribble out during sleep.

Merc. cyan. has much in common with *Lachesis* in its affinity for the throat and its toxic states. But a sufferer needs much more stability, for example too much fresh air would distress Merc. cyan., while invigorating Lachesis.

REMEDY SOURCE

Mercurius cyanatus is made from bicyanide of mercury ($HgCN_2$).

THE MERCURIUS CYANATUS PERSONALITY

Like Mercurius vivus, the Mercurius cyanatus personality is characterized by the urge to find a balance while feeling that everything is flying away. The poet W. B. Yeats' well-known line, 'Things fall apart, the centre cannot hold,' might have been written to describe the Mercurius state. In Mercurius cyanatus, the patient's feelings are more powerful.

***Mercury is also the source of bicyanide of mercury, which is itself the source for* Mercurius cyanatus. *There is a family of mercury remedies, and this is one of the more important after* Mercurius vivus.**

Natrum muriaticum

- **May follow a loss, a grief, rejection, unrequited love or a reprimand**
- **Often worse from 10–11am**
- **Discharge from mucous membranes is watery or thick like white of egg**
- **Awful bursting headaches**
- **Thirst for cold drinks throughout**
- **Mucous membranes are dry**

INTRODUCTION

This is a very powerful remedy made from a very simple source. It is not recommended for acute conditions. Natrum mur., Nat. mur., *and* Nat. m. *are the abbreviations for this remedy.*

THE MAIN SYMPTOM PICTURE

Complaints often follow a **loss**, **grief**, **a rejection**, **unrequited love or a reprimand**. Patients hold their feelings in and rarely weep in front of others. They may be sensitive to a change of weather. There may be weakness, nervous prostration, and nervous irritability. They desire solitude when they are ill; consolation makes them worse. They are greatly disturbed by excitement, and can be extremely emotional. The whole nervous system may be in a state of fret and irritation. Worse for sudden noises, may feel weak and ill afterwards, worse for music.

REMEDY SOURCE

Natrum muriaticum is made from sodium chloride (NaCl), common salt. Sea or rock salt is the usual source.

Worse from 10–11am. Worse lying down. Pains are stitching, electric shock-like, and shooting, with twitching, jerking and trembling.

Patients catch cold easily when sweating or when in a draft but are in general better in the open air, though worse if they get hot. They are usually quite warm-blooded people.

Discharge from mucous membranes is watery or thick like the white of an egg. May also come from ears and eyes too.

Awful headaches: feel as if head is bursting or being crushed in a vice. Hammering and throbbing pains; pains in the morning on waking. Great nervousness. They fall asleep late and wake with a headache. Headache at 10 or 11am. Periodic headaches.

A bursting headache during chills and fever with copious thirst, relieved by sweating. Other headaches are not relieved by sweating.

Headache from the inability to focus the eyes rapidly enough, and from eye-strain.

Chills at 10 or 11am; starting in the extremities, with a throbbing head and flushed face.

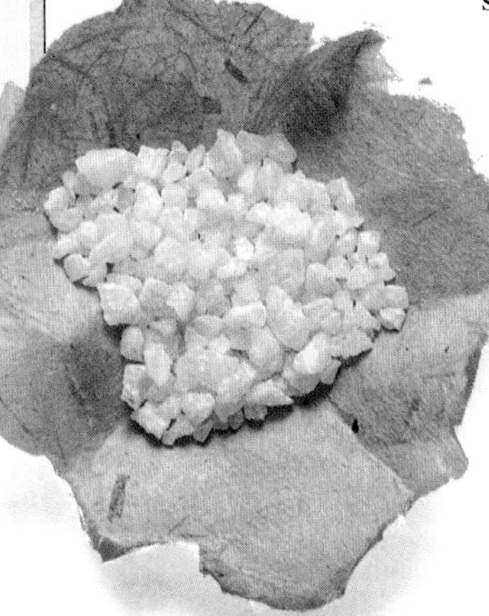

Rock salt, a source for* Natrum muriaticum. *A proving appears in the first edition of Hahnemann's* Chronic Diseases. *It is one of the 12 tissue, or mineral, salts identified by Dr Wilhelm Schuessler (1821-98).

Thirst for cold drinks throughout. During chills patients are not better with heat or by covering up, and they will still want cold drinks despite chattering teeth and aching bones. Tossing and turning. In fevers they may become very hot and go into a congestive stupor or sleep.

Mucous membranes are dry. Lips dry and cracked, split in the center. Cold sore on the lips. Throat dry, red, and patulous with a splinter sensation. Chronic dryness without ulceration. Much catarrhal discharge, with dryness at other times. There may be a sense of dryness without actual dryness, as in Merc. A bitter taste at times.

Slow digestion, sensation of a lump in the stomach after eating, which disagrees. Bowels distended with gas. Stools hard and difficult. Stitching, tearing pains in the liver, with fullness.

Cough from a tickle low in the throat. Bursting pain in the forehead. Stitches all over the chest.

THE NATRUM MUR. PERSONALITY

The Natrum mur. subject is emotionally sensitive and may exhibit inappropriate emotional responses, laughing when solemnity is indicated, for example. Averse to fuss, comfort or cuddles, independent and unpredictable; prefers to suffer slights, injuries or disappointments in silence.

Natrum sulphuricum

- **Tissue salt**
- **Thick yellow catarrh**
- **Dirty tongue**
- **Biliousness**
- **Sadness**
- **Much thirst and urination**
- **Diabetes**
- **Worse in damp weather or damp conditions**
- **Sudden violent symptoms**
- **Skin conditions with pus**

INTRODUCTION

Natrum sulphuricum *is a tissue salt whose main use is in promoting elimination of toxins from the body. This remedy is characterized by an intolerance of sea air or edible plants growing near water. Symptoms may be precipitated by emotional strain after nursing relations for long periods.* Natrum sulph., Nat. sulph., *and* Nat. s. *are the abbreviations for this remedy.*

THE MAIN SYMPTOM PICTURE

In colds and flu there is a **thick yellowish catarrh** which may be fluent from the nose, particularly at night, or drop down the throat. The mouth feels slimy and burning, especially the **tongue,** which **has a dirty coating**. Toothache and ear ache give burning pains.

In stomach disorders there is a **bilious quality** with the Nat. sulph. symptoms of yellowish-green vomit and diarrhea, and burning pains. The liver is sore and congested, and there may be a low fever.

Frequent urination occurs in keeping with this remedy's eliminative qualities, often combined with a **great thirst** for cold water. *Nat. sulph.* is an important remedy to consider in diabetes.

This disturbance in the balance of body fluids shows up as a **poor ability to deal with damp conditions**. It is useful in illness that comes on during damp weather, when living in a damp room or close to a river or pond. Watery fruit and vegetables disagree with the patient. Despite feeling thirsty, cold drinks also tend to cause indigestion.

REMEDY SOURCE

Natrum sulphuricum is made from sodium sulphate ($NaSO_3$), also known as Glauber's salts. This is one of the salts found in mineral water.

Where Natrum mur. has a dryness that absorbs fluid into the body, Natrum sulph. is the balancing condition that requires excretion.

Natrum sulph. may be needed in skin conditions or injuries where a watery, yellowish-green pus has gathered, for example whitlows and acne.

Acute conditions are sudden and violent and may even come on after a fall or blow to the head. Such an injury may also bring on severe mental symptoms, even mania, but the general Natrum sulphuricum mental picture is of melancholy sadness.

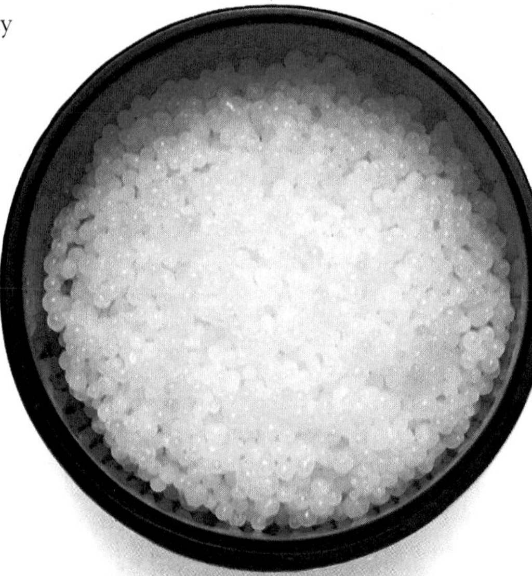

Sodium sulphate, the source for* Natrum sulphuricum. *It was proved by Schieler and Nenning and the results were published in Hering's* Materia Medica. *It is one of the 12 tissue, or mineral, salts identified by Dr Wilhelm Schuessler (1821-98).

THE NATRUM SULPHURICUM PERSONALITY

The person who needs *Natrum sulph.* is restless and discontented with life, even suicidal; he or she may brood on thoughts of hate and revenge. Depression is worse in the morning and the patient may feel he or she will never recover.

Nitricum acidum

- **Headache**
- **Winter colds**
- **Mouth ulcers**
- **Sore throat with sharp splinter pains**
- **Anal warts**
- **Skin cracks and fissures**
- **Sharp sticking splinter-like pains**
- **Offensive discharges**
- **Worse for touch, jarring, cold air, morning milk**
- **Better for gliding motion, mild weather, warmth, pressure**

INTRODUCTION

Nitricum acidum *is a particularly good remedy for cracked and fissured skin, anal warts with burning sticking pain, also burning, sticking piles. It is very effective around orifices where mucous membranes merge with skin (nose, mouth, anus, urethra, genitals), and for warts and growths with characteristic sticking, splinter-like pains which are worse for touch. It is also useful for severe acne.* Nit. ac. *is the abbreviation for this remedy.*

THE MAIN SYMPTOM PICTURE

Headaches. Crushing head pains **worse for** the pressure of hat, noise, or **jarring**. Sensation of band around the head. Scalp is very sensitive and hair may fall out. **Better for gliding motion** (car or train ride).

Winter colds. Person may suffer from deafness and catarrh in the ears. Worse for noise. Susceptible to winter colds with chronic offensive nasal catarrh with excoriating **discharge**. The nose is obstructed at night and green casts are blown out in the morning. May sneeze in cold air, and may have a nosebleed. **Worse for cold** and **cold air**.

Ulcers in mouth on tongue and soft palate in **throat**, giving sharp **splinter-like pains** which are worse on swallowing. Pains are sharp and extend into the ears. Thick mucus in the throat, which person tries to clear constantly. Patients often have swollen gums, putrid breath and increased salivation; corners of mouth very sore.

This is the number one remedy for **fissures** in the rectum giving agonizing sharp, cutting, splinter-like pains. Rectum feels torn and stools tear the anus (even if soft) giving prolonged pain for hours afterwards. Patient experiences great straining to pass stools and is in agony afterwards. May be constipated with painful bleeding piles. May have nausea and occasional vomiting; **worse for milk**, craves fat and salt. Very useful remedy for **anal warts** with burning, sticking pain; also burning, sticking piles which are agony during or after passing stools. Strong-smelling urine which is cold when passed; offensive urine, breath and stools; leucorrhea; foul sweat and body odor.

Warts on hands which are often large, moist and bleeding. Herpes between fingers. Yellow curved nails with sensation of splinter underneath; distorted nails; cracks and fissures of skin and skin ulcers; all with **sharp splinter pain. Worse for touch**.

REMEDY SOURCE

Nitricum acidum is prepared from nitric acid (HNO_3) an extremely corrosive acid also know as *aqua fortis*, or strong water.

THE NITRICUM ACIDUM PERSONALITY

People who need this remedy are irritable (particularly in the morning) and may be vindictive and hateful. They tremble with anger and are full of anxiety about their health and fear of their death. Sensitive because of their own thoughts, they are also physically sensitive to every little noise and disturbance. They are unhappy, dissatisfied and unforgiving, so engrossed in their own miseries that they have no time for things outside themselves. Always chilly, they crave fat and salt.

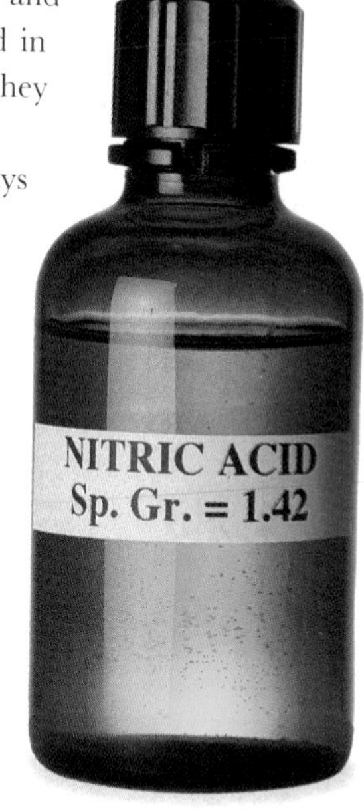

Nitric acid, the source for **Nitricum acidum.** *It was proved by Hahnemann and appears in the second edition of his* **Chronic Diseases.**

Nux vomica

- **Complaints coming from overindulgence in food, drink, spicy foods, stimulants of all sorts, or from mental overwork**
- **Problems following exposure to cold, dry winds**
- **Digestive upset**
- **Marked oversensitivity**
- **Severe chills in a fever**
- **When vomiting there is much retching, gagging and straining**
- **Much straining but only scanty stools**
- **Worse for cold**

INTRODUCTION

Nux vomica *is probably best known as the hangover remedy, but it is very suitable for over-medicated urbanites, particularly sedentary people who work with their brains and are prey to mental or emotional strain rather than physical exhaustion.* Nux vom. *and* Nux v. *are the abbreviations for this remedy.*

***The poison-nut plant, the source for* Nux vomica. *It was first proved by Hahnemann and appears in the third edition of the first volume of his* Materia Medica Pura.**

THE MAIN SYMPTOM PICTURE

Complaints coming from **over-indulgence in food**, **drink**, **spicy foods**, **stimulants** of all sorts, or from mental overwork. Problems following **exposure to cold**, **dry winds**.

The complaints are often accompanied by some sort of **digestive upset** (as in Pulsatilla).

Marked oversensitivity; irritable and touchy, never contented, never satisfied. Patients may be prone to arguments and quarrel over any imagined offence. They can feel hurried and driven, critical and quick to reproach. They may prefer to be left alone and hate having to depend on others who are less capable than themselves. They may be sleepless from an overactive mind, and sensitive to slight noises which disturb them.

A chilly person, sensitive to drafts. Sweats easily. Always catching cold which settles in the nose, throat or ears and goes to the chest. A warm room makes the coryza worse, followed by a fever; after the fever he or she must have heat.

Severe chills during the fever. Patients cannot get warm and cannot bear to be uncovered, for it sends waves of chills through them. They feel hot for a short time, then become extremely hot with hot sweat. Worse in the morning. A very red face during the fever.

Neuralgic headaches stick and tear, burn and sting; drawing pains especially likely. A sensation of tension in the muscles.

Headache worse for mental exertion, **anger**, open air, on waking, after eating, coffee, sun, light, noise, stooping, movement, stormy weather. Headache with constipation and a sour stomach. Patients may have a weak digestion and be intolerant of many foods, yet crave pungent, bitter, or spicy things, tonics or milk. Meat can cause nausea. When vomiting there is **much retching**, **gagging and straining** before they can finally vomit. Likewise there may be **much straining but only scanty stools**. The spasmodic, colicky abdominal pains are worse for motion and better for heat. Nux v. is **worse for eating** and suffers from dyspepsia, heartburn, nausea, fullness, constipation, bloating and gas.

A feeling of pressure one or two hours after eating.

Backache worse when lying down: must get up and walk.

Dry, teasing cough with great soreness of the chest. Spasmodic cough with retching; worse in cold, dry, windy weather. Tickling and pain in the larynx. Cough causes a bursting headache.

Worse in the cold, or cold dry weather; for uncovering; for eating and especially overeating; for stimulants; in the mornings; for anger or mental exertion.

Better in evenings, for resting, in wet weather, after passing stools.

REMEDY SOURCE

Nux vomica is made from *Strychnos nux vomica*, the poison-nut plant native to the East Indies and northern Australia. The remedy is made from the dried seeds of the plant.

THE NUX VOMICA PERSONALITY

The person who needs *Nux vomica* is tense, irritable and anxious, given to outbursts of rage which are taken out on the nearest object. Fussy, intolerant, unable to take criticism and takes on too much.

Petroleum

- **Headache**
- **Ear problems**
- **Inflammation of mucous membranes**
- **Travel sickness**
- **Skin complaints**
- **Worse for motion, thunder, in winter**
- **Better for warm, dry weather**
- **Sense of duality**

INTRODUCTION

Petroleum *is a very useful remedy for skin complaints, especially dry skin with cracks. Also useful for catarrhal conditions of mucous membranes, and gastric acidity. Useful for chilblains that itch, burn and become purple; useful for eczema and herpes, and cracks in the skin that will not heal.* Petr. *is the abbreviation for this remedy.*

THE MAIN SYMPTOM PICTURE

All complaints are **worse in winter**.

Headaches. Person may have vertigo on rising; back of head (occiput) feels heavy, as if made of lead. Scalp is sore to touch and numb. Worse for coughing, holds temple to relieve. May have deafness.

Ear problems. Dryness and cracked skin in ears; may have discharge of pus and blood from ears. Itching deep in ears. May have ringing in the ears.

Inflammation of mucous membranes everywhere, producing watery yellow discharges. Nose, chest, and eyes subject to catarrhal complaints; also complaints form catarrh of stomach and bowels. Dry hacking cough, worse at night. Very hungry but cannot eat without pain; diarrhea worse in the day or only happens in daytime. Worse for eating cabbage which produces watery, gushing diarrhea.

Motion sickness (sea and car), headache with vertigo, ravenous hunger which drives person to eat. Nausea worse for motion of car, train or boat.

Skin conditions with dryness and split cracks, deep cracks in folds behind ears and on fingertips. Deep, bleeding cracks which itch violently. Skin is rough, thickened like leather. Eruptions have yellow-green crusts which are raw on occiput and genitals. Eruptions itch violently and must be scratched until they bleed; affected part becomes cold after scratching. Worse in skin folds.

Better for warm, dry weather. Worse for thunder.

REMEDY SOURCE

Petroleum is derived from crude shale oil.

THE PETROLEUM PERSONALITY

People who need *Petroleum* are easily offended and irritable; they are easily angered and are fearful. There is a tendency to scold others and an aversion to company. There is a sense of physical duality, as if their body is divided or they are somebody's double. There can be confusion of mind, a sudden sense of disorientation, and the person may suddenly lose his or her way in well-known streets.

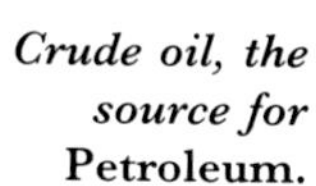

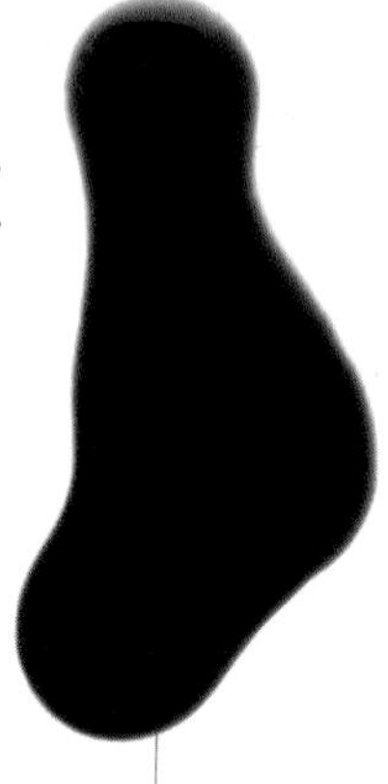

***Crude oil, the source for* Petroleum.**

Phosphorus

- **Sensitive to external stimuli; odors, touch, noise, cold etc.**
- **Flushes of heat**
- **Hemorrhages**
- **Headaches are congestive and throbbing**
- **Hunger**
- **Violent thirst for ice-cold and refreshing drinks**
- **Vomiting of warm drinks**
- **Hoarseness worse in evening**
- **Oppression and constriction in the chest**

***Bone ash, the source for phosphorus, itself the source for the* Phosphorus *remedy. A proving appears in the first edition of Hahnemann's* Chronic Diseases.**

INTRODUCTION

Phosphorus *is a very useful remedy for a variety of conditions resulting from malfunctioning cell or tissue metabolism. It is often used as a constitutional remedy and is particularly useful for young people exhausted after a rapid growth spurt. It is indicated for adolescents suffering from exam strain or fear of approaching exams.* Phos. *is the abbreviation for this remedy.*

THE MAIN SYMPTOM PICTURE

REMEDY SOURCE

Phosphorus used to be prepared from phosphorus derived from bone ash. *Phosphorus* is an essential element in the body for the transfer of energy between cells.

Complaints may come on from electric changes in the atmosphere.

Flushes of heat in people subject to palpitations and congestions.

Hemorrhages; anemia and relaxed conditions of muscles.

Burning pains, tearing and drawing pains. Sensation of intense heat running up the back.

May be very sensitive to all external stimuli. Great prostration of mind or body after any effort.

Trembling from slight causes; great excitability; can be restless and fidgety.

Vertigo and dizziness is common.

Headaches are congestive and throbbing; blood mounts to the head. Better for cold and rest, worse for heat, motion and lying down. Often patients have to sit up and apply pressure and a cold application to the head. Face flushed and hot. **Hunger** can precede or accompany the headaches.

Coryza; painful dryness in the nose; sneezing and running of the nose, maybe with blood. Yellow-green discharges too.

Swollen glands in weak, exhausted people.

Violent thirst for ice-cold drinks; dry mouth and throat. Sore, excoriated, bleeding mouth. Swollen tonsils; dysphagia and constriction.

Hunger may be violent; must eat during the chill, at night, with the headache; must eat or they will faint.

Vomiting of warm drinks when stomach is upset. Patients may desire cold food, sour or spicy things, wine.

Laryngitis with **hoarseness, worse in the evening**; larynx so painful they cannot talk; very sensitive to touch and cold air. Violent tickling in the larynx and behind the sternum. Colds may go to the larynx after a change of weather. A hard, dry, rasping cough. It is exhausting, and so painful that they suppress the cough. Anxiety, weakness, **oppression and constriction in the chest**; sensation as if a great weight were on the chest. Tightness. **Flushes of blood and heat** going upwards in the chest. Painful chest, especially in the lower right zone; better for pressure. Blood-stained sputum: salty, sour or yellow. Suffocation and constriction are better for pressure. Bursting headache with the cough. Cough worse for open air, going from a warm to a cold room or vice versa, twilight, lying on left side, talking, eating; better lying on right side.

Violent palpitations worse for lying on left side, motion. May sleep on right side for preference.

Stiffness on beginning to move in the morning.

THE PHOSPHORUS PERSONALITY

The mental picture of Phosphorus is one of intelligent cooperation, desiring and returning affection, but easily exhausted and liable to sink into apathy or become irritable. Outbursts of rage are balanced by remorse.

Phytolacca decandra

- **Headache**
- **Teething**
- **Sore throat**
- **Mastitis**
- **Stiff neck**
- **Worse for cold, drafts, motion, hot drinks, during menses**
- **Better for dry weather, lying on abdomen**

INTRODUCTION

Phytolacca decandra *is a frequently prescribed remedy for sore throats. It is an especially useful remedy for complaints of the breasts, neck and throat. It is also useful for diphtheria, quinsy and mumps.* Phytolacca *and* Phyt. *are the abbreviations for this remedy.*

THE MAIN SYMPTOM PICTURE

Headache with vertigo on rising. Head and brain feel sore as if beaten. Pains come on when it rains and are worse for eating.

Teething. There is an irresistible urge to clamp teeth and gums together.

Sore throat. Throat is dark or even bluish red. Pain is at the root of the tongue and extends to the ears. Worse for swallowing. Sensation of lump on swallowing. Throat feels rough, and dry with a hot pain like splinters. Tonsils swollen. Person feels chilly and wants to be covered. Pain on swallowing. **Worse for hot drinks** at night and on swallowing. Thick mucus in throat and there may be ulceration. Glands are swollen and hard (submaxillary and parotidal). **Useful for diphtheria, quinsy and mumps.** Much aching in body and restlessness may accompany the sore throat. Protrusion of tongue causes sharp pains at root of tongue; inability to swallow even water; throat feels full as if choked.

REMEDY SOURCE

Phytolacca decandra is made from *Phytolacca decandra* or *P. americana*, a perennial bushy plant that grows in North America, North Africa and China. Its local names include American nightshade, pigeon berry, pokeroot and red ink plant.

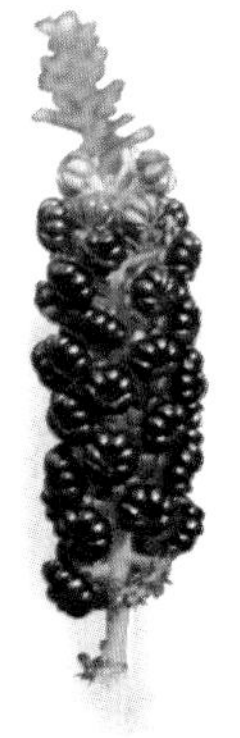

Mastitis. Breasts are heavy, stony, hard and very tender. Lumps in breast; glandular tumors that become hard. Breast is hard, painful and purple. Mammary abscess; nipples are cracked and very sensitive. In nursing mothers, when the baby feeds, pain goes from the nipple all over the body. Mastitis with aching back, bone pains, and shivering. Breasts sensitive before and during menses. *Phyt.* is useful for bloody, watery discharge from nipples.

Stiff neck. Pain on movement; **worse for cold and drafts**. Aching pain in lumbar and sacral region (lower back). Pain and stiffness in right shoulder with inability to lift arm. Pains fly around like electric shocks. Aching heels relieved by putting feet up.

THE PHYTOLACCA PERSONALITY

Patients who need this remedy have a gloomy outlook on life, are indifferent and can exhibit offensive behavior. They suffer from restlessness and prostration. May be aching and sore; often feel faint on rising. They have a compulsion to clench teeth and gums together. Interesting physical sensations have been recorded, such as eyes full of sand, bruised all over inside and out, scalded tongue. Patient feels weak and wants to lie down.

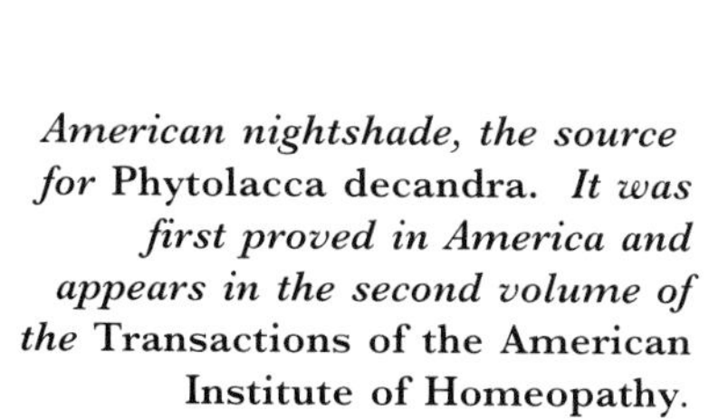

***American nightshade, the source for* Phytolacca decandra. *It was first proved in America and appears in the second volume of the* Transactions of the American Institute of Homeopathy.**

Podophyllum

- **Biliousness**
- **Diarrhea**
- **Worse in hot weather**
- **Better for lying on abdomen**
- **Better for massage to liver area**
- **Headache alternates with diarrhea**
- **Right-sided ovarian pain**

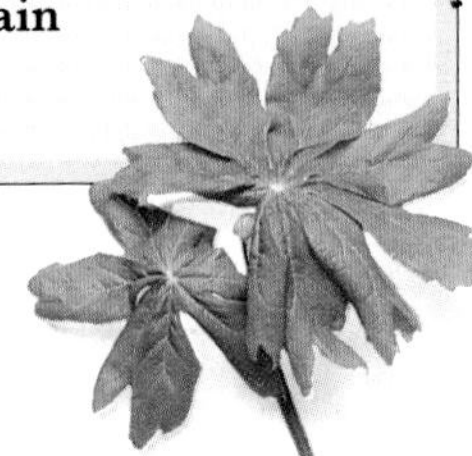

***Podophyllum peltatum, the source for* Podophyllum.**

INTRODUCTION

Podophyllum's *main area of use is in bilious conditions in the lower digestive tract.* Podophyllum *and* Podo. *are the abbreviations for this remedy.*

THE MAIN SYMPTOM PICTURE

Patients are **worse in hot weather**. This is a remedy for summer **diarrhea** (particularly after eating fruit), or during pregnancy.

Headaches have an association with the **diarrhea**: the two symptoms may alternate, or onset of diarrhea may relieve the headache. Toothache and teething respond to this remedy if the bowel disorder is also present.

There is a bitter taste in the mouth and a longing for sour food even though this aggravates the **biliousness**. The liver area is particularly sore. Rubbing or massaging the area brings relief, often in the form of profuse pale diarrhea. Sore rectum.

REMEDY SOURCE

This remedy is prepared from *Podophyllumi peltatum*, a hardy herbaceous perennial. The roots and rootstocks are poisonous.

In women, symptoms may be associated with pregnancy or the menses. **Ovarian pain** is likely to be on the right side and may shoot up to the shoulder or down the inner thigh. In men there may be prostate problems.

Lying on the abdomen brings some relief.

THE PODOPHYLLUM PERSONALITY

There is no marked psychological picture for Podophyllum, but patients may tend to babble.

Pulsatilla

- **A gentle, mild, yielding person desiring attention**
- **Changeable in mood**
- **Clingy, whiny child who evokes your sympathy**
- **Desires company and comforting which makes condition better**
- **Worse for heat, they desire cool, open air**
- **Flushes to the face**
- **Better for slow, gentle motion**
- **Thirstlessness**
- **Changeability is marked**
- **Catarrhs thick, yellow-green and bland**
- **Digestive complaints often accompany every illness**
- **Worse for rich and fatty foods**
- **Digestive complaints worse in the morning, mental complaints worse in the evening**
- **One-sided complaints**
- **Many catarrhal complaints of eye, ear and nose**

INTRODUCTION

Pulsatilla *is often chosen for children or for complaints starting in adolescence. It is often selected on its emotional picture, and has a special affinity with the mucous membranes.* Pulsatilla *and* Puls. *are the abbreviations for this remedy.*

THE MAIN SYMPTOM PICTURE

Complaints may follow getting the feet wet, or dietary indulgence, especially of rich foods which upset the patients.

Markedly worse for heat; **patients desire cool, open air**. The skin feels hot, even without a fever. **Flushes to the face**.

Better for slow, gentle motion, which is soothing both generally and for specific complaints such as pains, headaches etc.

Thirstlessness is usual, even with a fever or the dry mouth which is also commonly present.

Changeability is marked even on the physical level, for example diarrhea with no two stools alike. Pains may wander and symptoms change, or come on suddenly and be slow to go.

Catarrhs of any mucous membrane which is inflamed and can look purplish, are common. The discharges are **thick**, **yellow-green** and bland.

With nasal catarrh of some duration, there may be loss of smell or taste.

Digestive complaints often accompany every illness. Bloated and sensitive, worse especially after eating. Prefer cold things and are **worse for rich and fatty foods**, ice-cream, pork, fruit, cold things; they may crave the foods which make them worse. **Tongue coated**, bad taste in the mouth, especially early in the morning.

Digestive complaints are worse in the morning and mental complaints are worse in the evening.

Patients also worse at rest: become frantic. Better lying on the painful side. May not be able to sleep on the left side because of the palpitations and suffocation.

One-sided complaints: fever, headache, sweat, chill, etc.

Headache throbbing, and congestive. Better for cold, pressure, tying the head up tightly, slow motion. Worse in the evening and for stooping. Often has pains in the temples and sides. Headaches before menses (which are often scanty).

Many catarrhal complaints of eye, ear and nose. Itching eyelids. Styes are better for cold, worse for heat, with the typical discharge. The nose stuffs up in the evening and in a warm room. It is stuffed up on rising but can be cleared out. Nosebleeds are common.

Chills begin in the hands and feet with pains in the limbs, or down one side; numbness; fever. Thirst before the chill. Profuse sweat all over or on one side. Feel hot with distended blood vessels. Vomiting of mucus at times during chills.

Pains accompanied by constant chilliness and the more the pain, the worse the chilliness.

Dry cough at night, which is worse for lying down, and a loose cough in the morning. Thick yellow-green mucus.

Cough from tickling in the larynx, want fresh air. Coughing when breathing in; worse in evening and warm room.

The wind-flower, the source for **Pulsatilla**. *It was proved by Hahnemann and appears in the second volume of his* **Materia Medica Pura.**

THE PULSATILLA PERSONALITY

A gentle, mild, yielding person desiring attention. Nervous, fidgety, changeable in mood, easily led. A clingy, whiny child who evokes your sympathy. May be fussy and irritable but not like the tantrums of Chamomilla or the touchiness of Hepar. Desires company and comforting, which ameliorates. Moods may change easily from laughter to sadness; cries easily, even at the thought of pain. Tends to be sweet and loving when well, but self-pitying when ill. Indecisive. May not look ill.

REMEDY SOURCE

Pulsatilla is prepared from *Pulsatilla nigricans*, also known as the wind-flower, field anemone or pasque flower. It is native to the chalklands of Europe. The remedy is prepared from the entire fresh plant.

Pyrogenium

- **Septic fever**
- **Puerperal infection**
- **Varicose ulcers**
- **Septic wounds**
- **Worse for cold and damp**
- **Better for motion, heat, hot bath, pressure**

INTRODUCTION

Pyrogenium *is a nosode, a remedy made from diseased or putrid tissue. It is a wonderful remedy for septic states with intense restlessness. The person who needs* Pyrogen *is usually extremely ill and suffering from septicemia. Needs treatment by a qualified practitioner and possibly to go to hospital.* Pyrogenium *is active and very valid in the hands of a practitioner. It is a frequently indicated remedy for septic fevers, puerperal fever, recurrent abscesses and typhoid. Useful for obstinate, offensive varicose ulcers of the elderly.* Pyrogen *and* Pyrog. *are the abbreviations for this remedy.*

THE MAIN SYMPTOM PICTURE

The septic state shows intense restlessness; the heartbeat becomes weak and there is marked aching in the muscles which is **relieved by motion and heat**. Person feels bruised and sore all over, but is compelled to move for relief. **Worse for cold**. Discharges are horribly offensive – menstrual flow, lochia, diarrhea, vomit, sweat etc. Patients are very sick indeed, with an extremely rapid pulse and a high temperature, but not as correspondingly high as the rapid pulse warrants. Delirious, confused and irritable. Prostrated but must move even though they feel very sore and aching. May have throbbing head. Want to roll head from side to side; feel better for bandaging. Cold sweat on forehead, flaring nostrils. May sneeze every time hand moves from under covers. Often have horrible offensive breath. Vomit looks like coffee grounds or is putrid; mouth is putrid and tongue is coated and brown. If they have diarrhea it is watery, copious and putrid. Urination is scanty.

Septic fever. Patients are cold and chilly, the chill begins in the back and temperature rises rapidly. Great heat and sweat, which does not lower the temperature.

Frequently, patients have never recovered full health since a previous septic state such as pyemia, typhoid or infected wounds. There are palpitations and the pulse is abnormally rapid. Tremendous aching in all limbs, and must move to get relief. All secretions are foul.

Puerperal fever. Fever at each menstrual period. Menses horribly offensive; pelvic inflammation; septicemia following abortion.

Septic wounds, offensive varicose ulcers. Small cut or injury becomes very swollen or inflamed and septic. Painful varicose ulcers with foul discharge, slow to clear up.

REMEDY SOURCE

Pyrogenium, or *Pyrogen*, is made from lean beef allowed to putrefy before being boiled in water. It was first made in the 1870s.

THE PYROGEN PERSONALITY

The mind of the person who needs *Pyrogenium* is very active; the person is very anxious and has insane notions, may think himself very wealthy. Very talkative, talks very fast. Strange sense of duality; person feels 'as if crowded with arms and legs'; a state of irritability and delirium.

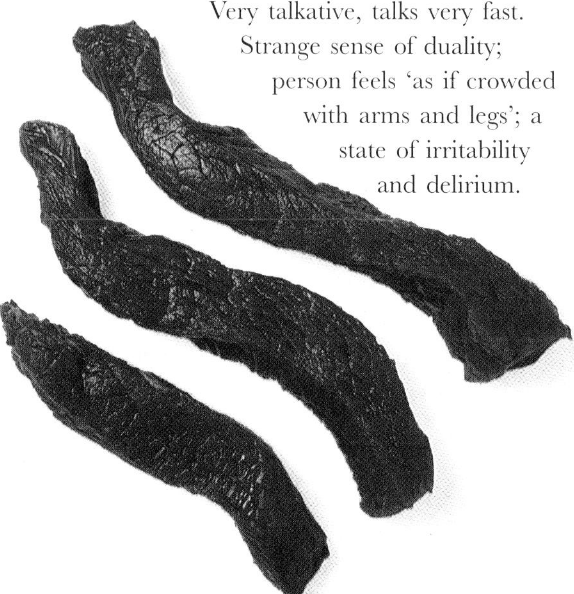

Raw beef, the source for **Pyrogenium**. *It was proved by Drysdale, Wyborn* **et al** *and the results appeared in* **Materia Medica of the Nosodes.**

Rhus toxicodendron

- **Affects the joints, ligaments, tendons and skin**
- **Worse for cold**
- **Better for heat and motion**
- **Restless, anxious**
- **Aching, sore and bruised pains, tearing pains**
- **Stupefying headaches**
- **Red, triangular tip to tongue**
- **Eruptions are red, itchy and often with blisters**

INTRODUCTION

Rhus toxicodendron *is indicated for symptoms which appear after getting wet, or by undue activity, or after a surgical operation. It has a wide range of applications and is useful in low but tenacious fevers which are accompanied by chilliness. It particularly affects the joints, ligaments, tendons and skin.* Rhus tox *and* Rhus t. *are the abbreviations for this remedy.*

REMEDY SOURCE

Rhus toxicodendron is prepared from both poison ivy (*Rhus toxicodendron*) or a variety of it called poison oak (*Rhus diversiloba* or *Toxicodendron quercifolium*), both natives of North America and Canada. The remedy is prepared from leaves gathered just before flowering.

THE MAIN SYMPTOM PICTURE

Complaints come on from **cold and damp weather, exposure, getting the feet wet or exposure whilst perspiring, overexertion, strained muscles**. Complaints often start at night.

Worse for cold in all complaints; worse for uncovering, in the evening and at night, for overexertion, getting wet.

Better for heat, motion, pressure, rubbing, perspiration.

First motion makes patients worse, but continued motion ameliorates; then they become exhausted and have to stop and rest, which makes them worse again; never at ease.

Restless, anxious; aching, sore, bruised and tearing pains. Pains often with numbness and weakness of the limbs.

Fever-type **headaches**, brain feels loose. **Stupefied** with buzzing in the ears. Sensation as if parts of the skull are screwed together. Sore muscles and sore skull. Occipital pain better when holding the head back; great restlessness and aching with this; better for motion.

Headaches may be worse for wetting the hair.

***Poison ivy, the source for* Rhus toxicodendron. *It was proved by Hahnemann and appears in the second volume of his* Materia Medica Pura.**

Low forms of fever, incoherent talking, answer hastily. Anxiety and mild delirium. All worse at night. Mild, persistent delirium; restless with laborious dreams.

Colds settle throughout the body and limbs. **Full of dizziness**. Violent coryza. Great soreness of the nostrils. Yellow, thick, offensive discharge.

Cold may go to the larynx, producing hoarseness; better for using the voice. Sore throat, with swollen glands and a stiff neck.

Thirst is usually marked but there can be dysphagia for solids from the constriction. Dry mucous membranes; dry or coated tongue with a **red, triangular tip**. Cold drinks can bring on chilliness or cough.

Dry, teasing, tickling cough before or during chills; racking cough. Cough during sleep; cough from the least uncovering. Pneumonia or pleurisy with sharp, stitching pains in the chest, much fever, aching bones, restlessness. Generally better for motion, but prostration comes on. Marked thirst and fever. Fevers with cold sores.

Sensation of hunger without appetite.

Stiff, lame back, better lying on a hard floor; sore joints and tearing pains down the limbs.

Eruptions are red, itchy and often with blisters. Urticaria during heat.

THE RHUS TOX. PERSONALITY

People who need *Rhus toxicodendron* are restless, especially at night, depressed and worried and plagued by unpleasant thoughts. They may be so suspicious that they fear the medicine they are given is poisoned, and may plan to 'escape' from their beds. They may cry pointlessly.

Rumex crispus

- **The respiratory symptoms are its main indication for use**
- **A hoarse, barking cough in attacks every night at 11pm, at 2 and 5am**
- **Cough from the slightest breathing of cold air**
- **Cough worse for lying down**
- **Very sensitive to cold air**
- **Sit very still**

INTRODUCTION

Rumex crispus does not have the febrile symptoms of Bryonia, Rhus tox. and Aconite, nor does it have the general disturbance, the aching limbs, the general soreness, the fever and thirst. The respiratory symptoms are its main indication for use. Rumex *is the abbreviation for the* Rumex crispus *remedy.*

REMEDY SOURCE

Rumex is prepared from *Rumex crispus*, known as curled dock or yellow dock. The fresh root is used to make the remedy. Curled dock is also used by herbalists for chronic skin complaints.

THE MAIN SYMPTOM PICTURE

Hoarse, barking cough attacks every night at 11pm, at 2 and 5am. Cough with pain behind the mid-sternum. Cough worse for lying down, which causes a more violent cough to appear a few moments later. **Cough from the slightest breathing of cold air**, as in Phosphorus and Spongia; from going from warm to cold. **Very sensitive to cold air**, must cover the mouth to protect against the cold air.

Copious, thin, frothy, white mucus is coughed up by the mouthful. There may also be a hard, dry, spasmodic cough at first. Watery expectoration that later becomes thick, yellow, stringy and tenacious. This often accompanies a brown, morning diarrhea. Cough with the loss of a little urine (as in Causticum).

Extreme rawness in the larynx and trachea; burning and smarting. Patients cannot endure any pressure on the pit of the throat. Tickling in the pit of the throat, or down the center of the chest to the stomach, causes coughing and maybe a congested head and wrenching pains in the right of the chest.

Sit very still: patients cannot breathe deeply or rapidly, because the burning is increased so much by any change in the pattern of respiration. Cough from changes of temperature.

Lachesis children cough in their sleep at 11pm, but if kept awake they will not cough. However, in Rumex they will cough in either case.

Sensitive to open air; sometimes a sensation of breathlessness as if passing rapidly through the air.

Intense itching of the skin when undressing to go to bed may be present.

THE RUMEX CRISPUS PERSONALITY

As it is primarily an acute remedy for respiratory troubles, there is no extensive psychological picture for Rumex crispus. There may be a generally low level of spirits and a disinclination to any mental activity.

A TRADITIONAL SOOTHER

Dock leaves have always been known in folk medicine as an antidote to the effects of stinging nettles.

***Curled dock, the source for* Rumex crispus.**

Ruta graveolens

- **First aid remedy**
- **Strained ligaments and tissues**
- **Bruised soreness**
- **Restlessness**
- **Weakness and weariness**

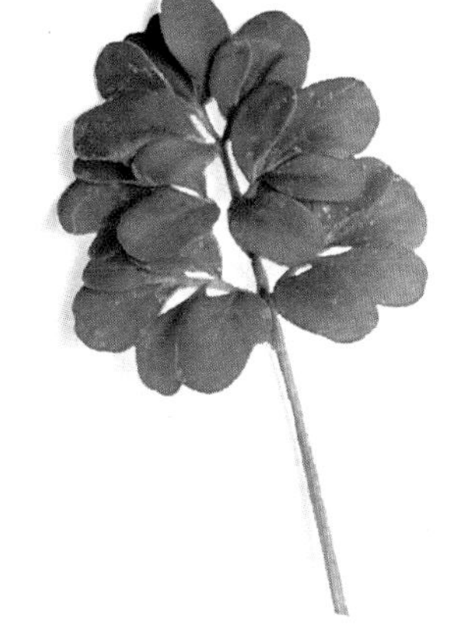

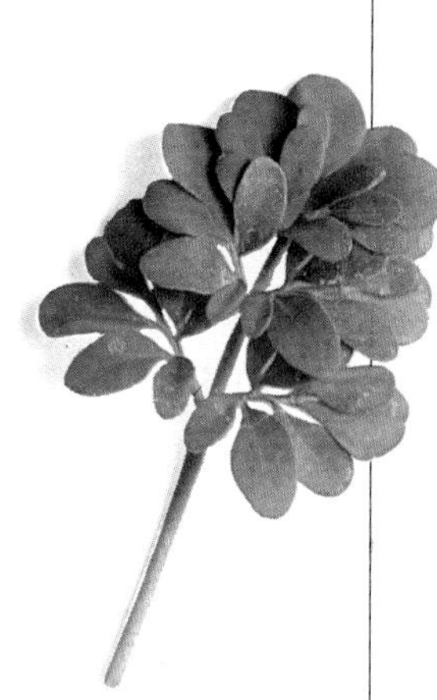

INTRODUCTION

Ruta graveolens *is a first aid remedy for strains to tissues around bony parts, often those brought on by overexertion, and for fracture or damage to bones. It is particularly useful for wrists, knees and ankles.* Ruta *is the abbreviation for this remedy.*

THE MAIN SYMPTOM PICTURE

Thighs in particular are weak and painful: it is difficult to get up when seated. Patients with backache feel better lying on the back.

Ruta is also useful for eyestrain where the eyes feel hot, bruised and sore after overuse, and vision deteriorates.

The body has a general **bruised soreness**, aching with **weakness**.

Symptoms are worse when lying or sitting still, the part lain on feels bruised, so patients are very **restless** (although not usually as restless as Rhus toxicodendron).

Pains are worse in the cold and damp, especially wet, windy weather. Any kind of **exertion is** painful and **exhausting**; going up and down stairs is particularly difficult.

JAIL FEVER

Bunches of rue were spread over the floors of sixteenth- and seventeenth-century courtrooms to prevent the spread of jail fever, or typhus, a disease carried by lice. Rue was considered particularly effective against lice and fleas.

In more long-term cases of painful joints and tissues, such as rheumatism, other aspects of the Ruta picture may be seen. These include sudden nausea and vomiting when eating, great thirst for cold water and a constant urge to urinate.

REMEDY SOURCE

Ruta is made from rue, *Ruta graveolens*, known as the herb of grace. The remedy is made from the whole plant, picked before the flowers have developed. Rue has a long history as a medicinal plant; warriors who smeared their sword blades with it considered themselves invulnerable and it was used as an antidote to poison. In the Middle Ages it was used to combat the plague.

THE RUTA PERSONALITY

People who need *Ruta* are troubled in their minds. They become quarrelsome and dissatisfied and, despite their restlessness, feel languid and despairing.

***Rue, the source for* Ruta graveolens. *A proving appears in the fourth volume of Hahnemann's* Materia Medica Pura.**

Sanguinaria

- **Flushes of heat**
- **Burning heat**
- **Headache over right eye**
- **Worse for sun**
- **Heavy periods**
- **Pain in right shoulder**
- **Menopausal problems**

INTRODUCTION

Sanguinaria *has an affinity with the circulation, the mucous membranes, and the uterus. It is useful for coughs and breathing problems during influenza.* Sanguinaria *and* Sang. *are the abbreviations for this remedy.*

THE MAIN SYMPTOM PICTURE

***Bloodroot, the source for* Sanguinaria. *It was proved in America and results are recorded in the* Materia Medica of American Provings.**

The **flushes of heat** characteristic of Sanguinaria make this a useful remedy for the **menopause**.

Burning sensations occur in various parts of the body. This congestion of the blood leads to **headaches** where the pain rises up and settles **over the right eye**.

The headache, and other symptoms, can be brought on or made **worse by the sun**, but symptoms also come on at night. Cool air ameliorates.

Periods are heavy, often due to polyps in the uterus, with discomfort in the breasts. There may be an unpleasant burning discharge between periods. These symptoms are found particularly at the time of the **menopause**.

All sorts of chest complaints occur, including asthma and a dry cough.

Sang. has a specific use in rheumatic arthritis of the **right shoulder joint**.

THE SANGUINARIA PERSONALITY

The mental picture of Sanguinaria is one of great anxiety, with lassitude and disinclination to physical or mental effort.

REMEDY SOURCE

Sanguinaria is made from *Sanguinaria canadensis*, a member of the poppy family native to North America. Its local names are bloodroot, red puccoon, Indian red paint, red root, snakebite and tetterwort. The remedy is prepared from the fresh root of the plant.

Sarsaparilla

- **Cystitis**
- **Painful urination**
- **Blood and pus in urine**
- **Colic and backache**
- **Old-looking skin**

INTRODUCTION

Sarsaparilla *is known as a blood purifier which cleans the skin but it is a remedy with a particular affinity for the genito-urinary tract. It was once a major allopathic remedy in syphilis, used to counteract the effects of mercury, the primary cure.* Sars. *is the abbreviation for this remedy.*

***Wild licorice, the source for* Sarsaparilla.**

THE MAIN SYMPTOM PICTURE

It is useful in cases of **cystitis** where **passing urine is** very **painful**. The last drops of urine are particularly painful and may contain drops of **blood or pus**.

Sometimes it may be difficult to pass urine, especially during the day, and standing up helps the urine to flow.

Other symptoms which may occur with the cystitis include **colic**, **backache** and constipation.

The skin can become cracked, blotchy or itchy, and in long-term cases **develops a shrivelled look** that makes the person seem older than he or she is.

REMEDY SOURCE

Sarsaparilla is prepared from *Smilax officinalis*, a vine plant native to tropical South America. Its roots are used to make the remedy. It is also used by herbalists for skin conditions and rheumatism.

THE SARSAPARILLA PERSONALITY

There is no outstanding mental picture for *Sarsaparilla*, although weariness and despondency may occur.

Sepia

- **Lack of emotion**
- **'Dragged-down' sensation**
- **Menstrual and menopausal problems**
- **Sallow skin**
- **Offensive sweat**
- **Chilly, better for warmth and sun**
- **Craves sweets, pickles, vinegar**
- **Nausea and morning sickness in pregnancy**

INTRODUCTION

Sepia *is usually considered a remedy that is useful for women, and is often needed in cases of menstrual disorders and menopausal problems. It is also useful for easily tired children.* Sep. *is the abbreviation for this remedy.*

THE MAIN SYMPTOM PICTURE

Women often feel generally '**dragged-down**'. This applies not only to their emotional state, but also to their physical body. This may be reflected in a woman's posture and give rise to the classic Sepia sensation of weight in the abdomen, where the patient feels the need to cross her legs 'or everything will fall out'.

Sepia states typically arise during and after pregnancy (particularly after many pregnancies), before or during **periods** and at the **menopause**. But any situation which leaves women feeling worn out, drooping and unable to rise to any kind of joy or emotion, may bring about the Sepia picture.

The Sepia woman needs a lot of stimulation before she can get back in touch with her physical, emotional and sexual energy. There is a look of droopiness and flabbiness about her, drooping eyelids, sagging shoulders, a pot belly.

The skin **has a sallow look**, particularly the 'Sepia saddle' which is a yellow tinge across the nose and cheeks. This is not always present, but when seen it is a good indication for the use of the *Sepia* remedy.

Hair feels coarse and there may be excessive bodily hair. There is much **offensive sweat**, particularly in armpits and genitals. The lower lip may be swollen.

She is **chilly** and feels **better for warmth**, especially warm sunshine, while cold and drafts aggravate symptoms.

She may have sudden cravings for certain foods, particularly **sweets and pickles**.

Constipation, piles and prolapse of rectum and vagina are part of the Sepia picture.

The smell, or even the thought, of food can cause nausea, so *Sepia* is often useful during **pregnancy**, particularly for **morning sickness**.

Although *Sepia* is often useful for minor ailments during pregnancy, such as **nausea**, it should not be taken in high potency or repeated frequently unless professionally prescribed. Experienced homeopaths sometimes use *Sepia* for certain conditions in pregnancy such as *placenta previa*, so care must be taken in home use not to 'prove' the remedy.

REMEDY SOURCE

Sepia is made from the fluid produced in the ink sac of the cuttlefish *Sepia officinalis*. It is said that Hahnemann first came across the remedy when he was treating an artist for depression and apathy. The artist had been sucking his brushes, loaded with sepia paint made from cuttlefish ink.

THE SEPIA PERSONALITY

The Sepia woman appears detached and unemotional, but can be hit by sudden spells of weeping, often without knowing what she is weeping about. Men who choose a detached, unemotional lifestyle may also show a Sepia picture.

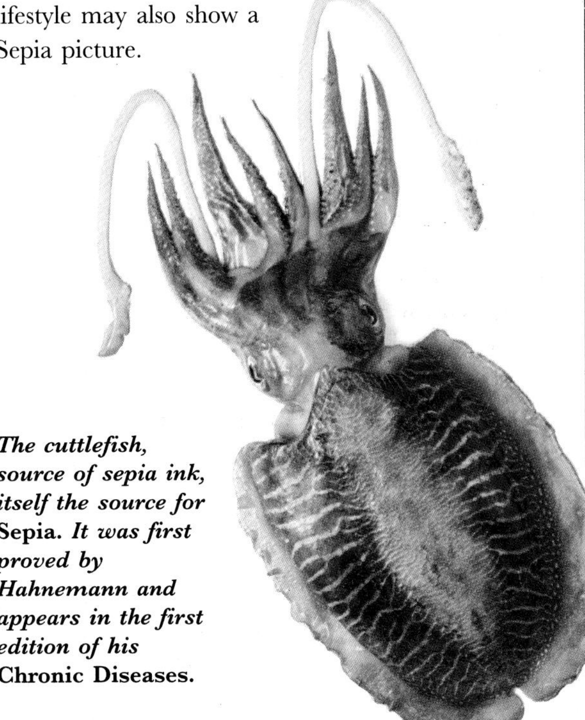

***The cuttlefish, source of sepia ink, itself the source for* Sepia. *It was first proved by Hahnemann and appears in the first edition of his* Chronic Diseases.**

Silica

- **Complaints after getting the feet wet; from suppressed discharges or sweat**
- **Catarrhs with a thick, yellow discharge**
- **Lymph nodes enlarge and become hard**
- **Worse in warm rooms and heat**
- **Sweat about the upper part of the body or head**
- **Headache from back of head, going over forehead**

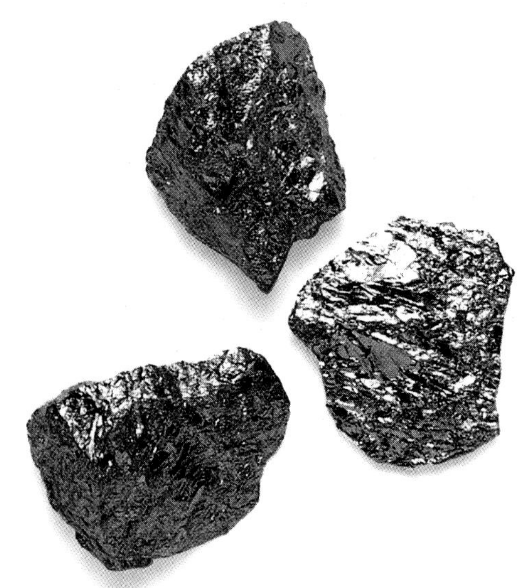

INTRODUCTION

Silica *has an affinity with the digestive system, where food is not properly assimilated. It is particularly useful in chronic disease. One remarkable feature is the ability of* Silica *to promote the extrusion of foreign bodies – splinters, glass shards, thorns – from body tissues. People with any kind of implants should avoid this remedy.* Sil. *is the abbreviation for this remedy, which is sometimes called* Silicea.

THE MAIN SYMPTOM PICTURE

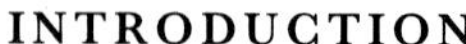

REMEDY SOURCE

Silica is prepared from silicon dioxide (SiO_2) which is found in quartz, flint, and sandstone.

Symptoms often come on in cold, damp weather and may be improved by cold, dry weather. Complaints after **getting the feet wet** (as Pulsatilla), from **suppressed discharges or sweat**. Patients are easily affected by extremes of temperature, easily overheat and sweat, then take cold.

Catarrh: a thick, yellow discharge.

Lymph nodes enlarge and become hard, especially in the neck; inflamed glands.

Acute illnesses are worse in warm rooms and heat; normally Silica is chilly and worse for drafts.

Offensive sweat about the upper part of the body or head.

Headache from the back of the head, going over the forehead. Worse at night, for noise, cold air; better for heat and pressure.

Suppuration of eyelid margins with stinging, burning and redness. Photophobia is marked. Eyes inflamed from trauma or removal of foreign bodies.

Chronic ear discharges: offensive, thick, yellow; roaring and hissing in the ears; Eustachian catarrh. Hearing returns with a snap. Better for gaping or swallowing.

Hard crusts accumulate in the nose, with loss of taste and smell. Nosebleeds.

Cracked, peeling, rough lips, crusty at the margins of the mucous membranes; encrusted ears.

Nausea, vomiting and hiccups, with aversion to warm food and desire for cold food. Hot drinks cause sweating and hot flushes of the face and head. Milk aggravates and causes diarrhea and vomiting. Sour vomiting; sour curds in the stools.

Colic, stomach feels sore when touched; the patient feels worse after eating and better for heat and application of heat.

Silicon, the source for* Silica. *It was proved by Hahnemann and appears in the first edition of his* Chronic Diseases. *It is one of the 12 tissue, or mineral, salts identified by Dr Wilhelm Schuessler (1821-98).

THE SILICA PERSONALITY

Silica people are self-willed yet lack self-confidence and fear to undertake anything; they are chronically tired and want to sit and do nothing. They grumble angrily if they are questioned about their lack of drive, and find intellectual work almost impossible.

Spigelia anthelmia

- **Intense pains that are shooting, burning, stabbing, tearing, neuralgic**
- **Pains that increase from sunrise to midday, and decrease as the sun goes down and sets**
- **Worse for motion**
- **Headaches are often one-sided, beginning in the occiput and extending forward and settling over the left eye**
- **Neuralgia**

INTRODUCTION

Spigelia anthelmia *has an affinity with the brain and spinal cord. It is known by its pains and is useful in trigeminal neuralgia. It is also used for heart problems.* Spigelia *and* Spig. *are the abbreviations for this remedy.*

THE MAIN SYMPTOM PICTURE

Spigelia is known by its pains.

There are shooting, burning, stabbing, tearing, neuralgic pains; **intense pains.**

Pains that increase from sunrise to midday, and decrease as the sun goes down and sets (as in Natrum mur.). Run-down people may feel pain on catching cold.

Worse for motion; even mental exertion makes the pains worse.

Worse for eating, in the morning, for noise, cold, damp rainy weather.

Better for quiet, and dry air.

Pains in the neck and shoulders are better for heat. Patients often cannot move because of pain.

Pains about the eyes are better for cold.

Head pains are worse for heat, and are temporarily better from cold applications. **Trigeminal neuralgia**, especially of the left side.

Painful parts can become red, inflamed and sensitive. Pulsating and stitching pains in the head may be better lying with the head held high; worse for motion, stooping, noise.

Pains in the extremities like hot wires; usually better for keeping still. So sore that any jarring is unbearable. Vertigo from looking downward, therefore they sit and look straight ahead.

Headaches are often one-sided, beginning in the occiput and extending forward and settling over the left eye (right eye for Sanguinaria, Silica etc.). The eye of the affected side may water with tears. There may be aversion to coffee and tobacco smoke. Appetite may disappear but there is violent thirst.

REMEDY SOURCE

Spigelia is made from *Spigelia anthelmia,* also known as pink root and annual wormgrass, a perennial herb native to the West Indies and South America. The remedy is made from the freshly dried plant.

THE SPIGELIA PERSONALITY

The mental state of Spigelia patients is one of hypersensitivity and intolerance. They cannot bear to be touched. They may be restless, easily irritated and anxious. There is a peculiar fear of pointed objects such as pins, needles etc.

Pink root, the source for **Spigelia anthelmia.** *It was proved by Hahnemann and appears in the fifth volume of his* **Materia Medica Pura.**

THE POWDERS OF SUCCESSION

Pink root is extremely poisonous and shares the fatal qualities of strychnine. It was used as a basis for *Les Poudres de Succession* (the Powders of Succession), a highly effective poison used by the infamous Madame de Brinvilliers, among others, for eliminating political enemies and inconvenient but rich relatives in seventeenth-century France.

Spongia tosta

- **Similar to Aconite but lacks its febrile excitement and is slower in pace**
- **Worse for warm room and heat, but better for warm drinks**
- **Remedy for croup**
- **Brought on by exposure to dry, cold winds**
- **Roughness and dryness of the mucous membranes**
- **Dry cough with no rattling**

INTRODUCTION

Spongia tosta is similar to Aconite but lacks its febrile excitement and is slower in pace, its onset taking several days and often beginning in the evening. It is another remedy with an affinity for the respiratory tract. Spongia *and* Spong. *are the abbreviations for this remedy.*

THE MAIN SYMPTOM PICTURE

Worse for warm room and heat, but is **better for warm drinks**.

A main **remedy for croup**, especially if it follows catching cold, or exposure to dry, cold winds one or two days previously. First there appears a **roughness and dryness of the mucous membranes**. Sneezing and croup comes on before midnight with a dry, hoarse, barking cough, like a saw being driven through a plank of wood, and dry air passages. The more rattling there is, the more likely it is that *Hepar Sulph.* is indicated, especially if patient is inclined to get worse after midnight or in the morning hours. **A dry cough with no rattling** is Spongia, and it may follow Aconite if the croup continues after midnight and into the next day. Patients wake from sleep with suffocation, alarm, anxiety and a loud cough. Later, tough mucus may form which is difficult to expectorate.

Dyspnea is worse for lying down, with the head low; better for warm food. Cough better for warm food and drink; worse for talking, singing, swallowing.

Hoarseness with loss of voice, great dryness of the larynx from a cold. Coryza, sneezing, the whole chest rings, and is very dry. Voice is hissy, croupy and dry.

After catching a cold, rawness of the larynx and trachea come on, then spasmodic constriction of the larynx at night. The larynx is sensitive to touch (as in Phosphorus). If the symptoms recur or get more croupy every evening, then Phosphorus may be indicated and should be studied.

Violent basilar headaches, worse when lying down; must sit up and keep still.

In adult laryngitis and bronchitis, *Spongia* is as useful as it is for children's croup. Patients are very hoarse, with some soreness and burning in the throat. The cough is worse for talking, reading, singing, swallowing.

Cough worse for cold air, in the evening and morning; better for drinking and warm food.

This remedy may come up after a Belladonna sore throat has gone down to the chest.

REMEDY SOURCE

Spongia is made from the marine sponge, *Euspongia officinalis,* after it has been roasted and powdered. In the fourteenth century, the sponge was used as a cure for thyroid problems.

THE SPONGIA PERSONALITY

Mentally there may be marked anxiety, even to the fear of death and suffocation. Palpitations and uneasiness in the heart region; pain and a sense of fullness or stuffiness in the heart region or chest. People may wake from sleep with great fear, agitation and anxiety, and a sense of suffocation, as in Lachesis.

Sea sponge, the source for **Spongia tosta.** ***It was first proved by Hahnemann and appears in the sixth volume of his*** **Materia Medica Pura.**

Staphysagria

- **Ailments from indignation, grief, anger**
- **Headaches**
- **Styes**
- **Toothache**
- **Injuries from sharp instruments**
- **Post-operative pain**
- **Chronic diarrhea**
- **Urinary problems**
- **Cystitis**
- **Eczema**
- **Head lice**
- **Worse for emotion, touch, cold drinks, tobacco**
- **Better for warmth, rest, breakfast**

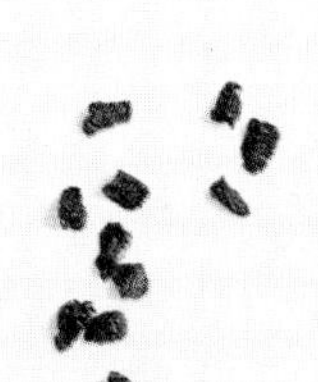

INTRODUCTION

Staphysagria *was used in the time of Hippocrates as an emetic. It is a good remedy for head lice, also stinging pains in clean-cut surgical wounds. It is also the sovereign remedy for 'honeymoon cystitis' and useful for prostate trouble, salpingitis or amenorrhea from emotional excitement.* Staph. *is the abbreviation for this remedy.*

THE MAIN SYMPTOM PICTURE

Nervous afflictions with trembling. Patients shake all over with indignation, feel a heart attack is imminent. Sleepless for many nights. Hypersensitive to touch, noise, smell; are **better for warmth and rest**.

Headache compressive, stupefying; brain feels squeezed or torn. There is the sensation of a heavy ball in the forehead. Better for yawning, worse for emotions such as anger or vexation. There may be moist encrustations on the head.

Eyes feel dry and sunken, and there may be **styes**, for which Staph. is a good remedy.

In Staphysagria **toothache**, teeth may be loose, black and crumbling. Gums are pale and bleeding. Toothache gets worse during menses; teeth are sensitive after filling. Infant teeth decay as soon as they come through. Toothache is worse for the least touch and for drink.

Stinging pains in clean-cut surgical wounds from operations, particularly abdominal operations. *Staphysagria* is recommended for **injuries from sharp instruments**.

Colic pains in abdomen, diarrhea from drinking cold water. Worse for food or drink and anger. Flatus smells like rotten eggs. Cystitis brought on by excessive sexual intercourse; cystitis during pregnancy. Frequent desire to urinate with either scanty or profuse discharge of watery urine, passed drop by drop. Burning during and after urination. Worse for walking, better for urinating. Useful for prostate troubles, salpingitis or amenorrhea from emotional excitement.

Eczema of head, ears, face and body, with thick scabs which are dry and itch violently. Arthritic nodes on finger joints and numbness in fingertips.

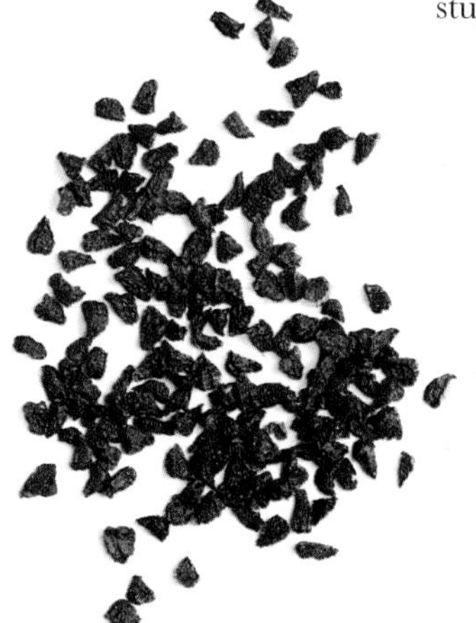

Seeds from the palmated larkspur, the source for **Staphysagria.** ***It was proved by Hahnemann and appears in the fourth volume of his*** **Materia Medica Pura.**

REMEDY SOURCE

Staphysagria is made from *Delphinium staphysagria,* also known as stavesacre or palmated larkspur. It is a biennial plant which flowers from early spring to late summer. The remedy is made from the seeds produced by the fruit of this herb.

THE STAPHYSAGRIA PERSONALITY

People who need *Staphysagria* suffer in silence, walling up their emotions. Yielding and mild on the surface, with an abhorrence of 'scenes', they are timid and sensitive with an exaggerated respect and fear for authority. They are eager to please and suppress all anger and resentment at injustice from others. Their buried anger eventually surfaces as trembling, silent rage. They are irritable, nervous and snappy. Overly worried about others' opinions; because they swallow indignation, they become powerless and a type of hardening occurs on the mental and then the physical plane. Often obsessed with sexual matters.

Sulphur

- **Healthy people who are emotionally thick-skinned**
- **Burning – pains, eruptions, sensations and discharges**
- **Offensive odors – sweat, discharges**
- **Aversion to washing**
- **Dry scaly skin**
- **Very thirsty**
- **Heat on top of the head; feet burn at night in bed; hot flushes rise up.**
- **Congestions**
- **Worse for heat, standing, at night, 12am or 12pm**
- **Hunger at 11am; feel faint and weak**
- **Catarrhs, especially lingering catarrhs**

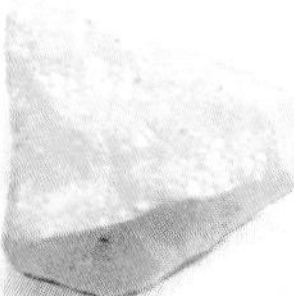

INTRODUCTION

Sulphur *is a very important homeopathic remedy. It is considered to drive out deep-seated toxins. There are a great many conditions in which* Sulphur *may be indicated, and it is also useful when the selected remedy is not performing as expected, or when the remedy picture is unclear. Its ability to bring out deep poisons will help clarify the remedy picture by revealing more readable symptoms.* Sulphur *can be used as both an acute and chronic remedy. It is often needed by robust, healthy people who are emotionally thick-skinned.* Sulph. *is the abbreviation for this remedy.*

THE MAIN SYMPTOM PICTURE

Burning **pains, eruptions, sensations and discharges**. The feet, eyes, ears, nose, throat, vertex of head, stomach, and chest all burn.

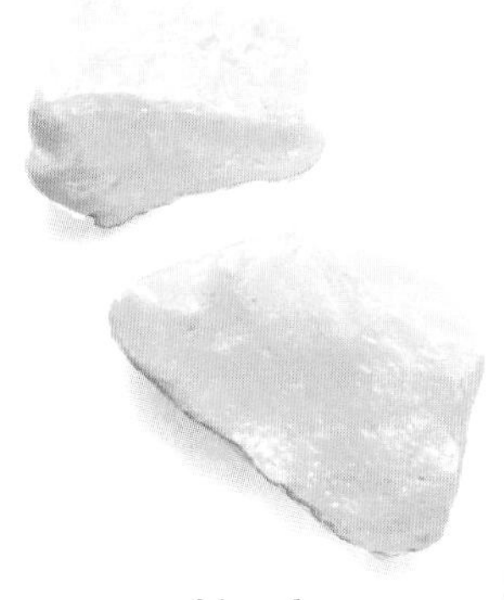

Offensive odors – sweat, discharges; the patient may be unaware of the smell.

Aversion to washing, which can make the skin worse. Worse for water and bathing.

Very thirsty usually.

Heat on top of the head; feet burn at night in bed; hot flushes rise up. Congestion. Patients feel so oppressed that they want the window open, especially at night. **Worse for heat.** Eruptions itch and burn. Warmth of the bed produces uneasiness.

Worse at noon or midnight.

Worse at night, with sinking and exhaustion.

Worse standing, and bathing. Better sitting, or lying.

Hunger at 11am; feels faint and weak.

Catarrhs of all mucous membranes; suppurations with burning discharges; ulcerations; acrid discharges.

Burning, stinging, itching eruptions, which are worse for heat. Inflammation from pressure; inflamed area can indurate (get hard). Skin affected easily by the atmosphere, becomes red from the wind and the cold. Flushes begin in the chest and rise up; patients become dusky red at the least provocation. Skin itching

REMEDY SOURCE

The remedy *Sulphur* is made from *sulphur,* which has always been an important medical aid.

***Sulphur, the source for* Sulphur. *It was proved by Hahnemann and appears in the fourth volume of his* Materia Medica Pura.**

worse for heat; scratching ameliorates but it turns to burning.

Ruddy, purple appearance which may alternate with paleness plus the hot flushes. Purplish throat, rash; a venous appearance.

Sleepless, yet patients are worse if they oversleep; extremely lethargic.

Diarrhea which drives them from bed in the morning, worse at 5am.

Dyspnea, especially on exertion, copious sweat, and very exhausted. Rattling in the chest; every cold goes to the chest or nose, and catarrh lasts for a long time. Patients do not convalesce, are slow to pick up, cannot muster the energy to get better. Lingering cough after a chest infection.

Problems improve temporarily and then recur and the previously effective remedy no longer works: a dose or two of *Sulphur* in this situation will often either clear up the problem or allow the indicated remedy to work again.

Red lips, red eyelids and redness around the orifices of the body.

A violent racking cough in bronchitis. Patients feel they are suffocating and want doors and windows open at night. Night cough. Cough with congested head. Burning in the chest etc.

A remedy commonly needed in measles, especially if the rash has not come out fully or has disappeared again and the patient becomes more ill.

They may be impatient, hurried and quick-tempered in an acute illness.

THE SULPHUR PERSONALITY

The Sulphur patient is selfish, self-centered and thinks he is the best despite evidence to the contrary. Sulphur is quick-tempered, takes offense easily and tends to be a shooting star – a flash of brilliance which then fades away. May be a hypochondriac, self-pitying and worry about his prospects. There is an aversion to water and washing and great sensitivity to smell.

***Comfrey, the source for* Symphytum.**

Symphytum

- **Broken bones**
- **Injured cartilage**
- **Backache**
- **Injury to the eyes**

INTRODUCTION

Symphytum *has the common name of knitbone, and is widely used in its herbal form as well as in homeopathic potency, to aid healing of broken or damaged bony tissue.* Symph. *is the abbreviation for this remedy.*

THE MAIN SYMPTOM PICTURE

After an accident, *Arnica* may be used for the initial trauma. When the **broken bone** has been set, *Symphytum* can be introduced to speed the knitting process of the bone.

Symphytum is also beneficial for joint pains, for example **damaged cartilage** in the knee or sciatica resulting from problems in the hip joint. The **spine** needs *Symphytum* when there has been injury or strain, or if there is disintegration of tissue.

The other use is for **injury to the eyes,** caused by a blow or knock. *Symphytum* tincture can be applied externally where there is swelling.

REMEDY SOURCE

Symphytum is prepared from comfrey (*Symphytum officinalis*) which has always been a herbal remedy for healing wounds. Its folk name is *knitbone*, because it was thought that comfrey, taken as a tonic helped the body, to heal itself more rapidly.

THE SYMPHYTUM PERSONALITY

As it is primarily a first aid remedy, there is no extensive psychological picture for Symphytum. It is mostly used in a short-term situation, so there has been no need to observe long-term psychological symptoms to add to the remedy picture.

Tabacum

- **Seasickness**
- **Nausea, vomiting, vertigo**
- **Palpitations**
- **Pallor and sweating**

INTRODUCTION

Tabacum's *main use is in travel-sickness. Good for travelers who are ill from any kind of motion, particularly in a boat, and need plenty of fresh air while avoiding any extremes of temperature.* Tab. *is the abbreviation for this remedy.*

THE MAIN SYMPTOM PICTURE

Patients suffer terrible **nausea**, **vomiting** and extreme **vertigo,** which all bring them out in a cold **sweat**. The mouth fills with saliva and the **face turns very pale**, perhaps with just one cheek red and hot.

The heart suffers violent **palpitations** and the skin itches.

Although this picture is most frequently found in seasickness, it might also arise in pregnancy, Ménière's disease or heart disease.

REMEDY SOURCE

Tabacum is made from *Nicotiana tabacum,* the tobacco plant. The remedy is made from the the leaves before the flowers develop. This is the same plant that is grown commercially for tobacco.

THE TABACUM PERSONALITY

As it is primarily a first aid remedy for travel-sickness, there is no extensive psychological picture for Tabacum. There may be impaired mental faculties, physical inertia and trembling dizziness. One peculiar symptom noted is 'silly talking' in boys.

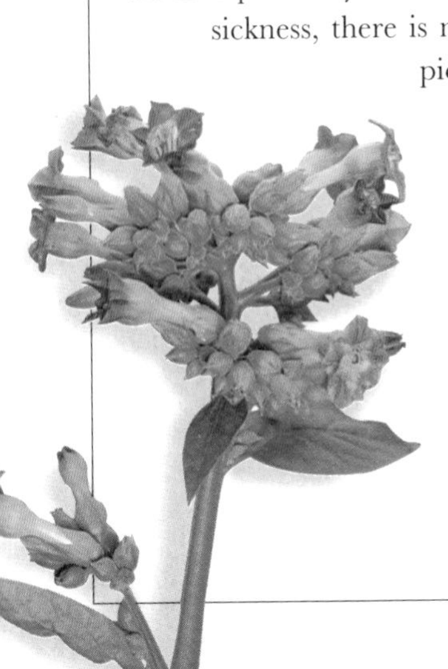

The tobacco plant, the source for **Tabacum.**

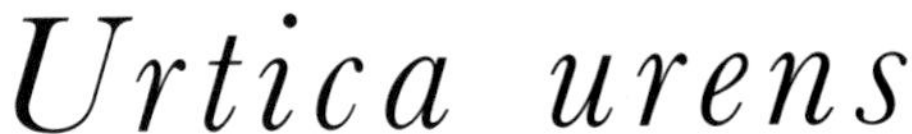

Urtica urens

- **First aid remedy**
- **Stinging and burning sensations**
- **Skin rashes**
- **Bee stings**
- **Painful breasts**
- **Cystitis**
- **Gout**

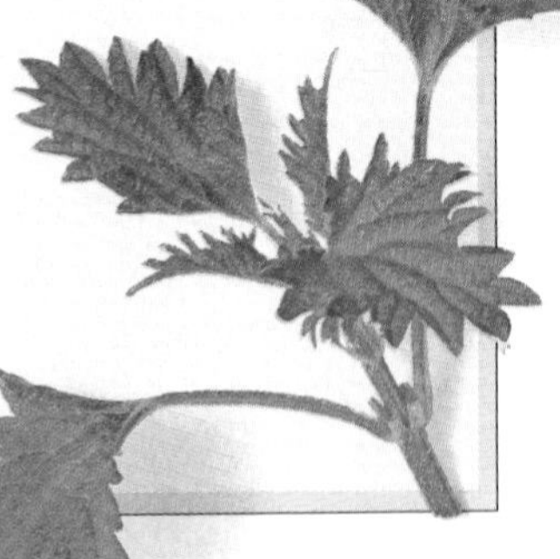

Stinging nettles, the source for **Urtica urens.** ***It was first proved by Hahnemann and appears in the first volume of his*** **Materia Medica Pura.**

INTRODUCTION

Urtica urens *is indicated if there is a rash that looks like nettle-rash (white marks on red skin), which has been caused by nervous problems. Dioscorides, the Greek physician, used the source, stinging nettles, as a purge and detoxicant.* Urtica *and* Urt. u. *are the abbreviations for this remedy.*

THE MAIN SYMPTOM PICTURE

Urtica pains are **stinging and burning,** and the skin develops weal-like eruptions similar to the effect of being stung by nettles. This remedy is useful in some cases of allergy, where the picture fits – for example, a rash after eating shellfish. It can also be used in cases of burns or **bee stings,** where the picture fits.

There is an affinity for the mammary glands. *Urtica* is useful for **painful breasts** when milk is suppressed and the pain is stinging and burning.

Urtica also affects the genito-urinary tract with stinging, burning and itching of the genitals, also on urinating.

Excess uric acid and **gout** may respond well.

Urtica urens is available as a lotion to apply direct to the skin or can be taken in tablet form.

REMEDY SOURCE

Urtica urens is prepared from the stinging nettle *Urtica dioica,* which has always been known as a herbal remedy for skin problems.

THE URTICA PERSONALITY

There is no outstanding mental picture for Urtica urens, but as it is a remedy for gout, impatience and irascibility may be expected.

Veratrum album

- **Sudden violent symptoms**
- **Very cold**
- **Fainting**
- **Collapse**
- **Dehydration**
- **Whooping cough**
- **Vomiting and diarrhea**
- **Restless anxiety**

INTRODUCTION

Veratrum album *is indicated when symptoms are strong: unbearable pain, extreme prostration, icy coldness, copious sweating. It is useful for the young and very old, and for emotional disturbance during menstruation. It should only be prescribed by a homeopathic practitioner.* Verat. alb. *and* Verat. *are the abbreviations for this remedy.*

THE MAIN SYMPTOM PICTURE

Veratrum album **symptoms come on rapidly** and are **strongly marked**. Noticeably, patients become **icy cold** and break out in a cold sweat, particularly on the head.

Verat. alb. is possibly the first remedy to think of for **fainting,** if the picture fits. In all cases there is a **state of collapse** or great prostration, and the weakness grows steadily worse.

Despite being so chilly, patients have a desire for ice-cold water. However, this is vomited straight back.

***White hellebore, the source for* Veratrum album. *It was proved by Hahnemann and appears in the third volume of his* Materia Medica Pura.**

Vomiting and **diarrhea** as seen in cholera. Although this disease is rarely seen in the West, a similar picture can still occur in gastric flu, etc. The violence of the vomiting and diarrhea leaves patients exhausted.

It is possible for the Verat. alb. picture to be brought on by hysteria, with a tendency to religious mania. In severe illness there may be delirium, mania and fear of dying. In other cases, the mental state is either brooding and sullen, or **restless and anxious**. This is a case that needs to be taken carefully, as the Verat. alb. patient has a tendency not to tell the truth.

Where the chest is affected, there is a violent cough, which makes this a useful remedy in **whooping cough** where the picture of coldness, prostration and sudden onset of **violent symptoms** fits.

REMEDY SOURCE

Veratrum album is made from white hellebore, a hardy perennial native to central and southern Europe. It is extremely poisonous, and dried powdered hellebore was used by the Romans to make the tips of their daggers and arrows more deadly.

THE VERATRUM ALBUM PERSONALITY

The Veratrum album picture shows an extreme restlessness, an urge for constant activity. There may be maniacal talking or malicious witty remarks, or sulky silence. People may consider themselves slighted or used, and tell dreadful lies. Hallucinations of many kinds noted.

***Veratrum album* is another remedy where the picture shows a patient with strong symptoms who may well need professional medical care.**

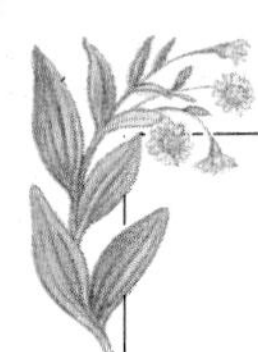
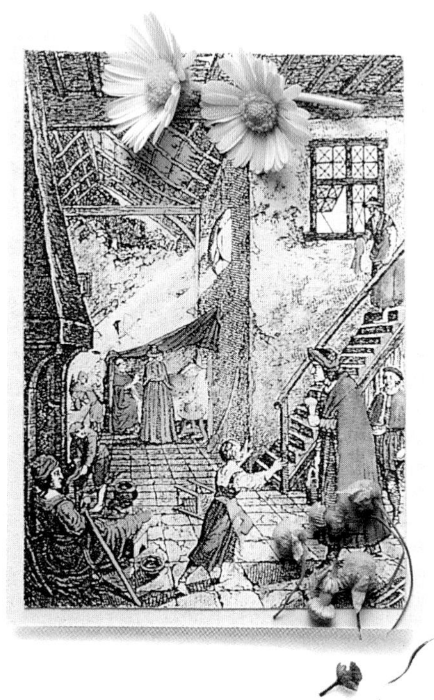
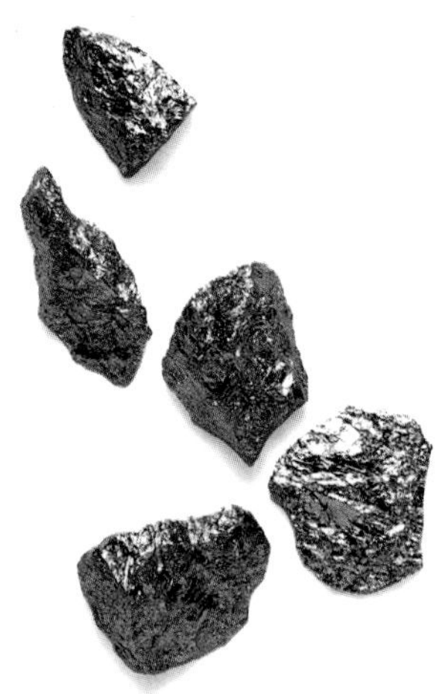
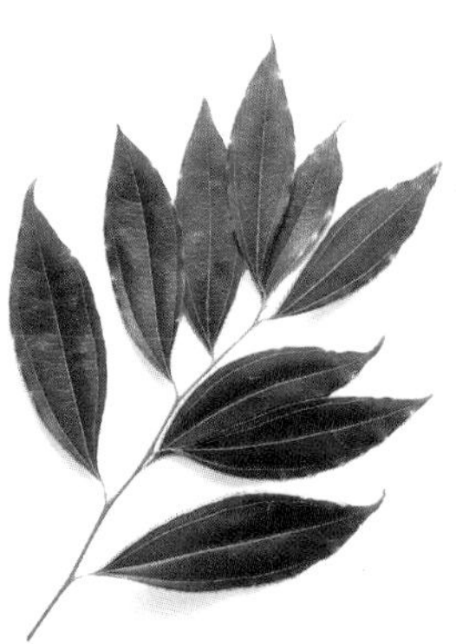
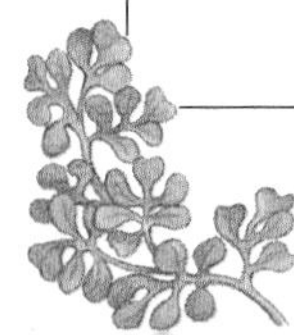

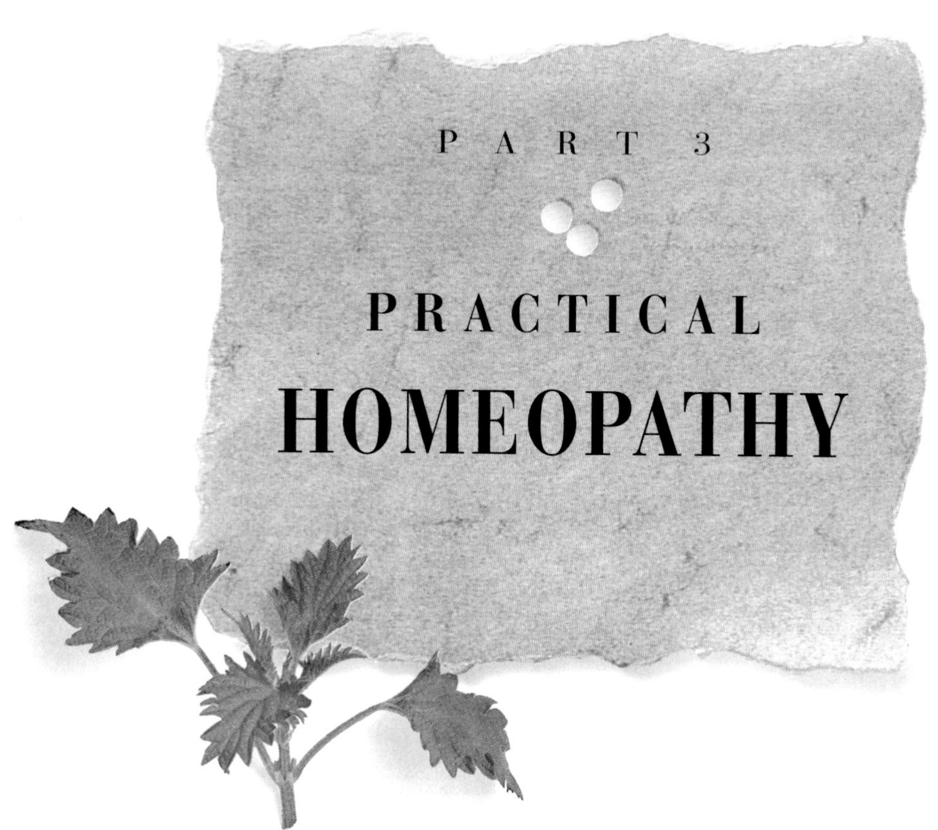

PART 3

PRACTICAL HOMEOPATHY

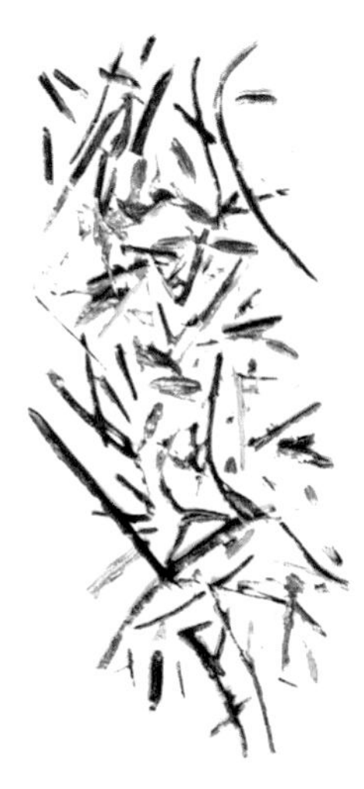

INTRODUCTION

Rue, the source for the Ruta graveolens *remedy.*

The essence of homeopathy is to match a remedy picture to the disease picture in an individual. A picture in this sense consists of the collection of symptoms which characterize the remedy or the patient with his or her illness. Symptoms are changes from the normal state of a person occurring at any level of his or her being and range from changes of mood or behavior to physical things such as pains, temperature reactions, color changes, sweats etc.

That which a remedy is capable of causing (that is, the picture of the remedy) is also able to be cured by that remedy. This is the Law of Similars – 'like cures like'. An explanation of why this should be is given in the first part of the book. However, homeopathy can be used for simple acute illnesses such as those described in this book, without a full understanding of its philosophy and theory. Remember the aim – to find the remedy with the most similar symptom picture to the picture of disease in the patient.

Raw coffee beans, the source for the Coffea cruda *remedy*

Charcoal, the source for the Carbo vegetabilis *remedy.*

Here arises the first problem: how completely must the picture of the disease and the remedy match in order to be assured of a beneficial result?

Black snake root, the source for the **Cimicifuga racemosa** *remedy.*

Clearly, the more complete the fit between the remedy and the illness, the more certain and the greater will be the success of the prescription. Only an expert, after much study and practical experience, will achieve consistently good responses. So how can the beginner maximize the chance of success? It was with this in mind that the book was written. This section shows clearly and simply how you go about taking a homeopathic case, what to observe, which questions to ask and how to use the information you obtain; four simple case studies are given as examples. Read together with Part Four, The Remedy Pictures, *it will enable anyone to make a start in finding, with a reasonable degree of accuracy, remedies to treat common family illnesses. And if you persevere in your prescribing, it will help you to develop a deeper knowledge and understanding of the many homeopathic remedies and their uses.*

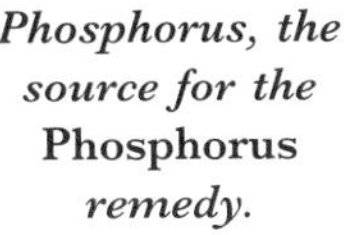

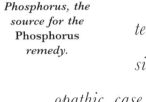

Phosphorus, the source for the **Phosphorus** ***remedy.***

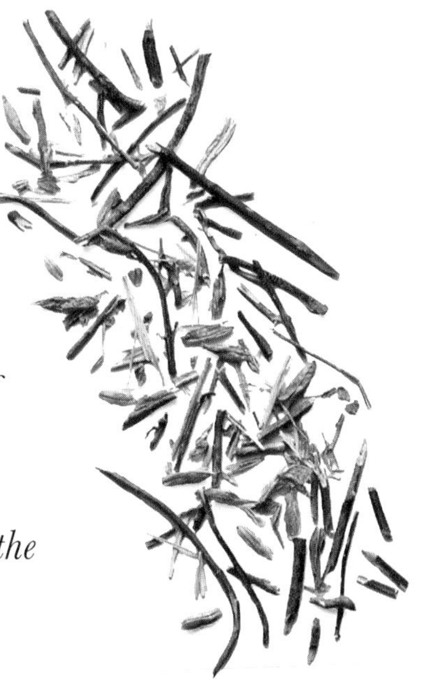

Dried eyebright, the source of the **Euphrasia officinalis** ***remedy.***

Taking the case

Firstly, the picture of the disease in the patient is needed. Obtaining this information is called 'taking the case'. There are only two requirements when taking a case and they are interdependent: observation and objectivity. In order to find the most similar remedy, we need to identify the symptoms that characterize the individuality of the disease process in each case.

Observation

Observation involves seeing, hearing, smelling, touching and, rarely, tasting! The vital clue to an individual's sickness may come through any of the senses, so use them all. Having observed something, just record it and do not reason it out as to why it is so. Best of all, record the patient's own words, especially for the important symptoms. The less thinking and interpreting that goes on the better. By all means make enquiries to aid observation. Indeed, the largest part of the case will be heard as the patient tells of his symptoms. However, try to allow the patient to speak of what they themselves notice to be wrong and try not to put words into their mouth. Use questions such as, 'What else?' and, 'Can you tell me more about that?' in order to extract more information.

What the patient tells you without prompting will usually be of greater importance. Of course, you have to take into account the basic personality of the patient; some will tell all without needing to be questioned, others need tact, diplomacy and perseverance to get any symptoms from them. This fact in itself may be a symptom of the illness, particularly if it is not usual for them to behave in that way. This would be an example of a mental symptom. The more marked the change in behavior or mental state, the more important it will be to find a remedy with that same mental picture.

Other things to be observed would be the patient's appearance, presence or absence of heat and sweat in different areas of the body, their behavior and mood, what they want in their surroundings and environment.

A FAMILY RECORD

YOU MAY like to keep a family or personal health record to note all relevant health matters – patterns of health, details of specific illnesses, their treatment and outcome, accidents, vaccinations and their effect, etc. It would be interesting to note also the stresses that occur from time to time, be they physical, mental or emotional and to observe their effect on health. One of the secrets of staying healthy is to discover what it is that tends to throw you out of balance and causes illnesses to appear. This will be very individual and may be important for your long-term health. When taking a case, even your own, write it down in whatever layout and form you find suits you. You may divide it into sections, record it just as it is spoken, or choose some other method, but do record it for later reference and to help you learn.

Curled dock, the source for **Rumex.**

USING YOUR SENSES

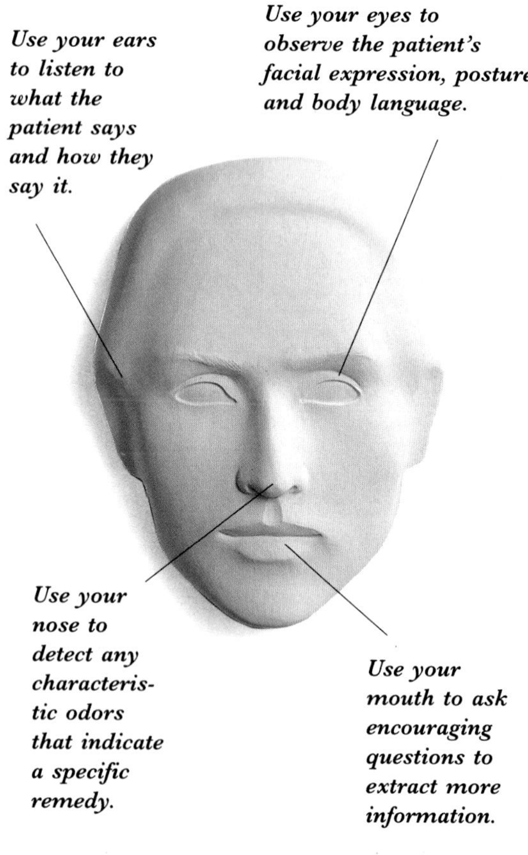

Use your ears to listen to what the patient says and how they say it.

Use your eyes to observe the patient's facial expression, posture and body language.

Use your nose to detect any characteristic odors that indicate a specific remedy.

Use your mouth to ask encouraging questions to extract more information.

Underline anything that is very prominent and strong. You may wish to underline some things two or three times. Make a special note of anything that is unexpected, such as a sore throat that is better for swallowing solid food – normally one would expect this to make it worse. Symptoms like this are called strange, rare and peculiar, and are often of prime importance in finding the remedy or group of remedies from which to make one's selection. Things which affect the person as a whole are of much greater importance than those affecting only a part. Mental and general symptoms carry greater weight when evaluating a case for homeopathic treatment.

Likewise symptoms that are indefinite, mild and nebulous. Unless, of course, all the symptoms are like that in which case it becomes a general symptom and might point towards a remedy like *Ferrum phos.* or maybe *Pulsatilla.*

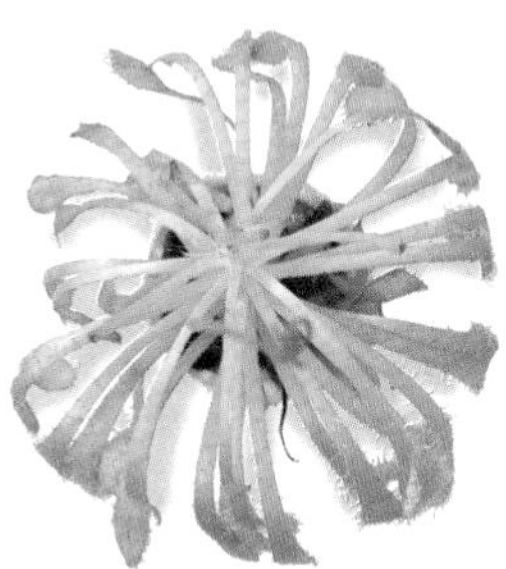

Round-leaved sundew, the source for the* Drosera rotundifolia *remedy.

So look out for the strong, the peculiar, the characteristic symptoms, any general symptoms that run through the case in different areas of the body and any changes in the mental state of the patient. Make sure that you have all the details of each symptom: any cause, the speed of onset, the site, the sensations, the modalities etc. Have you ascertained the strength and consistency of each symptom? This will help you to appreciate the unique state of the patient and just how the illness is affecting them.

There is no one way to take a case. It is a creative and individual process reflecting the relationship between yourself and the patient. This is why you should be as free from emotional upset and involvement as possible when taking it. With practice, you will discover different ways of obtaining the information to suit the different types of cases.

FOUR KINDS OF EAR ACHE

In the following four acute cases, all the children had painful ears and it is likely they would all have received the same antibiotic from an allopathic practitioner.

These simple case studied demonstrate how their presenting states were clearly observable and different from each other and how they all required different remedies and careful individualization.

Ears must be treated with gentleness and caution, and medical advice sought from a practitioner if symptoms persist.

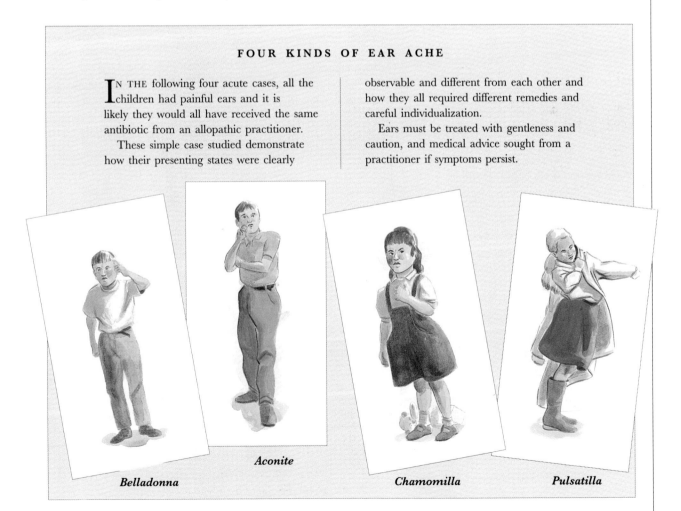

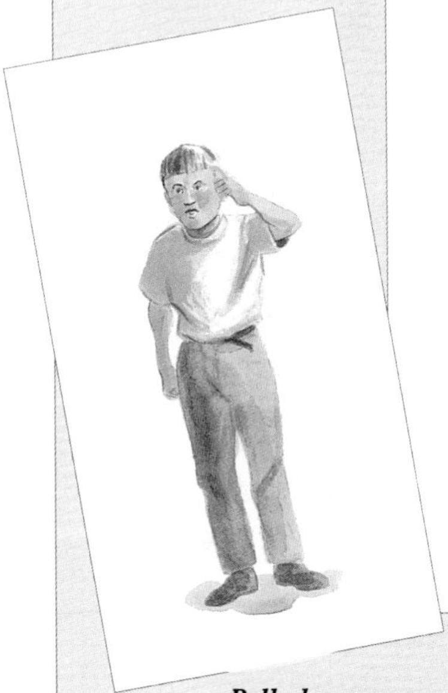

Belladonna

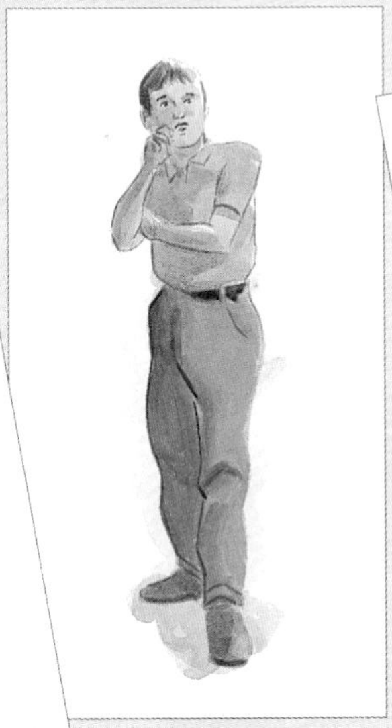

Aconite

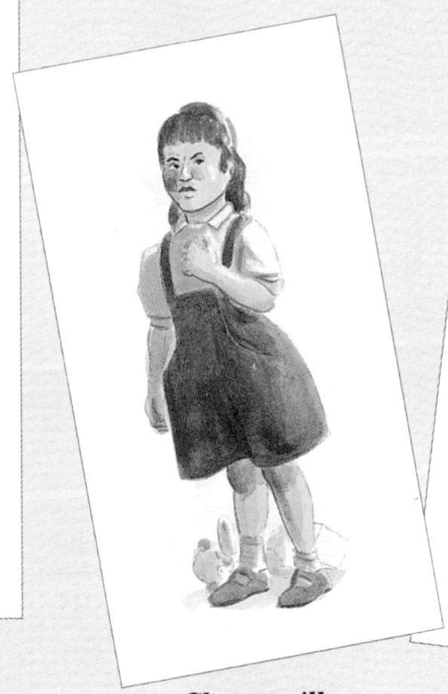

Chamomilla

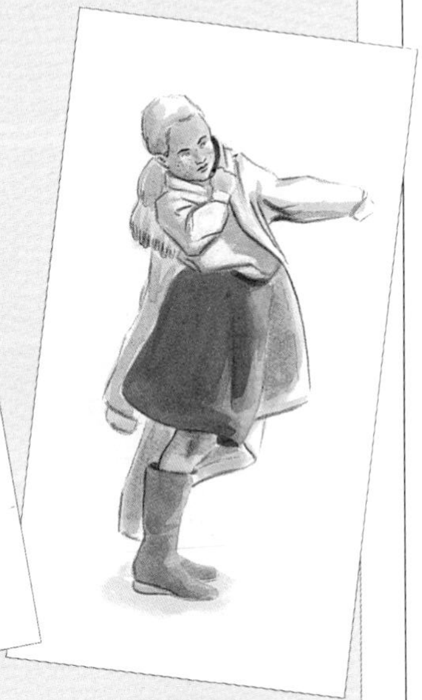

Pulsatilla

Four case studies

Each case study shows the most important symptoms written up as notes, with a résumé of the case history, the remedy selected and the results achieved given separately.

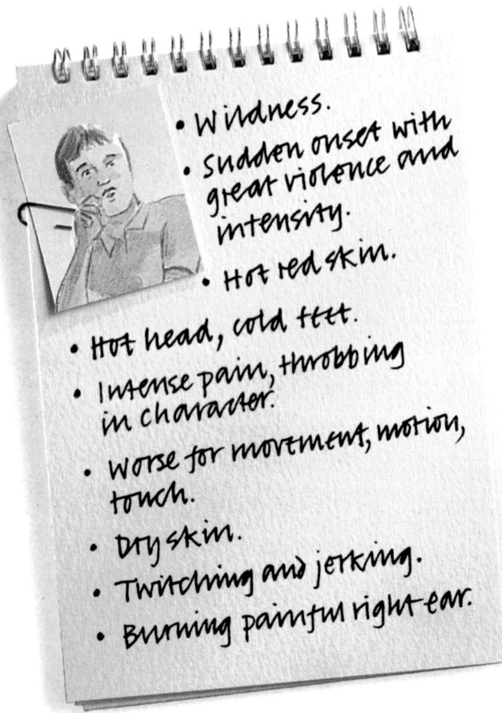
• Wildness.
• Sudden onset with great violence and intensity.
• Hot red skin.
• Hot head, cold feet.
• Intense pain, throbbing in character.
• Worse for movement, motion, touch.
• Dry skin.
• Twitching and jerking.
• Burning painful right ear.

CASE ONE

THE BELLADONNA CHILD

SAM, aged 7 years, is usually a quiet, well-behaved, robust child who likes to go at his own pace and will not be hurried. Parents were very worried as he appeared very ill indeed. He had woken up at 10 pm, suddenly, in great pain in his right ear. His right ear was bright red and hot to touch, as was his head. Blood vessels in the head and neck were pulsating and the skin was dry, red and hot to touch. His feet were cold. Mother was frightened by the look of him, his pupils shining and dilated, he was gnashing his teeth and looked 'wild'. The child said he saw a horrible face on the wallpaper. Twitching and jerking while lying down. Father accidentally bumped bed and he screamed in pain. Throbbing ear, severe pain, holding his right ear; did not want to move or be touched; wanted fizzy lemonade, had a very dry mouth.

REMEDY SELECTED: BELLADONNA

After remedy: slept; rather twitchy and jerky; awoke in the morning and asked for breakfast; red face but not hot; needed to rest in bed; ear pain less; ear pain subsided next day.

CASE TWO

THE PULSATILLA CHILD

FOUR-YEAR-OLD Laura sat on her mother's knee and refused to move. She would not play or be distracted by any toys. Mother says she is generally not clingy and plays happily by herself. Mother in a terrible state, completely drained and exhausted. She said child would not leave her for a minute. Child woke at 9 pm the previous night crying, with left-side ear ache. She was furious the babysitter was there and not her mother. Screamed and cried for mother. Babysitter telephoned the restaurant and mother came home. Child attached herself to mother and wanted to be carried and rocked gently. Slept with mother. Wanted a lot of fuss and sympathy. Would not be left alone in the morning when mother was trying to get older sister off to school; said, 'Don't leave me by myself'. Has had a cold for a few days with bland yellow-green discharge from nose. Child pointed inside left ear and said it hurt. Pain much worse at night, screaming and holding ear. Refused to drink anything. Wanted covers off in bed. Would not wear coat, wanted windows open in car.

REMEDY SELECTED: PULSATILLA

After remedy: child went home and lay down with mother; slept for four hours. Now drinking; let sister read her a story.

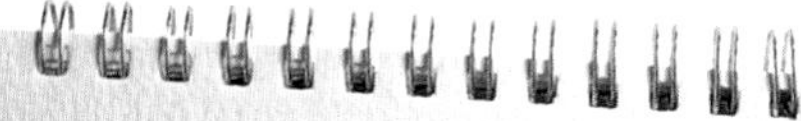
• Desires company - will not be left alone.
• Made better by comfort and fuss.
• Better for gentle rocking.
• Worse for slow gentle motion.
• Thirstless.
• Thick bland yellow-green discharge from nose.
• Worse for heat.
• Desires cool open air.
• Left-sided ear pain.

- Very irritable and angry.
- Terrible temper.
- Spiteful.
- Great sensitivity to ear pain.
- Wants things then rejects them.
- Demands to be carried.
- One cheek red, one pale.
- Better for being carried.

CASE THREE
THE CHAMOMILLA CHILD

JENNY, aged 2 years, had been in pain all day and at 7 pm mother said she could bear the child's behavior no longer, said she felt murderous towards her. Child was holding on to right ear and screeching with pain. Ear lobes were red. She had one red cheek and the other cheek was pale. Mother said child did not know what she wanted, asked for a drink then threw it on the floor; asked for her favorite doll then hit mother over the head with it. Mother said she had been in the most terrible temper, angry and screaming and then moaning and crying. Mother felt everything she did was wrong and said the child was really spiteful to her and baby brother. Demanding to be carried by mother then father, Jenny could not keep still with the pain, in a real frenzy. Drinking beakers of cold water. Sweating about the head and feverish.

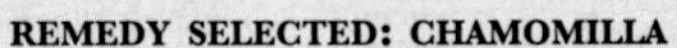

REMEDY SELECTED: CHAMOMILLA

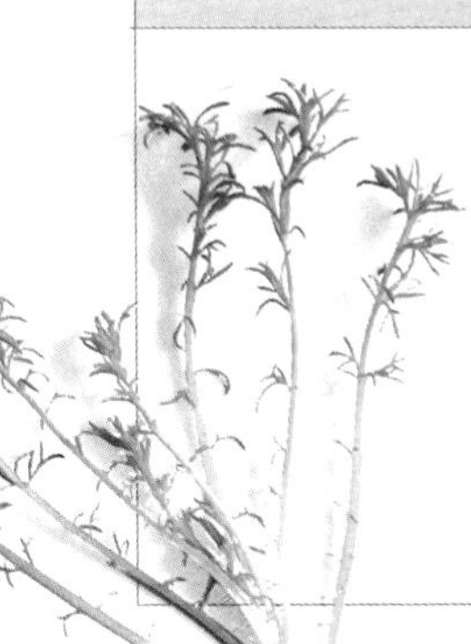

After remedy: slept until 5 pm; woke with ear pain. Remedy repeated. Slept for long periods. Temper much better. Watched TV and played with toys. Ear pain subsided; occasionally pulled at ear.

CASE FOUR
THE ACONITE CHILD

NINE-YEAR-OLD John's ear ache came on when he was in bed. Mother says the family had been out for a winter walk in the afternoon, it had been dry but a cold wind was blowing. She feared they had walked too long, but John seemed fine. He went to bed at 8 pm and awoke half an hour later suddenly complaining of terrible stinging, burning pains in both ears. He screamed with pain and could not bear his parents talking. His mother has never seen him so anxious and afraid. He is tossing about in the bed, unable to settle he is so restless. Holding both his ears, skin red on ears. So afraid he asked if he was going to die. Usually he is healthy and robust, hardly ever unwell. Skin on head dry and hot. John is very thirsty indeed for cold water; cannot bear bedclothes on him. Face is congested and red, and veins are visibly pulsating.

REMEDY SELECTED: ACONITE

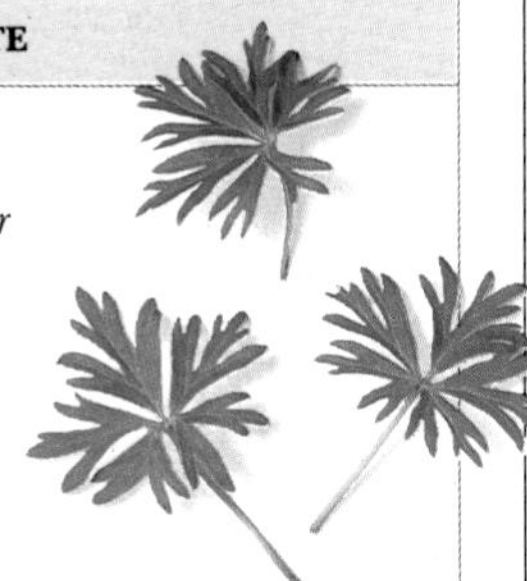

After remedy: went to sleep, woke 6 am less restless and anxious; ear pain less; needed to rest and sleep next day; ear pain subsided.

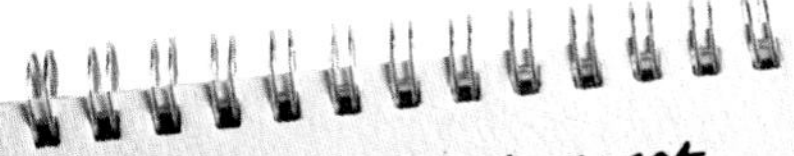

- Sudden violent onset.
- Exposure to cold, dry wind.
- Restlessness.
- Anxious.
- Fear of death.
- Intense burning, stinging pain.
- Worse for noise and covering.
- Very thirsty for cold water.
- Congested circulation.
- Dry, hot skin.

Analyzing the case

Now that you have 'taken the case' it needs to be analyzed. The most important features of the case should be clear, strong and characteristic of the patient's illness right now. Be quite sure the symptoms are new changes and do not relate to the patient's normal state of health. Changes of intensity may be included, although they are proportionally less significant.

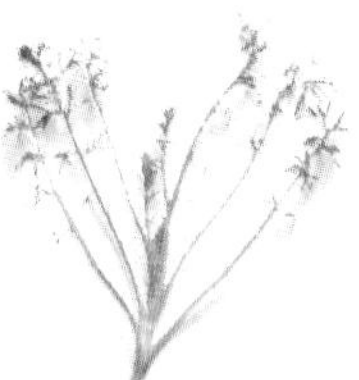

Wild chamomile, the source for the **Chamomilla** *remedy, often called for in children's cases.*

The evaluation of the importance of each symptom mainly arises from a combination of three factors. Firstly, the depth of the symptom – that is, at what level of the person's being it is taking place; secondly, the strength of the symptom; and thirdly, how uniquely characteristic is the symptom of the patient's state.

A useful guide to the first two is to see what effect a symptom has on the patient's ability to function as a whole, creative, happy, loving human being, taking into account their normal state, of course! It is clear that anything which affects the mind will be of prime importance in this, as will anything that affects the person as a whole. Mental and general symptoms are therefore ranked high.

Particular symptoms which relate to the separate parts are usually of less significance.

NOTES IN PROGRESS

QUESTIONS

1) Where is pain?
2) What sort of pain is it?
3) How does it make you feel?
4) How is it different from normal?
5) When did it start? Hours... days?
6) What was happening at the time?
7) What makes it better?
8) What makes it worse?
9) Any other changes?
10) Has this occurred before?
11) Are you taking any drugs?

Bad breath, sweating and stinking green discharge ears? Merc.?

Clingy, won't be put down, won't drink, green discharge nose? Puls.?

Premenstrual, emotional shock, fright, etc?

Pressure, heat, cold, motion, noise?

Regularly? The first time?

Allopathic or homeopathic?

Irritable, much worse movement, stitch pains in chest? Bryonia?

Location? Where did it start? Has it extended?

Going from bed to bed, anxious? Arsen.?

Burning hot and red skin, worse for jar? Belladonna?

This notebook shows the typical questions that you should ask when taking a case. The jottings at the side indicate the thinking that leads to the selection of a particular remedy.

Nevertheless, if the patient is mentally and emotionally unaffected but has, for example, a pain somewhere, then the details of the pain will make up the whole case, or 'totality' as it is called, for which a similar remedy must be found. This can also happen if a pain is so severe and strong that it makes all the other symptoms pale into insignificance.

Peculiar symptoms fall outside this method of evaluation because they may be very debilitating or make little difference to the patient's ability to function. Their high ranking stems from the individuality of the symptom to that patient. If the peculiar is also strong and consistent then this will increase its importance even occasionally to the point where it will override any mental and general symptoms when evaluating the case. Peculiars are by definition uncommon but they are worth searching for and if present in a case would strongly favor any remedies showing that same symptom. Examples of peculiar symptoms would be 'dry mouth without thirst' or 'symptoms affecting one half of the body only'.

Clearly the strength of each symptom needs to be taken into account. How the patient speaks of their symptoms, their tone of voice, gestures and expressions will tell of the intensity. At first, you may like to employ a points system to help in your evaluation of symptoms.

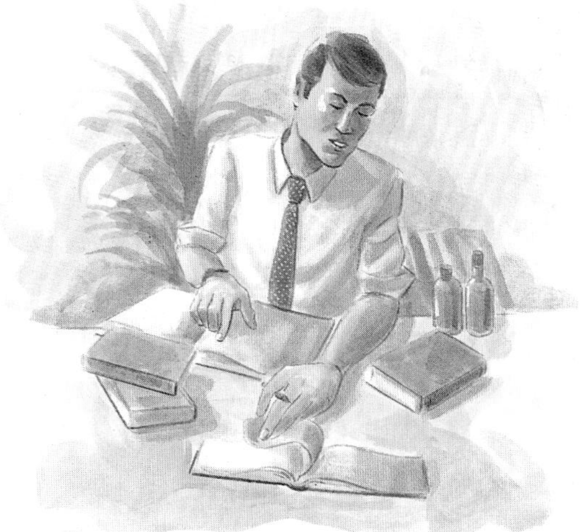

It takes time, patience and experience to analyze a case well.

- Assign 3 points to mental symptoms.
- Assign 2 points to physical symptoms that are generals (symptoms that can be expressed 'I am . . .').
- Assign 1 point to particular symptoms that relate to the separate parts of the body.
- Rank peculiars according to their degree of peculiarity on a scale of 1 to 3.
- Rank the strength and intensity of each symptom on a scale of 1 to 3.
- Add up the points for each symptom; the higher the sum, the more important and characteristic the symptom.

THE LAW OF CURE

OBSTACLES TO HEALTH
Factors that can stand in the way of recovery
POOR LIVING CONDITIONS
BAD NUTRITION
DESTRUCTIVE PERSONAL RELATIONSHIPS
OVERWORK OR WORKAHOLISM
UNHEALTHY WORKING ENVIRONMENT
PREVIOUS DISEASE UNRESOLVED
A NEGATIVE ATTITUDE

WITH a view to aiding the assessment of a patient's progress, there are a few simple guidelines that can be followed; for cure to be taking place the disease should go from within to without, from organs of greater importance to lesser importance, from above to below and to disappear in the reverse order to their original appearance. The last is probably the most important since it has been observed time and again that, during constitutional treatment, old symptoms reminiscent of previous states of health tend to recur, until a state of health can sometimes eventually be achieved where the only illnesses experienced are those common to childhood, such as coughs, colds, sore throats, and skin rashes.

There may also be external factors which adversely influence health (see left) and they must be considered when monitoring the patient's progress.

Selecting the remedy

To select a remedy that matches the symptoms you have noted, turn to the section of the book called *The Remedy Pictures* (pages 136 to 237), which is arranged in the form of charts. The main area or areas of complaint will indicate the first charts you should consult. Look along the sections of the tables and match the main features of the case with the features of the remedies. The remedy picture may include a lot of other symptoms that are not in the case itself. Do not worry about this so long as all or most of the important symptoms of the case are in the remedy. Construct a list of matching remedies.

Podophyllum peltatum the source for the* Podophyllum *remedy.

You may find that reference to more than one set of charts will help you. For instance, someone with a sore throat may well also have a fever and you will get a fuller picture by looking at the remedies in both sections.

If you find that none is a good match then you are probably including too much detail and are not selecting the most important features. Go back to the case and review critically the main characteristic symptoms, eliminating those that are not strong, are vague, have perhaps only occurred once or twice and are not really important features of the illness. Use the points system (see page 127) to help you.

If you find six or more remedies are matching, then you have probably included too many common symptoms, those that are characteristic of the disease in general in everyone and not the disease in the individual. Review the case looking for the more individual features. Ideally you should end up with less than six and probably more than one or two remedies to consider in greater detail.

Only add those things of which you are quite sure. If there is a doubt, pencil in the remedy and wait for confirmation from your own experience.

Refining your choice

The second stage in the selection process is to refine the match. Is there a remedy picture which most closely resembles the important features of the case? Do many or most of the important symptoms of the remedy (which appear in bold type) match the strongest symptoms of the case? Are the more minor symptoms of the case to be found in

TWO APPROACHES TO SELECTION

SELECTING a remedy is part science, part art. Commonly, it begins as a scientific process in which all the different features of the case are evaluated and carefully compared with the most likely remedies. This is the logical, step-by-step, scientific approach. The artistic approach involves a more intuitive, creative way of thinking, and comes from experience. This is also a valid way and can produce better results than the scientific method. However, it does require a certain knowledge of the remedies. Commonly the prescriber will be familiar with the remedies and will 'just know' the remedy as the case is taken, or may only need to look up one or two symptoms to confirm the remedy.

The process of evaluating and matching remedy pictures as a whole, which takes place in this more intuitive process, might be compared to the difference between a mathematician and a child when presented with a simple sum: the child works it out on his or her fingers, whereas the mathematician will look at it and simply know the answer.

This process must not be confused with guessing or wishful thinking. It is very different and, as you can see, must be based on some knowledge or understanding. As this knowledge of the remedies grows in you, do not be surprised if you sometimes 'just know' which is the right remedy and know it without any doubts. Sometimes there is something about the 'image' of a remedy which just seems to fit the patient. Have a good look at that remedy and see if your intuitive feelings can be justified.

Mercury, the source for the* Mercurius *family of remedies.* Mercurius vivus *and* Mercurius solubilis *are the most used.

TREATING WHOLE PERSON

Homeopathy looks at the person as a whole. It is important to note all the symptoms wherever they appear. They all influence the final choice of remedy.

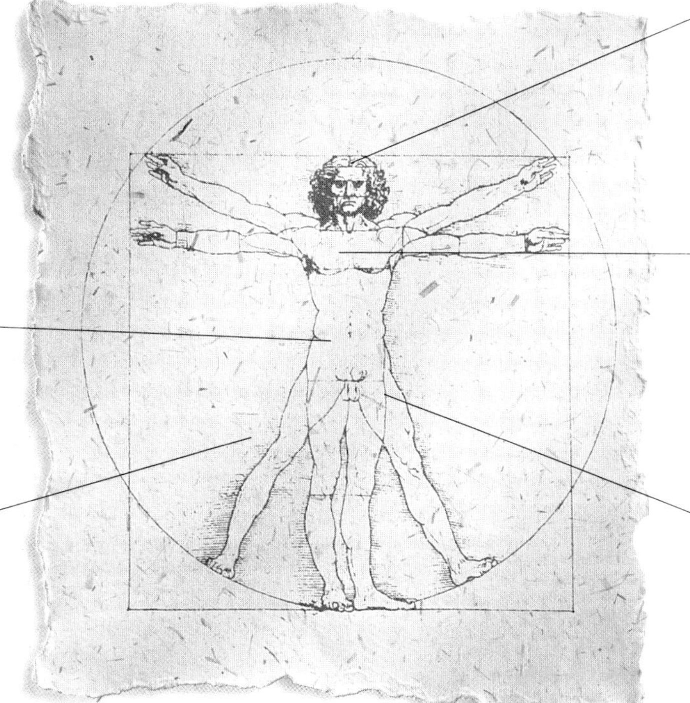

Headache with stiff neck, dizzy when looking down: **Spigelia** *a possible remedy.*

Cold spreads rapidly to chest: **Ipecacuanha** *a possible remedy.*

Violent, clutching, cramping pains after overeating: **Colocynthis** *a possible remedy.*

Icy cold blood seems to flow in the veins during a stuffy cold: **Arsenicum** *a possible remedy.*

Great weight and tiredness of body and limbs with a sore throat: **Gelsemium** *a possible remedy.*

the remedy? This is less important but may confirm your choice or help to differentiate between two equally close remedies. Read the whole case again, read all the symptoms of the remedy and refer to the *Materia Medica* (pages 36 to 117) for the final comparison.

When comparing the symptoms of the case and the remedy, you should make sure that the most important symptoms do not clash or contradict. For example, Belladonna has a rapid, vigorous and violent fever coming on quickly. If the patient's fever took several days to appear then the remedy is unlikely to be *Belladonna* no matter how much the rest of the picture looks like it. You will also find that some remedies have opposite symptoms, for example Belladonna may be thirstless or thirsty in its fever.

A warning should be issued here. You hardly ever find all the symptoms of the case in a remedy picture and you will never find all the symptoms of a remedy in the disease picture of the case, so do not look for them or try to fit them all in. It is much more important to look out for those strong, peculiar, characteristic symptoms and any mental or general or concomitant symptoms and let those be your guide.

However you work in selecting a remedy, find the way that suits you and gives you results as shown by a good response to its administration. The accuracy of your selection can only be proved by giving the remedy and seeing the patient getting better. In this sense, every homeopathic prescription is an experiment, even those of the most experienced professional.

Do not try more than four or six different remedies without success before seeking more expert homeopathic advice. Obviously, this will vary with the circumstances of each case and the experience of the prescriber. This is not a guide as to when to call on expert medical advice, which should always be determined by the condition of the patient and carried out at whatever stage you would normally call upon such help. Homeopathic treatment should always be an addition to whatever advice you would normally seek, never a substitute for it.

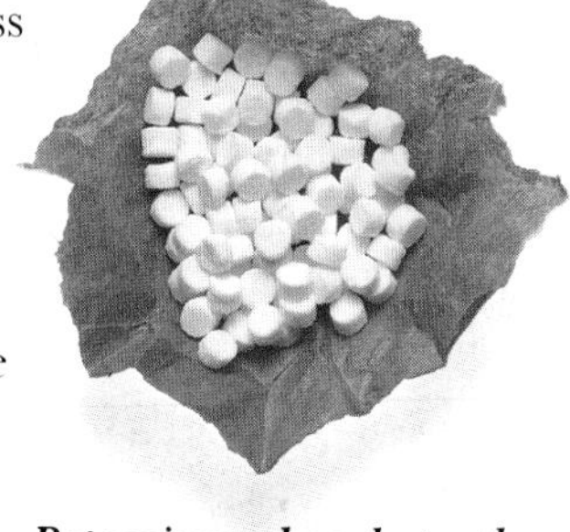

Potassium phosphate, the source for the tissue salt remedy, **Kali phosphoricum remedy.**

Giving the remedy

Once you have chosen a remedy, you must give it, but first I would like to offer a little reassurance to novice prescribers who may be nervous.

What if it is the wrong remedy? In treating acute illnesses there are only two outcomes to giving the wrong low-potency remedy. Firstly, there may be a partial response which does not last long, and secondly, there may be no response at all. In order to bring about a deterioration in the patient's condition with low-potency remedies, one would have to keep on repeating the wrong remedy many times and even then it is unlikely that much would happen unless the patient were particularly frail and weak, in which case they should be having constitutional treatment to boost their overall state and not 'first aid' treatment for the little bits that go wrong. Someone who has much chronic ill-health should not be treated except by an experienced practitioner. Nevertheless, it is very difficult to do any harm with 'first aid' homeopathy using low-potency remedies. They are very safe.

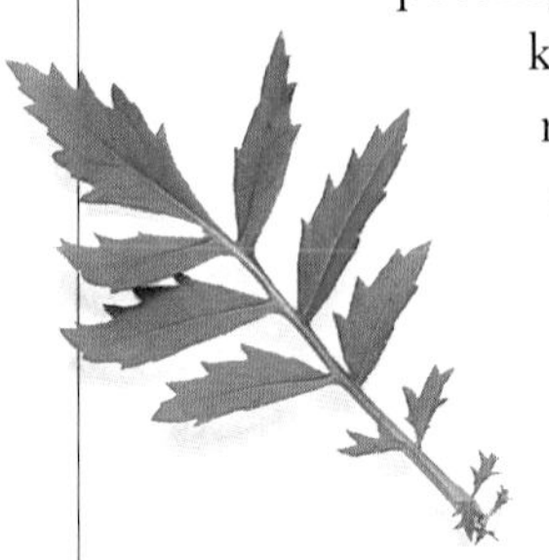

Marigold leaves, part of the source for the **Calendula** *remedy.*

Even if a child took a whole bottle full of remedies, it would not be harmed. This is because in homeopathy the important factor is the frequency of repetition of the remedy and not the quantity given.

SUCCEEDING WITH CHILDREN

When treating illness in children there are two very good signs that you have hit on the correct remedy: firstly, if the child vomits shortly after having the remedy, assuming he was not already vomiting all the time! You should not worry if part of the pill comes out as well, just wait and watch the child's condition.

The second is if the child goes off to sleep. Do not disturb unless there are other indications that the child is not sleeping a peaceful, healing sleep.

SAFETY MEASURES

The pills themselves, if stored tightly capped, out of the sun, and away from strong smells, can be kept for years without loss of potency. Keep them in their original containers and if you need to transfer them, make sure they go into a new, labelled bottle or clean paper envelope. **Only open one remedy bottle at a time.** Never re-use old remedy bottles or envelopes for a different remedy or potency.

Although they are much safer than allopathic or conventional drugs, it is obviously advisable to store them out of children's reach.

No more than one pill at a time is needed and the effect is not stronger by giving a full bottle. With homeopathy, the quantity does not matter, it is the quality that is important.

During pregnancy, low-potency remedies can be taken for acute illnesses without risk to mother or child.

Which potency?

The more a remedy is potentized, the quicker and deeper its action. It also becomes more specific and for the higher potencies the remedy selection has to be more accurate for the remedy to work.

Low potencies are usually regarded as being those up to and including the 30c or 30x. The letters 'c' and 'x' refer to the dilution factor used in

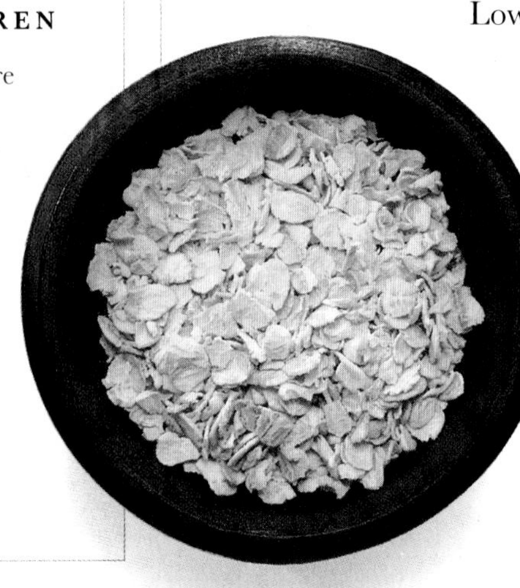

Grain cereal, the source for magnesium phosphate, itself the source for the **Magnesia phosphorica** *remedy.*

the preparation of the remedy and it need not concern us here, as to all practical intents and purposes, for home prescribing the difference is negligible. Commonly, one can readily obtain the following potencies; 6x, 6c, 12x, 12c, 30x and 30c. The higher the number the greater the potency of the remedy.

For the conditions described in this book it is the selection of the remedy that is of far greater importance than the specific potency used. As a general rule, if the sick person requires a remedy and you only have it available in one potency then that is the correct potency no matter what it is!

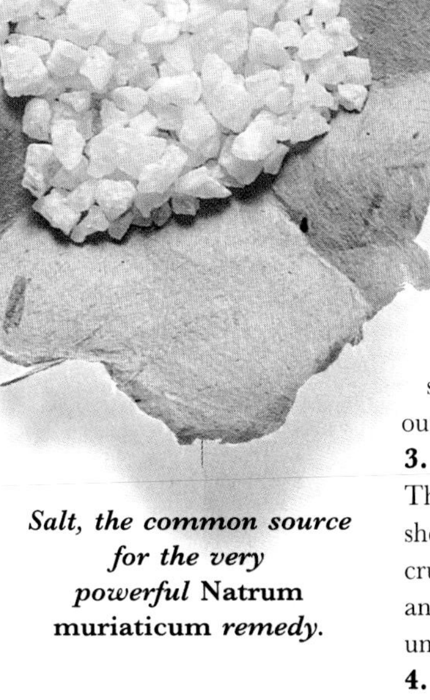

Salt, the common source for the very powerful* Natrum muriaticum *remedy.

If you are going to stock your medicine cupboard with only one potency of each remedy, my personal choice would be 12x or 12c. This will go a little further than a 6c but is not quite so specific as a 30c. If you have built up some experience using the remedies, then you will find the 30c an excellent potency for acute illness. If you are new to homeopathy and do not intend to follow case-taking and evaluation guidelines as given in this chapter, then a set of 6x remedies will serve you best.

In the vast majority of cases the 6th potency will work just as well as the 30th and does not require such accuracy.

One point that may help you is that the lower the potency the more frequently it is likely to need repeating.

Remedies should be kept in dark glass bottles and phials to protect them from sunlight.

TAKING THE MEDICINE

THE REMEDY may come as a liquid potency, when the dose is one drop, as granules, when the dose is 10 or 20 grains (like sugar strands or the 'hundreds and thousands' used to decorate cakes) or, most commonly, as tablets, when the dose is one tablet.

1. Do not touch the pills. The patient himself may pick one up with clean hands, but no one else. You may also use a clean spoon or piece of paper.
2. Do not return pills to the stock bottle if accidentally tipped out. Discard them.
3. Suck the pill under the tongue. They are made from sugar and should easily dissolve. If it is slow, crush it with the teeth and then suck the pieces under the tongue.
4. Ideally the mouth should be clean with no flavors, food or drink for 10 or 15 minutes before or after taking the pill.
5. While receiving homeopathic treatment, patients should avoid anything with a strong smell, scent, aroma or perfumes: no aromatic oils, vapor rubs, smelly nasal decongestants such as menthol or eucalyptus. Some homeopaths will also advise you to avoid coffee and toothpaste; others will not.
6. Children can either take remedies as a powder, by crushing the pill between two clean teaspoons, or dissolved in a little clean, fresh water in a glass.

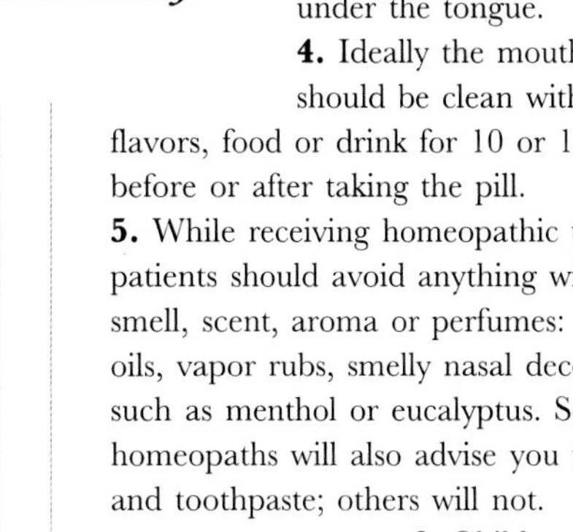

Results and reactions

Once you have administered the first dose, the homeopathic rule is not to repeat or change the remedy until the action of the previous dose has ceased. The four most common reactions to a remedy are listed in the panel on page 133.

What happens next

The patient may improve after each dose and gradually needs the remedy less frequently until they are better.

He or she may get better after each dose but requires it more and more frequently in order to sustain the benefit. This may well indicate the need for the next higher potency of that same remedy. If you don't have one then try plussing (see page 133). If this fails, then review the case and see if there have been any changes or if new information has come to light that would enable you to select a remedy which could carry on the work of the first remedy.

The patient may improve at first but is now slipping back and a different set of symptoms has appeared. Your first prescription was right but a new remedy is now needed. Base your selection on the new symptoms.

After initial improvement there is no response to the remedy and the same symptoms are still present. This probably means that the remedy was close but not quite close enough to give any sustained relief. Reassess the case and choose another remedy in a higher potency. If there has really been no response, wait for a time depending on the vigour and severity of the illness. If no changes occur then repeat the same remedy and wait again. Do this once or twice more before giving up on that remedy. If there is no response after three or four pills then either the prescription is wrong or the remedy is no good and has lost its potency. If you have some experience and were expecting the remedy to work, then mark on the bottle. If you find next time you need that remedy that it does not work, put another mark on the bottle and give it one more chance before discarding the whole batch.

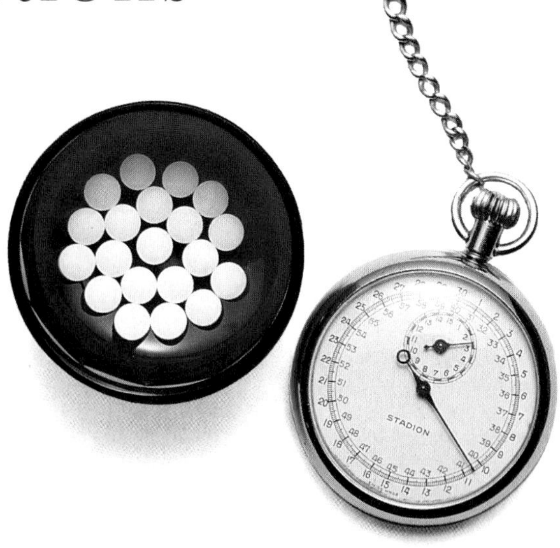

Remedy dosage should be carefully timed, especially at the beginning of the course.

Often changes in the patient's state are marked and obvious, and there is no doubt about what to do. Sometimes when the changes are slower it can be more difficult because allowance has to be made for the natural variations that occur hour by hour in an illness, even without any treatment. Here it is important to remember that vigorous, severe illnesses respond to remedies in a vigorous way. They also tend to 'use up' remedies quickly which may need repeating several times an hour at first but always according to the changes in the symptom picture. Cases of this severity are likely to be the ones which would lead you to seek expert medical advice from your local health care practitioner. While you are waiting for the expert help to arrive, there is no reason why you should not take the person's case and find a remedy for him. Very often the more severe and acute the illness, the clearer the disease pic-

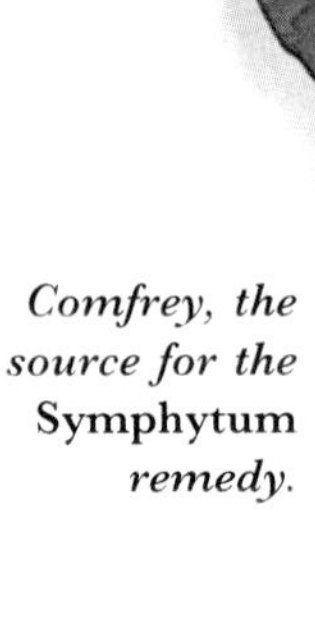

Comfrey, the source for the **Symphytum** *remedy.*

FOUR COMMON REACTIONS

1. The patient gets better. Do not repeat the remedy whilst improvement is still occurring. Nothing more to be done!
2. The symptoms get slightly worse straight after the remedy is given. This is a common reaction to the effect of the remedy and you should wait and expect to see an improvement over the next few minutes or hour or so depending on how severe the illness is. The more vigorous and acute the illness is the quicker things change. So in a lingering, slow fever you might wait several hours for a response to a remedy, whereas in a delirious, high, raging fever you would expect to see changes within 10 or 15 minutes.
3. The patient improves for a time, say an hour or more, then either stops getting better and the picture becomes more or less static, or begins to slip back again with the same symptoms. Your prescription has worked and now is the time to repeat the same remedy.
4. No effect. Often the first change is that the patient begins to feel better in themself but still has all the symptoms. This is a very important sign of a good response and must not be overlooked. You should wait and look for other improvements to follow.

ture so that the similar remedy may actually be easier to select. If the picture is clear, give the remedy. If you follow the guidelines given here, it can only help and certainly will not harm.

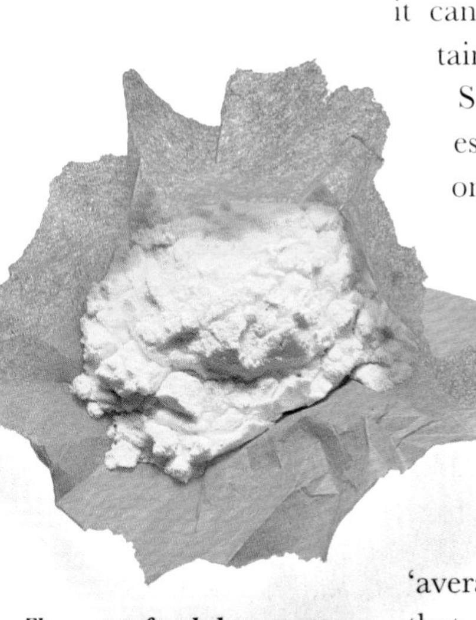

Flowers of sulphur, part of the source of the **Hepar sulphuris calcareum** *remedy.*

Slow lingering illnesses may require only one remedy a day or less. The patient will tell you by their symptoms what needs to be done, when to wait and when to treat.

As a rough guide the 'average' illness, the kind that will put a person in bed, is likely to need a remedy between three and eight times a day, needing more at the beginning of the illness than later on. A less severe cough, cold, throat or stomach upset etc. may need a dose two or three times a day. It is imperative that you let the patient tell you, through their symptoms, what needs to be done. The less rigid and routine your prescribing, the better the result will be.

One further thing that will help you to be a successful prescriber is to enjoy yourself. Homeopathy can be very satisfying if you do not get weighed down by the 'burden' of finding a remedy. Keep it light and sometimes when things are not as clear as you would like them to be, just trust and give the remedy you judge to be nearest. Homeopathy is very safe and forgiving especially to honest beginners. Even a prescription of the wrong remedy can sometimes affect the picture of symptoms so as to make the right remedy more obvious and easily discerned.

Dried eyebright, the source for the **Euphrasia officinalis** *remedy.*

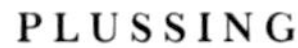

PLUSSING

In a very acute illness the remedy may need to be repeated every hour or two at first until sustained improvement sets in. In this situation, it is often worth dissolving two or three tablets, or their equivalent, in a clean glass of fresh water and taking a teaspoonful when needed. Between doses the water is best agitated by lifting a spoonful up in the air and allowing it to splash back in the glass 10 or 20 times. This is called plussing and it slightly alters the potency of the remedy in the glass which helps to maintain its effectiveness.

Remedies and pharmacies

> *....recognize the spirit-like force, which, hidden in the intimate essence of the medicines, gives them the power to change the way people feel and thereby cure disease.*
>
> SAMUEL HAHNEMANN

How can you be sure of the quality of the remedies on sale? When buying remedies there are several things to look for which will indicate a high quality product. Ask your local or usual supplier.

How are the remedies themselves actually prepared? Are they successed by hand or by machine? Succussion is part of the process of potentizing a remedy which involves vigorous shaking (succussion) and a series of dilutions. The most important change in this process is not the material one of dilution but is concerned with the change in energy, vital force, *ch'i*, consciousness or whatever you may be used to calling it. At any rate, practical experience teaches that the most 'potent' remedies are prepared by hand. Those prepared by mechanical succussion tend to be less effective. This is, therefore, the single most important question to ask.

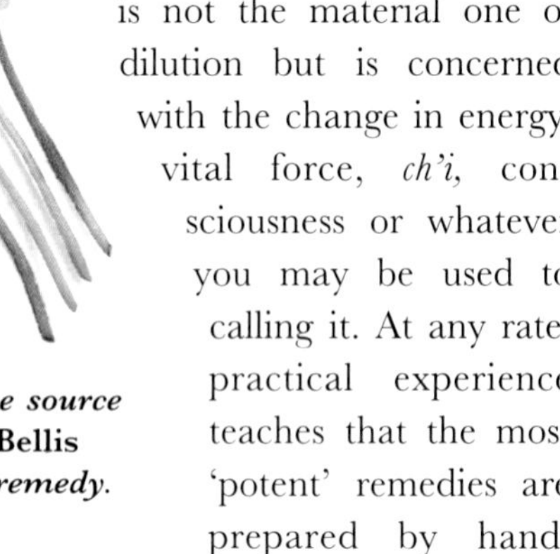

Daisies, the source for the* Bellis perennis *remedy.

What are the circumstances in which the remedies are prepared? Are they prepared quietly, calmly, methodically by someone paying attention to what they are doing? The greater the attention and awareness of the preparer, the more active the end product.

What safeguards are taken to ensure that one remedy does not, by its dust or vapor, contaminate another remedy during the preparation process?

Are the raw ingredients of the highest quality? For instance, with remedies prepared from plants, are the plants picked at the best time of the year, the best time of the day and in the best weather conditions to produce a high-quality plant tincture from which to prepare the remedy? All the specific conditions for growing, picking and preparing remedies are described precisely in the various homeopathic pharmacopeia used by the pharmacist.

Homeopathic tablets are made from milk sugar infused with the potentized remedy.

How much care is taken to ensure that the remedies are not handled?

Are they stored away from direct sunlight (which inactivates remedies) and preferably in secure, glass bottles?

It is not always the largest manufacturers who take the greatest care in preparing potentized remedies. Some do, but often you will find that remedies prepared by small homeopathic pharmacies are much more potent.

Which remedies do I need?

This is really an impossible one to answer because each person's health demands are different. However, the most basic kit should contain at least 24 remedies in one potency. This may be thought by some beginners to be too many to start with, so 12 of the most commonly required remedies have been suggested as a starter kit. More

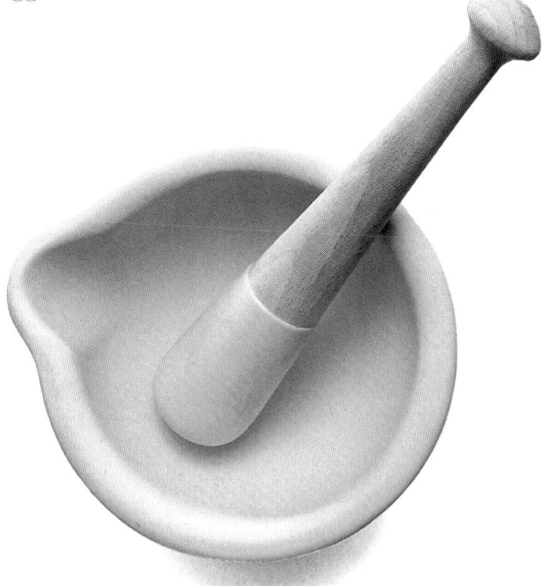

Insoluble remedy sources are ground up in a mortar before potentization.

comprehensive kits containing a further 24 remedies each time, are also suggested up to a total of 72. On the assumption that you already possess the basic 24 remedies, a few additional remedies are suggested to meet specific needs. Most of the additional remedies are amongst the total of 72. The question of potency is dealt with in the sections on pages 32 to 33 and 130 to 131. The 12c potency was recommended but the suitable range is from a 6x to a 30c.

These are suggestions to help the beginner get started. You may find that your family, or whoever you treat, will tend to have more of one type of illness than another and you will probably need to customize your remedy kit with remedies particularly suited to that type of condition. Be flexible in your approach and confident in your ability to choose what is specific to you and your families' needs. Buy only what you think you will need and use.

A HOME PHARMACY

REMEDY KITS

Starter kit of 12 remedies: *Aconite, Apis, Arnica, Belladonna, Bryonia, Chamomilla, Ferrum phosphoricum, Gelsemium, Ipecacuanha, Pulsatilla, Rhus toxicodendron, Sulphur.*

A useful addition to the kit would be some *Calendula* ointment or tincture, which can be diluted in water 1 part in 25 to bathe, clean, and dress cuts, scrapes, wounds, burns, ulcers etc.

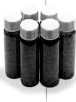

Basic kit (includes all the remedies in the starter kit and 12 more): *Aconite, Allium cepa, Apis, Arnica, Arsenicum, Belladonna, Bryonia, Chamomilla, Colocynthis, Dioscorea, Euphrasia, Ferrum phosphoricum, Gelsemium, Hepar sulphuris, Hypericum, Ipecacuanha, Ledum, Lycopodium, Magnesia phosphorica, Mercurius, Nux vomica, Pulsatilla, Rhus toxicodendron, Sulphur.*

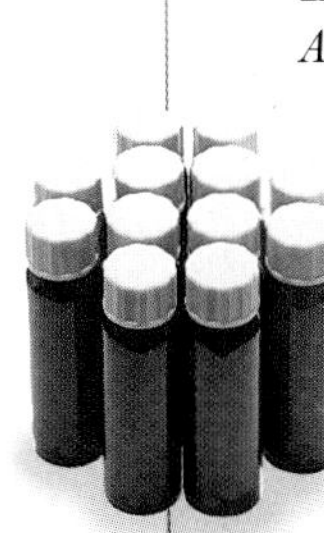
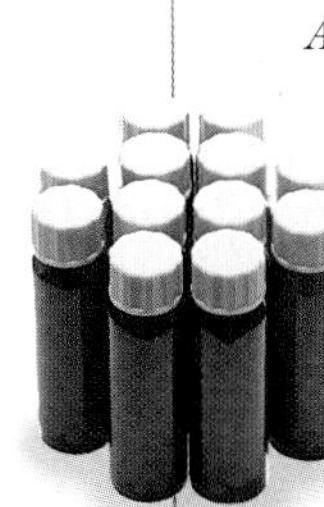

Intermediate kit (additional 24 remedies): *Antimonium tartaricum, Argentum nitricum, Bellis perennis, Calcarea carbonica, Causticum, Drosera, Dulcamara, Eupatorium perfoliatum, Jaborandi, Kali bichromicum, Lac caninum, Lachesis, Natrum muriaticum, Nitricum acidum, Phosphorus, Phytolacca, Podophyllum, Pyrogen, Ruta, Sanguinaria, Silica, Spigelia, Spongia, Urtica urens.*

Comprehensive kit (final 24 remedies): *Antimonium crudum, Baptisia, Calcarea phosphorica, Camphora, Carbo vegetabilis, Cantharis, Cinchona officinalis, Cocculus, Coffea, Cuprum, Glonoin, Hyoscyamus, Ignatia, Iris, Kali carbonicum, Kreosotum, Mercurius cyanatus, Natrum sulphuricum, Petroleum, Rumex, Staphysagria, Sepia, Symphytum, Tabacum, Veratrum album.*

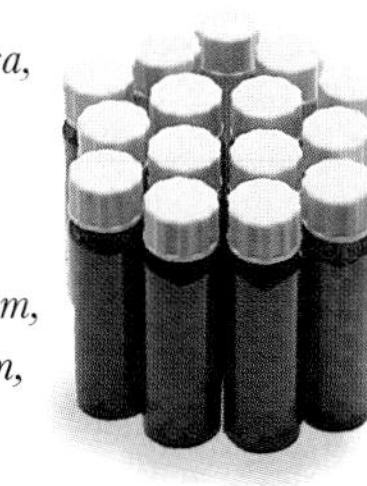

SPECIAL ADDITIONS

Measles, mumps and chicken pox: *Antimonium tartaricum, Camphora, Carbo vegetabilis, Jaborandi, Kali bichromicum, Phytolacca.*
Travel sickness: *Cocculus, Petroleum, Sepia, Staphysagria, Tabacum.*
First aid: *Bellis perennis, Calcarea phosphorica, Cantharis, Causticum, Cuprum, Eupatorium perfoliatum, Glonoin, Lachesis, Natrum muriaticum, Phosphorus, Silica, Staphysagria, Symphytum, Urtica urens.*
Diarrhea and vomiting: *Antimonium crudum, Antimonium tartaricum, Carbo vegetabilis, Cinchona officinalis, Dulcamara, Natrum sulphuricum, Phosphorus, Podophyllum, Sepia, Veratrum album.*
Cystitis: *Cantharis, Causticum, Kali muriaticum, Kali phosphoricum, Natrum muriaticum, Sarsaparilla, Staphysagria.*
Period pains: *Calcarea fluorica, Calcarea phosphorica, Cocculus, Conium, Kali phosphoricum, Lachesis, Sepia.*

REMEDIES FOR MOTHER AND BABY

Giving birth: *Aconite M, Arnica 200, Bellis perennis M, Caulophyllum 10M, Ipecacuanha 200, Kali phosphoricum 12x, Pulsatilla 200.*
Breast feeding: *Castor equi 3x, Hydrastis 6x or 12x, Phytolacca 6x or 12x.*
Mastitis: *Belladonna,* Bryonia,* Hepar sulphuris,* Mercurius,* Phytolacca.*
Milk supply: *Calcarea carbonica, Lac defloratum, Pulsatilla*.*
After pains: *Arnica,* Conium.*
Baby colic: *Chamomilla,* Colocynthis,* Dioscorea,* Magnesia phosphorica.**

(*in basic kit).

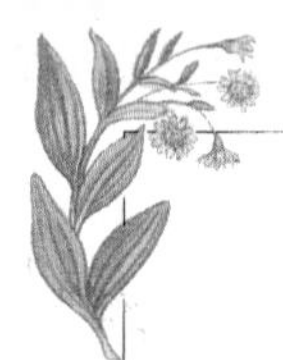

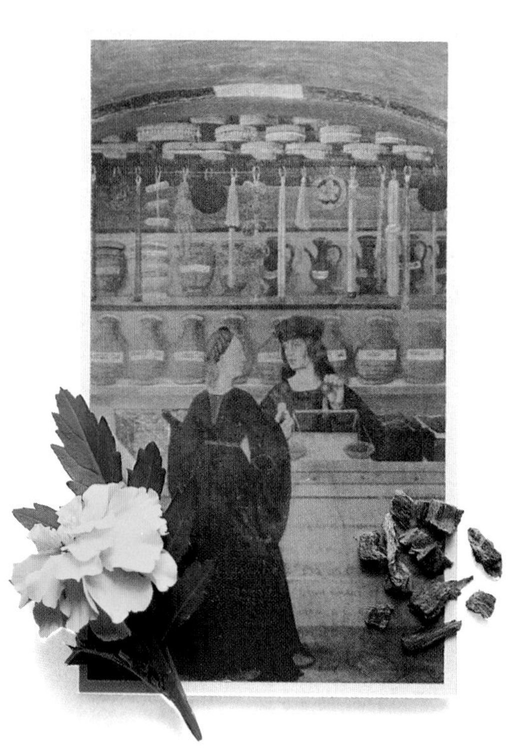

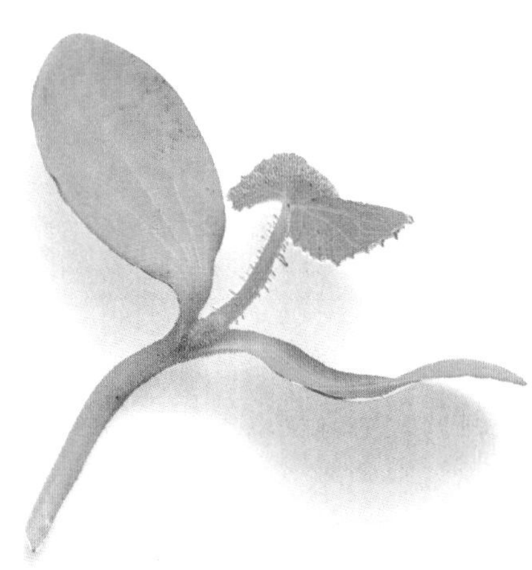

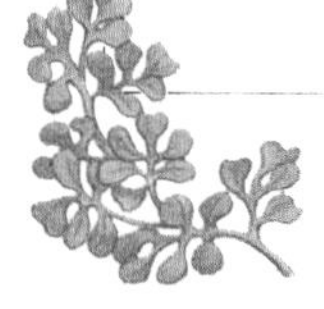

PART 4

THE REMEDY PICTURES

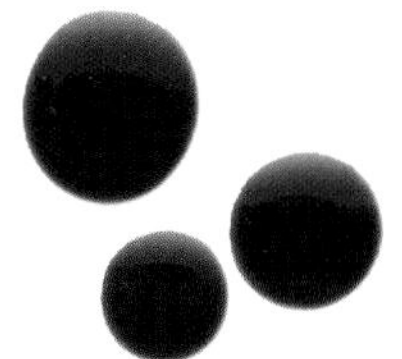

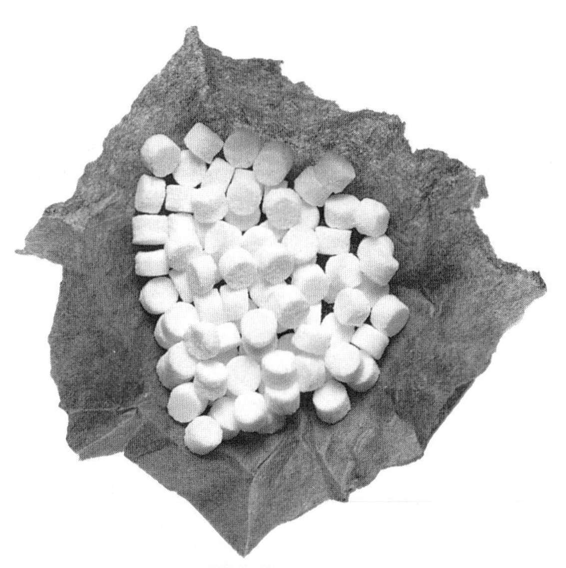

Looking at the remedy pictures

This section of the book is designed to help you find the remedies that match the case you have taken following the guidelines given in the Practical Homeopathy section. It is set out in the form of charts, one for each kind of complaint. Fevers are listed first as they affect the whole body, otherwise the charts are set out in accepted homeopathic order, from the head downwards; childrens' illnesses are grouped together at the end.

The way the charts are arranged will also help you take a case. Make enquiries into each of the sections covering the particular complaint. Under **cause** and **onset**, look at what has been happening in the preceding hours or days to the onset of the illness and consider the speed with which the illness came on and the order of events.

Next, ask for details of **sensations**, where they are situated, where they move to, how they start and change, find out what the pattern is but take care to use open-ended questions if possible, questions that cannot be answered by a simple 'yes' or 'no': ask, 'How does your head feel?' rather than, 'Do you have a headache?'

Be sure to ask about the **modalities** of the symptoms – these are the factors which make it better or worse. As can be seen from the tables, just about anything may affect a symptom. The stronger, more definite and consistent it is, the more important it will be as a symptom.

Concomitant symptoms are symptoms not directly related to, but arising at the same time as, the main complaint such as a headache with diarrhea or cold sores with a fever – things which are repeatedly associated, so that the patient might say, 'Whenever I get this problem I always get a stomach upset'.

Peculiar symptoms are any unusual bodily sensations, urges, fears or desires. They are often the key to the remedy that is needed, so take particular note of them.

Mentals and **generals** usually come last on the charts. They relate to the mood, behavior, speech pattern etc., of the patient. Characteristics of the patient when well that are still present when ill are not actually a part of the picture of the acute illness and are therefore not important when selecting a remedy for the acute disease. (This applies to any symptom, not just to mental conditions.) If someone who is normally very placid and kind became ill, say with an ear ache, and at the same time became uncharacteristically irritable and bad-tempered, then this would be a highly significant symptom. That patient would need a remedy capable of causing just such an irritability. Mental symptoms arising in this way are generally of the greatest importance when selecting the most similar remedy.

On each page of the chart, an explanatory panel tells you how to use the chart.

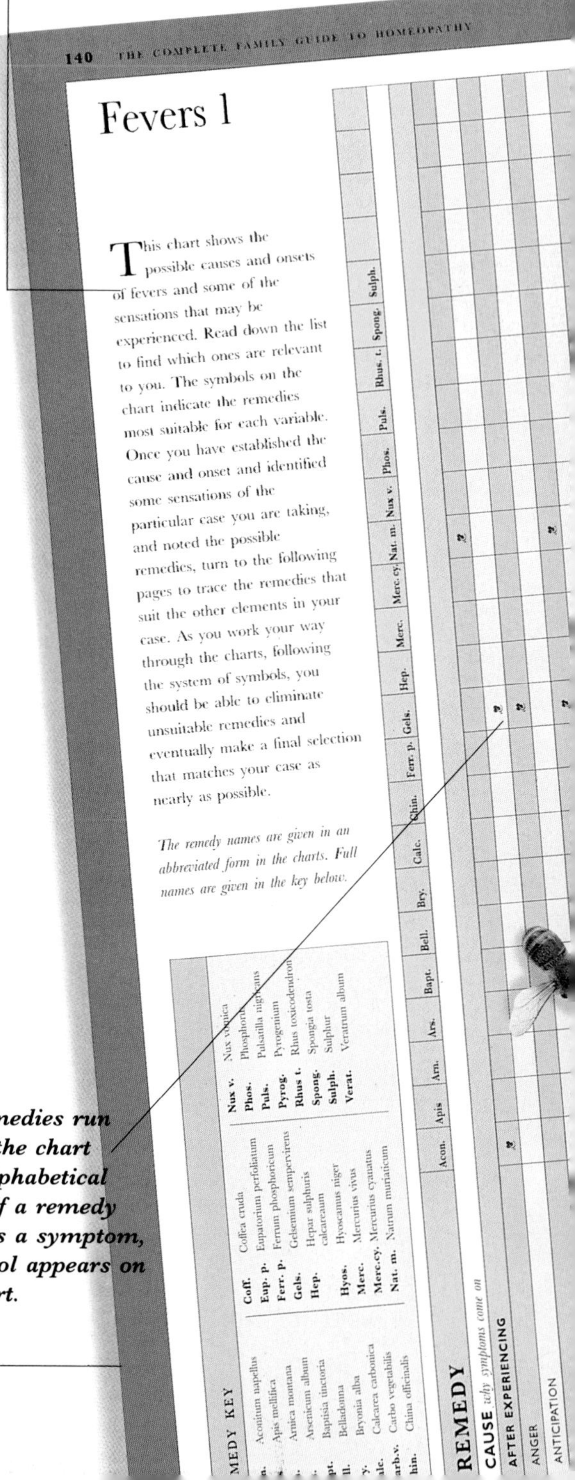

The remedies run across the chart in in alphabetical order. If a remedy matches a symptom, a symbol appears on the chart.

General symptoms can be preceded by the words 'I am', as in 'I am thirsty, hot, tired, lacking energy or burning all over'. The opposite of a general symptom is a particular symptom. This relates only to an isolated part of the person and is usually preceded by the word 'my', such as 'my head hurts, my throat is dry'.

Using this information, you should be able to discover which are the most significant symptoms in your case and choose a satisfactory remedy from the charts.

Find a symptom that matches your case, and look across the chart to see which remedy matches it.

Within the charts the symptoms are listed vertically under classic homeopathic categories: cause and onset, sensations, modalities, concomitants, peculiars and mentals and generals.

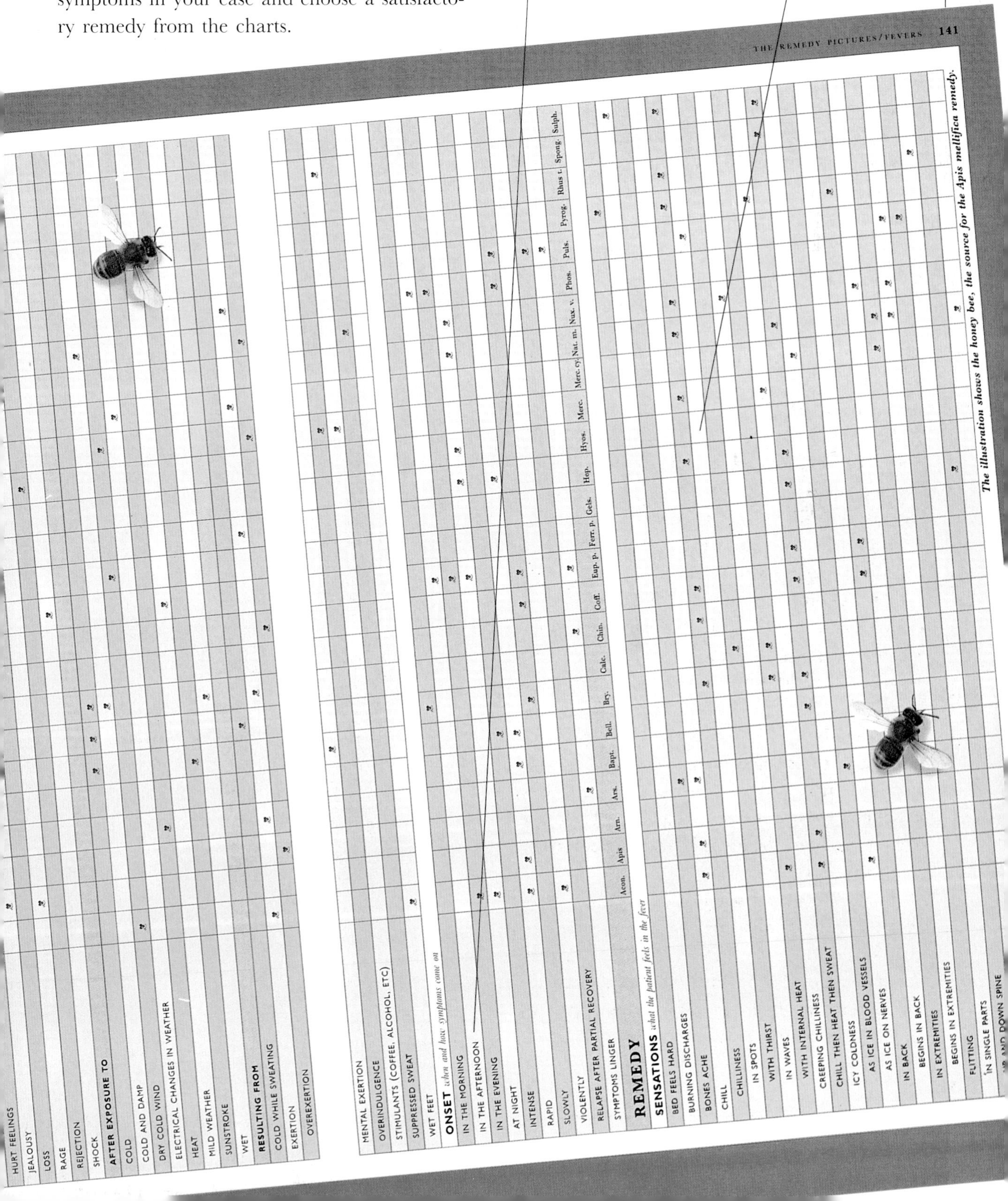

Fevers 1

The first part of this chart shows the **possible causes and onsets** of fevers and **some of the sensations** that may be experienced. Read down the list to find which ones are relevant to you. The symbols on the chart indicate the remedies most suitable for each variable. Once you have established the cause and onset and identified some sensations of the particular case you are taking, and noted the possible remedies, turn to the following pages to trace the remedies that suit the other elements in your case. As you work your way through the chart, following the system of symbols, you should be able to eliminate unsuitable remedies and eventually make a final selection that matches your case as nearly as possible.

The remedy names are given in an abbreviated form in the charts. Full names are given in the key below.

REMEDY KEY					
Acon.	Aconitum napellus	**Coff.**	Coffea cruda	**Nux v.**	Nux vomica
Apis	Apis mellifica	**Eup. p.**	Eupatorium perfoliatum	**Phos.**	Phosphorus
Arn.	Arnica montana	**Ferr. p.**	Ferrum phosphoricum	**Puls.**	Pulsatilla nigricans
Ars.	Arsenicum album	**Gels.**	Gelsemium sempervirens	**Pyrog.**	Pyrogenium
Bapt.	Baptisia tinctoria	**Hep.**	Hepar sulphuris calcareaum	**Rhus t.**	Rhus toxicodendron
Bell.	Belladonna	**Hyos.**	Hyoscamus niger	**Spong.**	Spongia tosta
Bry.	Bryonia alba	**Merc.**	Mercurius vivus	**Sulph.**	Sulphur
Calc.	Calcarea carbonica	**Merc.cy.**	Mercurius cyanatus	**Verat.**	Veratrum album
Carb.v.	Carbo vegetabilis	**Nat. m.**	Natrum muriaticum		
Chin.	China officinalis				

REMEDY	Acon.	Apis	Arn.	Ars.	Bapt.	Bell.	Bry.	Calc.	Chin.	Ferr. p.	Gels.	Hep.	Merc.	Merc. cy.	Nat. m.	Nux v.	Phos.	Puls.	Rhus. t.	Spong.	Sulph.
CAUSE *why symptoms come on*																					
AFTER EXPERIENCING																					
ANGER	●														●						
ANTICIPATION											●										
BAD NEWS											●										
DISAPPOINTMENT		●																			
EMOTION											●				●						
FEAR	●																				
FRIGHT	●	●									●										
GRIEF															●						
HURT FEELINGS							●														
JEALOUSY		●																			
LOSS															●						
RAGE		●																			
REJECTION															●						
SHOCK											●										
AFTER EXPOSURE TO																					
COLD						●	●	●													
COLD AND DAMP								●											●		
DRY COLD WIND	●											●				●					
ELECTRICAL CHANGES IN WEATHER																	●				
HEAT				●																	
MILD WEATHER											●										
SUNSTROKE						●															
WET								●													
RESULTING FROM																					
COLD WHILE SWEATING							●														
EXERTION	●			●				●					●				●			●	

REMEDY	Acon.	Apis	Arn.	Ars.	Bapt.	Bell.	Bry.	Calc.	Chin.	Coff.	Eup. p.	Ferr. p.	Gels.	Hep.	Hyos.	Merc.	Merc. cy.	Nat. m.	Nux. v.	Phos.	Puls.	Pyrog.	Rhus t.	Spong.	Sulph.
OVERINDULGENCE																●									
STIMULANTS (COFFEE, ALCOHOL, ETC)																●								●	
SUPPRESSED SWEAT																			●						
WET FEET	●																								
ONSET *when and how symptoms come on*																									
IN THE MORNING							●																		
IN THE AFTERNOON											●									●					
IN THE EVENING	●										●									●					
AT NIGHT	●										●			●	●			●	●						
INTENSE						●																			
RAPID	●	●			●	●								●											
SLOWLY							●			●	●									●	●				
VIOLENTLY	●																								
RELAPSE AFTER PARTIAL RECOVERY																					●				
SYMPTOMS LINGER				●					●		●										●				
SENSATIONS *what the patient feels in the fever*																									
BED FEELS HARD																						●			
BURNING DISCHARGES																									●
BONES ACHE				●																					
CHILL	●	●		●																					
CHILLINESS							●		●	●				●		●		●	●			●	●		●
IN SPOTS																					●				
WITH THIRST								●																	
IN WAVES																			●						
WITH INTERNAL HEAT	●						●	●																	
CHILLINESS (CREEPING)																●						●			
CHILL, THEN HEAT, THEN SWEAT	●	●				●	●			●	●		●	●				●						●	●
ICY COLDNESS																	●								
AS ICE IN BLOOD VESSELS				●																					
AS ICE ON NERVES	●																								
IN BACK										●	●											●			
BEGINS IN BACK																			●						
IN EXTREMITIES																	●	●							
BEGINS IN EXTREMITIES																		●	●		●				
FLITTING																					●				
IN SINGLE PARTS																							●		
UP AND DOWN SPINE													●												
TEETH CHATTER																		●							

The illustration shows the honey bee, the source for the Apis mellifica remedy.

Fevers 2

This part of the chart shows **further possible sensations** experienced in fevers. Read down the list to find which ones are relevant to you. The symbols on the chart indicate the remedies most suitable for each variable. Once you have identified the sensations experienced in the particular case you are taking, and noted the possible remedies, turn to the following pages to trace the remedies that suit the other elements in your case. As you work your way through the chart, following the system of symbols, you should be able to eliminate unsuitable remedies and eventually make a final selection that matches your case as nearly as possible.

The remedy names are given in an abbreviated form in the charts. Full names are given in the key below.

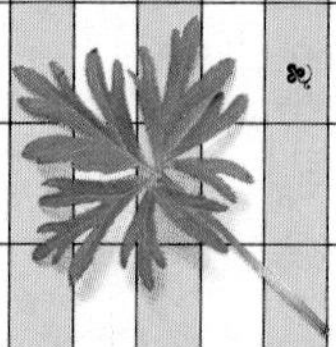

REMEDY KEY

Acon.	Aconitum napellus	**Coff.**	Coffea cruda	**Nux v.**	Nux vomica
Apis	Apis mellifica	**Eup. p.**	Eupatorium perfoliatum	**Phos.**	Phosphorus
Arn.	Arnica montana	**Ferr. p.**	Ferrum phosphoricum	**Puls.**	Pulsatilla nigricans
Ars.	Arsenicum album	**Gels.**	Gelsemium sempervirens	**Pyrog.**	Pyrogenium
Bapt.	Baptisia tinctoria	**Hep.**	Hepar sulphuris calcareum	**Rhus t.**	Rhus toxicodendron
Bell.	Belladonna			**Spong.**	Spongia tosta
Bry.	Bryonia alba	**Hyos.**	Hyoscyamus niger	**Sulph.**	Sulphur
Calc.	Calcarea carbonica	**Merc.**	Mercurius vivus	**Verat.**	Veratrum album
Carb.v.	Carbo vegetabilis	**Merc.cy.**	Mercurius cyanatus		
Chin.	China officinalis	**Nat. m.**	Natrum muriaticum		

REMEDY	Acon.	Apis	Arn.	Ars.	Bapt.	Bell.	Bry.	Calc.	Chin.	Coff.	Eup. p.	Ferr. p.	Gels.	Hep.	Hyos.	Merc.	Merc. cy.	Nat. m.	Nux. v.	Phos.	Puls.	Pyrog.	Rhus t.	Spong.	Sulph.
SENSATIONS (CONTINUED)																									
CHILL (CONTINUED)																									
WORSE FOR COLD DRINKS								•											•						
MOTION		•																	•						
UNCOVERING	•	•	•					•		•													•		
SLIGHTEST UNCOVERING														•					•				•		
NOT BETTER WARM WRAPPING																		•							
7-9AM											•														
10-11AM																		•							
4PM												•									•				
EVENING AND NIGHT										•						•									
DEBILITY									•																
DELIRIUM				•			•			•				•	•				•				•		
DRYNESS	•																							•	
DRYNESS OF MUCOUS MEMBRANES																								•	
FEVER														•											
ALTERNATES SHIVERING				•				•								•									
CONTINUED		•	•	•			•	•					•	•	•	•				•	•		•		•
HIGH					•		•															•	•		
RELAPSING																									•
VERY HIGH						•									•										
HEAT																									
BETTER FOR HEAT				•																					
BURNING	•	•		•		•	•						•	•	•						•			•	
BURNING ALL OVER											•														
BURNING WITH SLEEPLESSNESS															•										
BURNING (INTENSE)																							•		
BURNING IN BLOOD VESSELS				•			•	•							•		•								

EXTERNAL HEAT										•															
FLASHES OF HEAT																•									•
HEAT THEN CHILL																•									
HEAT AND CHILL ALTERNATE								•							•						•				
HOT DRY SKIN		•																							
ALTERNATES WITH SWEAT		•																			•				
HOT TO TOUCH						•					•														
INTENSE AND CONGESTIVE																		•							
INTENSE		•	•			•				•				•				•		•					
INTERNAL							•	•															•		•
NIGHT										•											•				
RUNNING UP BACK																				•					
HUNGER 11AM																									•
JERKINGS															•										
MENTAL SYMPTOMS																									
ALERT	•											•								•					
DAZED													•												
DELIRIOUS																				•					
DULL WHEN TIRED												•													
FRIGHTENED	•																								
LABORIOUS DREAMS																							•		
MUTTERING																							•		
TALKS AS IF DELIRIOUS													•												
MOUTH DRY							•											•			•				
MOUTH FOUL																•					•				
MOUTH HAS METALLIC TASTE																•									
MOUTH HAS SWEET TASTE																•									
NUMBNESS	•	•				•						•	•												
PAINS																									
BURNING				•																•					•
FLIT ABOUT							•														•				
RAWNESS																	•								
SEVERE						•																			
SORE AND BRUISED																						•	•		
SORENESS																	•								
SPLINTER LIKE														•											
STINGING		•																							
THROBBING						•																			
VIOLENT, PULSATING																						•			

The illustration shows monk's hood, the source for the Aconitum napellus remedy.

Fevers 3

This part of the chart shows **further possible sensations** experienced in fevers and some of the **modalities** that may make the patient feel better or worse. Read down the list to find which ones are relevant to you. The symbols on the chart indicate the remedies most suitable for each variable. Once you have established the sensations experienced and identified some of the modalities in the particular case you are taking, and noted the possible remedies, turn to the following pages to trace the remedies that suit the other elements in your case. As you work your way through the chart, following the system of symbols, you should be able to eliminate unsuitable remedies and eventually make a final selection that matches your case as nearly as possible.

The remedy names are given in an abbreviated form in the charts. Full names are given in the key below.

REMEDY KEY

Acon.	Aconitum napellus	**Coff.**	Coffea cruda	**Nux v.**	Nux vomica
Apis	Apis mellifica	**Eup. p.**	Eupatorium perfoliatum	**Phos.**	Phosphorus
Arn.	Arnica montana	**Ferr. p.**	Ferrum phosphoricum	**Puls.**	Pulsatilla nigricans
Ars.	Arsenicum album	**Gels.**	Gelsemium sempervirens	**Pyrog.**	Pyrogenium
Bapt.	Baptisia tinctoria	**Hep.**	Hepar sulphuris calcareum	**Rhus t.**	Rhus toxicodendron
Bell.	Belladonna			**Spong.**	Spongia tosta
Bry.	Bryonia alba	**Hyos.**	Hyoscamus niger	**Sulph.**	Sulphur
Calc.	Calcarea carbonica	**Merc.**	Mercurius vivus	**Verat.**	Veratrum album
Carb.v.	Carbo vegetabilis	**Merc.cy.**	Mercurius cyanatus		
Chin.	China officinalis	**Nat. m.**	Natrum muriaticum		

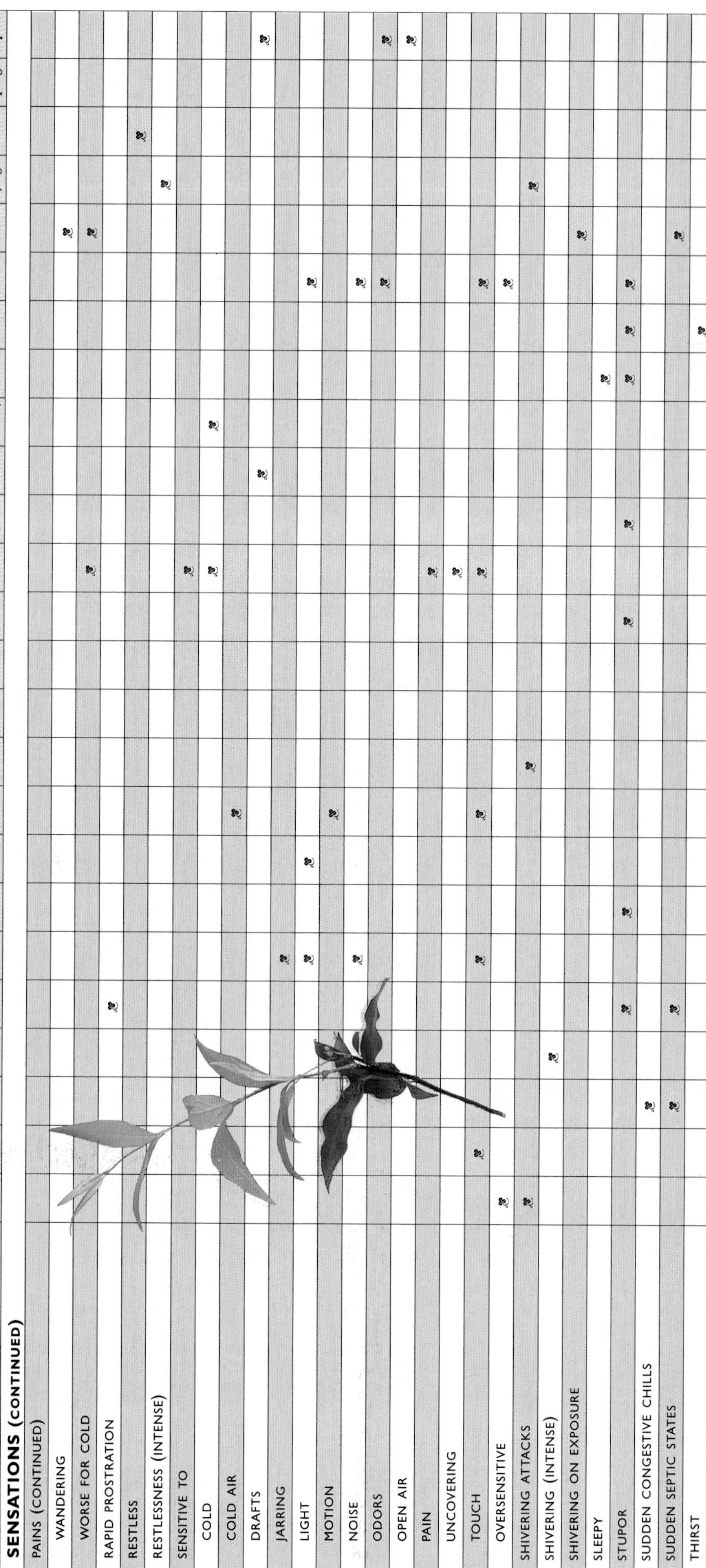

REMEDY	Acon.	Apis	Arn.	Ars.	Bapt.	Bell.	Bry.	Calc.	Chin.	Coff.	Eup. p.	Ferr. p.	Gels.	Hep.	Hyos.	Merc.	Merc. cy.	Nat. m.	Nux v.	Phos.	Puls.	Pyrog.	Rhus. t.	Spong.	Sulph.
SENSATIONS (CONTINUED)																									
PAINS (CONTINUED)																									
WANDERING																					•				
WORSE FOR COLD														•							•				
RAPID PROSTRATION					•																				
RESTLESS																							•		
RESTLESSNESS (INTENSE)																						•			
SENSITIVE TO														•											
COLD														•			•								
COLD AIR									•																
DRAFTS																•									•
JARRING						•																			
LIGHT						•		•												•					
MOTION									•																
NOISE						•														•					
ODORS																				•					•
OPEN AIR																									•
PAIN														•											
UNCOVERING														•											
TOUCH		•				•			•					•						•					
OVERSENSITIVE	•																			•					
SHIVERING ATTACKS	•									•												•			
SHIVERING (INTENSE)				•																					
SHIVERING ON EXPOSURE																					•				
SLEEPY																		•							
STUPOR					•		•						•		•			•	•	•					
SUDDEN CONGESTIVE CHILLS			•																						
SUDDEN SEPTIC STATES			•		•																•				
THIRST																			•						

EXTREME	❀																								
FEVER												❀													
FOR COLD DRINKS	❀	❀		❀			❀											❀		❀			❀		
HOT DRINKS DURING CHILL				❀							❀														
LARGE QUANTITIES							❀																		
LEMONADE						❀																			
MILK		❀																					❀		
SIPS				❀																					
WARM DRINKS																									❀
GREAT			❀			❀	❀													❀					
GREAT DURING CHILL ONLY			❀															❀							
GREAT DURING HEAT ONLY						❀																			
GREAT DURING SWEAT									❀																
HEAT BRINGS ON THIRST														❀						❀					
LITTLE THIRST													❀			❀									
LONG INTERVALS BETWEEN DRINKS							❀																		
THIRSTLESS		❀				❀							❀												
THIRSTLESS IN FEVER																					❀				
WORSE FOR DRINKING											❀														
THUMPING HEART																						❀			
TINGLING	❀	❀				❀																			
VOMITS WARM DRINKS																				❀					
MODALITIES *what makes the patient or symptoms better or worse*																									
WORSE																									
TIME																									
MORNING														❀					❀						
AFTERNOON													❀												
EVENING	❀						❀							❀			❀			❀	❀		❀		
NIGHT	❀			❀			❀		❀							❀					❀		❀		
DAYTIME																									❀
ALTERNATE DAYS									❀																
12AM																									❀
1-2AM				❀																					
10AM													❀												
10-11AM																		❀							
12PM	❀					❀																			❀
3PM						❀																			
3-5PM		❀																							
4PM																					❀				
9PM							❀																		

The illustration shows false jasmine, the source for the Gelsemium sempervirens remedy.

Fevers 4

This part of the chart shows **further possible modalities** in fevers that may make the patient feel better or worse. Read down the list to find which ones are relevant to you. The symbols on the chart indicate the remedies most suitable for each variable. Once you have identified more of the modalities in the particular case you are taking, and noted the possible remedies, turn to the following pages to trace the remedies that suit the other elements in your case. As you work your way through the chart, following the system of symbols, you should be able to eliminate unsuitable remedies and eventually make a final selection that matches your case as nearly as possible.

The remedy names are given in an abbreviated form in the charts. Full names are given in the key below.

REMEDY KEY					
Acon.	Aconitum napellus	**Coff.**	Coffea cruda	**Nux v.**	Nux vomica
Apis	Apis mellifica	**Eup. p.**	Eupatorium perfoliatum	**Phos.**	Phosphorus
Arn.	Arnica montana	**Ferr. p.**	Ferrum phosphoricum	**Puls.**	Pulsatilla nigricans
Ars.	Arsenicum album	**Gels.**	Gelsemium sempervirens	**Pyrog.**	Pyrogenium
Bapt.	Baptisia tinctoria	**Hep.**	Hepar sulphuris calcareum	**Rhus t.**	Rhus toxicodendron
Bell.	Belladonna	**Hyos.**	Hyoscamus niger	**Spong.**	Spongia tosta
Bry.	Bryonia alba	**Merc.**	Mercurius vivus	**Sulph.**	Sulphur
Calc.	Calcarea carbonica	**Merc.cy.**	Mercurius cyanatus	**Verat.**	Veratrum album
Carb.v.	Carbo vegetabilis	**Nat. m.**	Natrum muriaticum		
Chin.	China officinalis				

REMEDY	Acon.	Apis	Arn.	Ars.	Bapt.	Bell.	Bry.	Calc.	Chin.	Coff.	Eup. p.	Ferr. p.	Gels.	Hep.	Hyos.	Merc.	Merc. cy.	Nat. m.	Nux v.	Phos.	Puls.	Pyrog.	Rhus. t.	Spong.	Sulph.
MODALITIES (CONTINUED)																									
TEMPERATURE AND WEATHER																									
AIR (COLD)									●																
AIR (DRY, COLD OPEN)																			●						
AIR (OPEN)												●													
CHANGEABLE WEATHER																									●
CHILL																					●				
CLOSE ROOM																					●				
COLD						●		●				●		●		●							●		
COLD (EXCEPT HEAD)				●																					
DRAFTS				●		●										●									
HEAT	●	●					●									●					●				●
HEAT (IN FEVER)																		●							
SUN							●																		
WARM COVERS								●																	
MOVEMENT																									
BEGINNING TO MOVE																						●	●		
EXERTION				●				●				●		●											
OVEREXERTION																							●		
JARRING	●		●			●	●																		
MOTION			●	●		●	●		●		●			●					●						
RISING UP	●					●	●																		
STANDING												●													
GENERAL																									
COVERING	●																								
DAMP																							●		
EATING							●											●							
EVERYTHING																●									
FATTY RICH FOOD																					●				
LIGHT	●					●																			
LYING (COUGH)																					●				

LYING ON PAINFUL SIDE																			●						
LYING ON RIGHT SIDE																●									
MUSIC																		●							
NOISE						●	●					●						●	●						
PART HANG DOWN (LETTING)						●																			
PRESSURE		●												●											
REST																							●		
SLEEP (AFTER)		●																							
SOUR FOOD												●													
STIMULANTS																			●						
SWEATING (HEADACHE)											●														
TOUCH	●	●	●			●			●																
UNCOVERING				●		●										●			●						
VITAL FLUIDS (LOSS OF)									●																
WARM COVERING										●															
WASHING																									●
BETTER																									
AIR (OPEN)		●					●														●				●
IN BED															●										
COLD		●					●																		
COLD DRINKS																				●					
COLD FOOD																				●					
COMPANY				●																					
COOL																					●				
EVENING																			●						
HEAT														●									●		
HEAT (EXCEPT HEAD)				●																					
LYING DOWN						●										●									
LYING ON ABDOMEN						●																			
LYING ON PAINFUL SIDE																					●				
LYING PROPPED UP													●												
MOTION		●																							
MOTION (CONTINUED)																							●		
MOTION (GENTLE)												●									●				
PERSPIRING	●						●																		
PRESSURE																							●		
PRESSURE (FIRM)							●																		
RUBBING																				●			●		
SITTING (COUGH)																					●				
SITTING IN BED																			●						
SLEEP																			●	●					
STILL						●	●																		

The illustration shows deadly nightshade, the source for the Belladonna remedy.

Fevers 5

This part of the chart shows **further possible modalities** in fevers and **some concomitants** that may appear with the fever condition. Concomitants are listed in body order, that is from the head downwards. Read down the list to find which ones are relevant to you. The symbols on the chart indicate the remedies most suitable for each variable. Once you have identified the modalities and observed some of the concomitants in the particular case you are taking, and noted the possible remedies, turn to the following pages to trace the remedies that suit the other elements in your case. As you work your way through the chart, following the system of symbols, you should be able to eliminate unsuitable remedies and eventually make a final selection.

The remedy names are given in an abbreviated form in the charts. Full names are given in the key below.

REMEDY KEY

Acon.	Aconitum napellus	**Coff.**	Coffea cruda	**Nux v.**	Nux vomica
Apis	Apis mellifica	**Eup. p.**	Eupatorium perfoliatum	**Phos.**	Phosphorus
Arn.	Arnica montana	**Ferr. p.**	Ferrum phosphoricum	**Puls.**	Pulsatilla nigricans
Ars.	Arsenicum album	**Gels.**	Gelsemium sempervirens	**Pyrog.**	Pyrogenium
Bapt.	Baptisia tinctoria	**Hep.**	Hepar sulphuris calcareum	**Rhus t.**	Rhus toxicodendron
Bell.	Belladonna	**Hyos.**	Hyoscamus niger	**Spong.**	Spongia tosta
Bry.	Bryonia alba	**Merc.**	Mercurius vivus	**Sulph.**	Sulphur
Calc.	Calcarea carbonica	**Merc.cy.**	Mercurius cyanatus	**Verat.**	Veratrum album
Carb.v.	Carbo vegetabilis	**Nat. m.**	Natrum muriaticum		
Chin.	China officinalis				

REMEDY	Acon.	Apis	Arn.	Ars.	Bapt.	Bell.	Bry.	Calc.	Chin.	Coff.	Eup. p.	Ferr. p.	Gels.	Hep.	Hyos.	Merc.	Merc. cy.	Nat. m.	Nux v.	Phos.	Puls.	Pyrog.	Rhus. t.	Spong.	Sulph.
MODALITIES (CONTINUED)																									
STIMULANTS													●												
SWEATING													●					●					●		
TEMPERATURE (EVEN)																●									
UNCOVERING	●																								
URINATING													●												
WALKING IN OPEN AIR																				●					
WARM DRINKS																									●
WASHING		●																			●				
WET WEATHER														●											
CONCOMITANTS *other symptoms that come on with the fever*																									
HEAD																									
CATARRH			●	●																					
COLD SCALP								●																	
CONGESTED	●					●		●																	
HEADACHE (BURSTING)											●		●					●							
BETTER KEEPING STILL							●																		
BETTER FOR PRESSURE							●																		
FACE CONGESTED											●		●												
FLUSHED											●	●						●							
FLUSHED AND PALE ALTERNATELY	●											●													
HOT	●		●						●			●	●								●				
RED (DULL)					●																				
RED (DUSKY)													●												
RED (VERY)																			●						
RED PATCHES ON CHEEKS												●													
NOSEBLEED												●													
EYES SORE							●						●												
EYEBALLS SORE											●														
PUPILS CONTRACTED	●																								

MOUTH DRY	•																								
BREATH OFFENSIVE																•									
FEELS DRY AND THIRSTY																•									
FOUL																•									
INFLAMMATION WITH PUS					•											•									
LIPS DRY												•				•		•			•				
LIPS AND MOUTH DRY						•	•																		
LIPS AND MOUTH DRY AND RED																									
LIPS WITH COLD SORE																		•							
SALIVATION COPIOUS																•									
TONGUE COATED																					•				
TONGUE WHITE							•																		
STOMACH UPSET											•								•		•				
CONSTIPATION							•																		
FEARS WILL BURST		•																							
PAIN WORSE FOR COLD DRINKS	•																								
PAINFUL DISTENTION AFTER FOOD							•																		
TIGHTNESS		•																							
VOMITS BILE											•														
URINE COPIOUS													•									•			
SCANTY	•	•																							
SCANTY (FROM FEAR)	•																								
INCONTINENCE (FROM PARALYSIS)													•												
THROAT DRY																									
LARYNX SENSITIVE																									
RAWNESS																	•								
SOLIDS GAG (CAN SWALLOW FLUIDS)					•																				
SORE																				•			•	•	
TONSILS THICK WHITE COATING																	•								
ULCERATION																	•								
COUGH CROUPY														•											
DRY	•										•														
HACKING											•														
CHEST BURNING																									•
OPPRESSION																									•
STITCHES																									•
BACK AND NECK ACHING												•	•												
HOT													•												
PAIN BETTER LYING ON HARD SURFACE																							•		
STIFF																							•		
LIMBS																									
ACHING IN BONES											•														
BURNING DESIRE TO STRETCH									•																
CHANGE POSITION (WANTS TO)									•																
COLD			•			•						•	•			•		•							

The illustration shows mercury, the source for the Mercurius vivus remedy.

Fevers 6

This part of the chart shows **further possible concomitants** that may appear with the fever condition. Read down the list to find which ones are relevant to you. The symbols on the chart indicate the remedies most suitable for each variable. Once you have identified more of the concomitants in the particular case you are taking, and noted the possible remedies, turn to the following pages to trace the remedies that suit the other elements in your case. As you work your way through the chart, following the system of symbols, you should be able to eliminate unsuitable remedies and eventually make a final selection that matches your case as nearly as possible.

The remedy names are given in an abbreviated form in the charts. Full names are given in the key below.

REMEDY KEY

Acon.	Aconitum napellus
Apis	Apis mellifica
Arn.	Arnica montana
Ars.	Arsenicum album
Bapt.	Baptisia tinctoria
Bell.	Belladonna
Bry.	Bryonia alba
Calc.	Calcarea carbonica
Carb.v.	Carbo vegetabilis
Chin.	China officinalis
Coff.	Coffea cruda
Eup. p.	Eupatorium perfoliatum
Ferr. p.	Ferrum phosphoricum
Gels.	Gelsemium sempervirens
Hep.	Hepar sulphuris calcareum
Hyos.	Hyoscyamus niger
Merc.	Mercurius vivus
Merc.cy.	Mercurius cyanatus
Nat. m.	Natrum muriaticum
Nux v.	Nux vomica
Phos.	Phosphorus
Puls.	Pulsatilla nigricans
Pyrog.	Pyrogenium
Rhus t.	Rhus toxicodendron
Spong.	Spongia tosta
Sulph.	Sulphur
Verat.	Veratrum album

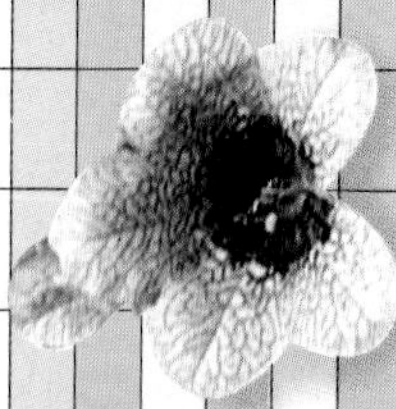

REMEDY	Acon.	Apis	Arn.	Ars.	Bapt.	Bell.	Bry.	Calc.	Chin.	Coff.	Eup. p.	Ferr. p.	Gels.	Hep.	Hyos.	Merc.	Merc.cy.	Nat. m.	Nux v.	Phos.	Puls.	Pyrog.	Rhus t.	Spong.	Sulph.
CONCOMITANTS (CONTINUED)																									
LIMBS (CONTINUED)																									
COLD AND BLUE																		✿							
FEET COLD												✿	✿			✿									✿
HANDS COLD AND PURPLE																			✿						
HANDS SWEATING														✿											
SOLES OF FEET BURN AT NIGHT																									✿
SWOLLEN, STIFF, PAINFUL							✿																✿		
WEARINESS									✿																
WHOLE BODY																									
BLEEDS EASILY												✿													
COLD	✿			✿																					
COLD IN SPOTS								✿																	
COLDNESS (EXTERNAL)				✿																					
COLDNESS OF PART LAIN ON			✿																						
COMATOSE					✿																				
DRUGGED, BESOTTED LOOK					✿																				
EDEMA		✿																							
GLANDS SWOLLEN								✿																	
HOT	✿		✿	✿		✿													✿						
INFLAMMATIONS (PUFFY)		✿														✿									
JOINT PAINS							✿																		
LYMPH NODES ENLARGED																✿									
ODOR (SOUR)								✿																	
PAINS RIGHT SIDED (WORSE LYING ON)							✿																		
PULSATIONS						✿																			
RESTLESS AND FIDGETY																				✿					
SORE (GENERALLY)																									

SORE BRUISED SENSATION							✿																		
SWELLING		✿																							
TEMPERATURE (HIGH)						✿								✿											
THROBBING						✿																			
TREMBLING																	✿								
WEAK													✿												
WEAK AND PROSTRATED																				✿					
SKIN BOILS														✿											
COLD AND MOIST																	✿								
DRY	✿	✿				✿												✿							
DUSKY						✿																			
DUSKY SPOTS (LIKE BRUISES)			✿																						
HOT		✿				✿																			
INFLAMMATION WITH PUS																✿									
ITCHING (WORSE FOR HEAT)																									✿
ITCHY ERUPTIONS																									
MOTTLED			✿																				✿		
RED (BRIGHT, FLUSHED)						✿																			
ULCERS														✿		✿									
WARM AND PALE															✿										
PULSE BOUNDING	✿																								
BLOOD VESSELS DILATED						✿									✿						✿				
BLOOD VESSELS DISTURBED			✿					✿							✿			✿							
SURGINGS OF BLOOD												✿													
PERSPIRATION																									
ABSENT		✿	✿			✿					✿				✿										
COPIOUS	✿																								
COVERED PARTS ONLY	✿					✿																			
EASY								✿						✿											
WITH HEAT																				✿					
WITH HEAT AND SHIVERING																							✿		
WITH THIRST				✿																					
HEAVY																✿									
HOT AND STEAMY						✿																			
NIGHT																✿									
NIGHT WITH HEAT														✿											
ALL NIGHT														✿											
EVENING AND NIGHT (WORSE)						✿																			
OFFENSIVE																✿									

The illustration shows hairy henbane, the source of the Hyoscyamus niger remedy.

Fevers 7

This part of the chart shows **further possible concomitants** that may appear with the fever condition, **peculiar symptoms** (which are often a key guide to the remedy you seek) and some of the **general mental symptoms** that may present. Read down the list to find which ones are relevant to you. The symbols on the chart indicate the remedies most suitable for each variable. Once you have established the concomitants and peculiars, and observed the general mental symptoms in the particular case you are taking, and noted the possible remedies, turn to the following pages to trace the remedies that suit the other elements in your case. As you work your way through the chart you should be able to eliminate unsuitable remedies and make a final selection.

The remedy names are given in an abbreviated form in the charts. Full names are given in the key below.

REMEDY KEY

Acon.	Aconitum napellus	**Coff.**	Coffea cruda	**Nux v.**	Nux vomica
Apis	Apis mellifica	**Eup. p.**	Eupatorium perfoliatum	**Phos.**	Phosphorus
Arn.	Arnica montana	**Ferr. p.**	Ferrum phosphoricum	**Puls.**	Pulsatilla nigricans
Ars.	Arsenicum album	**Gels.**	Gelsemium sempervirens	**Pyrog.**	Pyrogenium
Bapt.	Baptisia tinctoria	**Hep.**	Hepar sulphuris calcareum	**Rhus t.**	Rhus toxicodendron
Bell.	Belladonna			**Spong.**	Spongia tosta
Bry.	Bryonia alba	**Hyos.**	Hyoscamus niger	**Sulph.**	Sulphur
Calc.	Calcarea carbonica	**Merc.**	Mercurius vivus	**Verat.**	Veratrum album
Carb.v.	Carbo vegetabilis	**Merc.cy.**	Mercurius cyanatus		
Chin.	China officinalis	**Nat. m.**	Natrum muriaticum		

REMEDY	Acon.	Apis	Arn.	Ars.	Bapt.	Bell.	Bry.	Calc.	Chin.	Coff.	Eup. p.	Ferr. p.	Gels.	Hep.	Hyos.	Merc.	Merc. cy.	Nat. m.	Nux v.	Phos.	Puls.	Pyrog.	Rhus. t.	Spong.	Sulph.
CONCOMITANTS (CONTINUED)																									
PERSPIRATION (CONTINUED)																									
ONE-SIDED																					●				
PARTIAL		●																							
PROFUSE												●									●				
PROFUSE IN MORNING																					●				
PROLONGED				●																					
RELIEVES SYMPTOMS	●						●											●							
SCANTY											●														
SOUR				●										●											
UPPER PART OF BODY																									●
DISCHARGES																									
ACRID					●									●											
BLAND																					●				
BLOODY												●													
CHEESY														●											
CLEAR																		●							
EGG WHITE (LIKE)																		●							
EXCORIATING				●																					
OFFENSIVE					●									●		●									
PROFUSE														●											
THICK														●							●				
WATERY																		●							
YELLOW-GREEN																					●				
GENERAL																									
BED FEELS HARD				●																		●	●		
DESIRES FRESH AIR																					●				
DESIRES TO UNCOVER		●																			●				
EXHAUSTION				●																					
FALLS ASLEEP TALKING					●																				
LIES STILL							●																		
VERY RESTLESS	●			●												●									

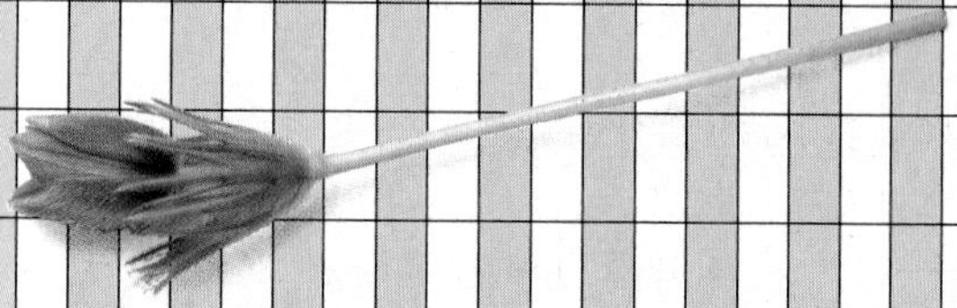

REMEDY	Acon.	Apis	Arn.	Ars.	Bapt.	Bell.	Bry.	Calc.	Eup. p.	Ferr. p.	Gels.	Hyos.	Merc.	Nat. m.	Phos.	Pyrog.	Puls.	Rhus. t.	Sulph.
PECULIARS *unusual symptoms*																			
BILIOUS VOMITING BETWEEN CHILL AND HEAT									✿										
DESIRES COLD DRINKS WHEN CHILLED														✿					
HEADACHE BETTER FOR COPIOUS URINATION											✿								
METALLIC TASTE													✿						
PARTS OF BODY FEEL SCATTERED (CAN'T GET HIMSELF TOGETHER)					✿														
SENSATION AS IF																			
BURNING IN BLOOD VESSELS				✿			✿	✿				✿		✿				✿	
CRAWLING IN SPINE AFTER CHILL	✿																		
ICE IN BLOOD VESSELS				✿															
RED HOT NEEDLES				✿															
SYMPTOMS																			
LEFT SIDED															✿				✿
ONE SIDED			✿			✿	✿			✿					✿		✿		✿
RIGHT SIDED		✿				✿				✿									
RIGHT MOVING TO LEFT		✿																	
TEMPERATURE AND PULSE OUT OF NORMAL RELATIONSHIP																✿			
TRIANGULAR RED TIP TO TONGUE																		✿	

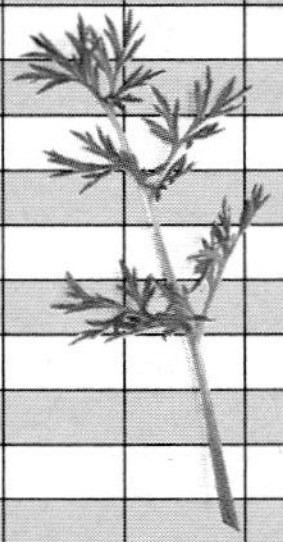

REMEDY	Acon.	Apis	Arn.	Ars.	Bapt.	Bell.	Bry.	Calc.	Chin.	Coff.	Eup. p.	Ferr. p.	Gels.	Hep.	Hyos.	Merc.	Merc. cy.	Nat. m.	Nux. v.	Phos.	Puls.	Pyrog.	Rhus. t.	Spong.	Sulph.
GENERALS *symptoms that affect the whole person*																									
MENTALS																									
ALONE (DESIRES TO BE)			✿										✿												
APATHETIC		✿																							
ANXIOUS				✿																	✿		✿	✿	
CLINGING																					✿				
COMPANY (DESIRES)				✿																✿					
CRITICAL																			✿						
CUDDLY (CHILDREN)																					✿				
DESPAIR (DRIVEN TO BY PAIN)	✿																								
DISCONTENTED														✿											
DISTURBED (DOES NOT WANT TO BE)							✿																		
DISORGANIZED AND MESSY																									✿
DULL MIND							✿						✿												
FASTIDIOUS				✿																					
FEARFUL	✿			✿																			✿		
FEAR GREAT ON WAKING																								✿	
OF DEATH																								✿	
OF SUFFOCATION																								✿	
PANICKY	✿																								
TO BE ALONE				✿																					
WITH NIGHTMARES			✿																						
FEARS (MANY)	✿																			✿					
FURIOUS DELIRIUM						✿																			

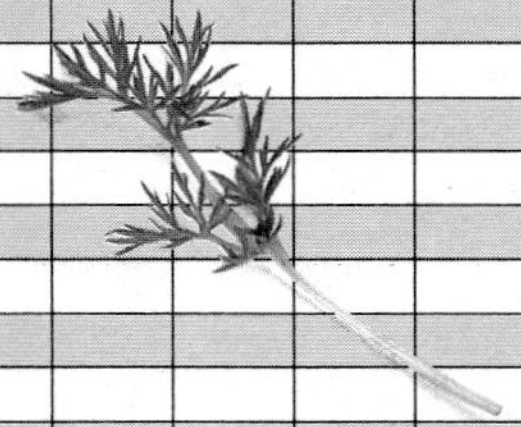

The illustration shows the wind-flower, the source for the Puslatilla nigricans remedy.

Fevers 8

This part of the chart shows **further possible general mental symptoms**, the **appearance of the patient** and **the characteristics of both the patient and their state**. Read down the list to find which ones are relevant to you. The symbols on the chart indicate the remedies most suitable for each variable. Once you have established the general mental symptoms and observed the patient carefully in the particular case you are taking, and noted the possible remedies, turn to the following pages to trace the remedies that suit the other elements in your case. As you work your way through the chart, following the system of symbols, you should be able to eliminate unsuitable remedies and eventually make a final selection that matches your case.

The remedy names are given in an abbreviated form in the charts. Full names are given in the key below.

REMEDY KEY

Acon.	Aconitum napellus	**Coff.**	Coffea cruda	**Nux v.**	Nux vomica
Apis	Apis mellifica	**Eup. p.**	Eupatorium perfoliatum	**Phos.**	Phosphorus
Arn.	Arnica montana	**Ferr. p.**	Ferrum phosphoricum	**Puls.**	Pulsatilla nigricans
Ars.	Arsenicum album	**Gels.**	Gelsemium sempervirens	**Pyrog.**	Pyrogenium
Bapt.	Baptisia tinctoria	**Hep.**	Hepar sulphuris calcareum	**Rhus t.**	Rhus toxicodendron
Bell.	Belladonna	**Hyos.**	Hyoscamus niger	**Spong.**	Spongia tosta
Bry.	Bryonia alba	**Merc.**	Mercurius vivus	**Sulph.**	Sulphur
Calc.	Calcarea carbonica	**Merc.cy.**	Mercurius cyanatus	**Verat.**	Veratrum album
Carb.v.	Carbo vegetabilis	**Nat. m.**	Natrum muriaticum		
Chin.	China officinalis				

REMEDY	Acon.	Apis	Arn.	Ars.	Bapt.	Bell.	Bry.	Calc.	Chin.	Coff.	Eup. p.	Ferr. p.	Gels.	Hep.	Hyos.	Merc.	Merc. cy.	Nat. m.	Nux. v.	Phos.	Puls.	Pyrog.	Rhus. t.	Spong.	Sulph.
GENERALS (CONTINUED)																									
MENTALS (CONTINUED)																									
GENTLE, MILD																					●				
HOMESICK							●																		
IMAGINES OFFENCES																			●						
IMPATIENT, HURRIED																			●						●
INDIFFERENT													●												
IRRITABLE		●					●							●					●		●		●		
MOROSE			●																						
NERVOUS EXCITABILITY						●															●				
OVEREXCITED																				●					
POSSESSIVE				●																					
QUARRELSOME														●											
RESTLESS	●		●	●																			●		
SCREAMS (CHILD)			●																						
STARTLED (EASILY)																				●					
SUSPICIOUS AND JEALOUS		●																							
WEEPS EASILY		●								●				●							●				
PHYSICAL AND PSYCHOLOGICAL FACTORS																									
ANEMIC, PALLID, WEAK									●																
INTENSE FEVER, DELIRIUM																		●							
INTENSE SUFFERING (OUT OF PROPORTION)				●										●											
DELICATE SENSITIVE PERSON														●						●					
NOT EMOTIONALLY SENSITIVE																									●
LOOKS WELL WHEN IS NOT																					●				
SAYS IS NOT ILL WHEN IS		●	●																						
SINKS RAPIDLY INTO STUPOR					●																				
RELAXED FLABBY BUILD								●																	
UNHEALTHY APPEARANCE																●									
FLUSHED, TIRED												●													

BETTER FOR MOTION																							❦		
CHANGEABLE																					❦				
INTENSE	❦																								
PERIODIC																		❦							
SLOW, CONGESTIVE													❦												
SUDDEN	❦																								
SUDDEN AND VIOLENT						❦																			
WORSE COLD (PAINS)																							❦		
MOTION (PAINS)																				❦					
MOTION (MUCH WORSE)							❦																		
FIRST MOTION																							❦		
NIGHT																							❦		
CHARACTERISTICS OF THE PATIENT'S STATE																									
AGITATED AND RESTLESS																❦									
BLEEDING (EASY)												❦													
CHEST (COLDS GO TO)																❦									
(FULLNESS IN)																								❦	
CHILLY				❦				❦																	
COLD OPEN AIR INVIGORATES																									❦
CONGESTIONS AND WEAKNESS								❦																	
DELIRIUM AND STUPOR			❦													❦									
DIZZY IN WARM ROOM							❦																		
DRIVEN OUT OF BED AT NIGHT																❦									
DROWSY DAY, RESTLESS NIGHT																									❦
DULL STUPOR						❦										❦									
EXERTION (WORSE FOR)								❦																	
EXHAUSTED EASILY												❦								❦					
FAINTS WITH PAIN														❦											
HEART REGION (UNEASINESS)																								❦	
HURRIED, IMPULSIVE																❦									
HYPERVENTILATION	❦																								
LETHARGIC (IF OVERSLEEPS)																									❦
PROSTRATION			❦																						
GREAT				❦	❦																				
RAPID																	❦								
RASHES SUPPRESSED		❦																							
UNDERDEVELOPED		❦																							
RESTLESS																				❦					
SORE AND BRUISED ALL OVER			❦																				❦		
SLEEPLESS							❦																	❦	
STARTING, TWITCHING, JERKING						❦																			
SWELLINGS						❦																			
TIRED												❦	❦												
TOUCH (AVERSE TO)			❦																						
WEAK (DISPROPORTIONATELY)				❦																					
(TIRES EASILY)													❦			❦				❦					
WEIGHT (SENSATION OF GREAT)													❦												

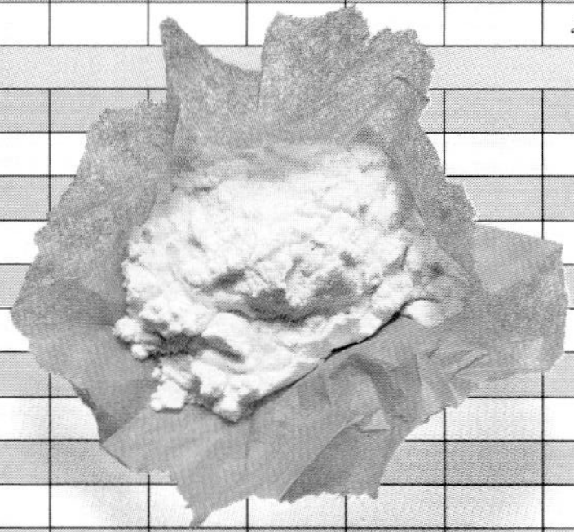

The illustration shows flowers of sulphur, the remedy for the Hepar sulphuris calcareum remedy.

Fevers 9

This part of the chart shows **further possible characteristics of** both the patient and their state. Read down the list to find which ones are relevant to you. The symbols on the chart indicate the remedies most suitable for each variable. It also indicates how remedies may compare when trying to diagnose this complicated picture. By assessing the data you have collected while consulting the chart, you should now be able to make a final selection to match your case as nearly as possible.

For further advice consult the panel on the right.

The remedy names are given in an abbreviated form in the charts. Full names are given in the key below.

REMEDY KEY					
Acon.	Aconitum napellus	**Coff.**	Coffea cruda	**Nux v.**	Nux vomica
Apis	Apis mellifica	**Eup. p.**	Eupatorium perfoliatum	**Phos.**	Phosphorus
Arn.	Arnica montana	**Ferr. p.**	Ferrum phosphoricum	**Puls.**	Pulsatilla nigricans
Ars.	Arsenicum album	**Gels.**	Gelsemium sempervirens	**Pyrog.**	Pyrogenium
Bapt.	Baptisia tinctoria	**Hep.**	Hepar sulphuris calcareum	**Rhus t.**	Rhus toxicodendron
Bell.	Belladonna			**Spong.**	Spongia tosta
Bry.	Bryonia alba	**Hyos.**	Hyoscamus niger	**Sulph.**	Sulphur
Calc.	Calcarea carbonica	**Merc.**	Mercurius vivus	**Verat.**	Veratrum album
Carb.v.	Carbo vegetabilis	**Merc.cy.**	Mercurius cyanatus		
Chin.	China officinalis	**Nat. m.**	Natrum muriaticum		

REMEDY	Acon.	Apis	Arn.	Ars.	Bapt.	Bell.	Bry.	Calc.	Chin.	Coff.	Eup. p.	Ferr. p.	Gels.	Hep.	Hyos.	Merc.	Merc.cy.	Nat. m.	Nux. v.	Phos.	Puls.	Pyro.g	Rhus. t.	Spong.	Sulph.
RELATIONSHIP OF REMEDIES																									
SIMILAR TO																									
ACONITE																								●	
BRYONIA											●														
PHOSPHORUS											●														
LESS RESTLESS THAN ACONITE												●													
LESS VIOLENT THAN BELLADONNA												●													
PULSATILLA MAY FOLLOW WELL		●																							
USE EARLY IN A FEVER	●											●													
OFTEN FOLLOWS BELLADONNA								●																	
NOT USED EARLY																				●					

WHEN TO SEEK ADVICE

Urgently, right now!

- If the fever is very high – approximately 41°C (106°F) or above, in any patient.
- For any fever in the young infant – less than four months. The very young can stop feeding and rapidly become very ill. The more lethargic, weak and ill the infant, the greater is the urgency and need for expert advice. If necessary you should be prepared to take your child to your health practitioner's surgery or even to hospital. Do whatever is necessary to get a very sick young infant seen.
- If the consciousness level of the patient is affected – drowsiness, confusion, lethargy and unresponsiveness.
- If there are fits or convulsions.
- If the neck becomes stiff.
- If the breathing is very rapid or labored.
- Look at the whole patient and ask yourself the question 'How sick?' If the answer is 'very' then seek advice, even if none of the above categories apply. With a young child the mother will often just know something is seriously wrong and she should trust this knowledge and act accordingly.

Within 24 hours

- If the fever is persistently above about 40°C (104°F) and will not respond to the following measures:
  1. Homeopathic treatment.
  2. Opening a window and keeping the room cool but not cold.
  3. Covering with only one blanket.
  4. Tepid sponging of the whole body. (Do not use cold water.)
- For fevers in children of four to six months and persistent fevers in older children. As a rough guide, if a fever persists more than a day or two in a child under two years then consider seeking advice. The older the child the longer you can wait so long as there are no other signs of serious illness.

Remember to give plenty of clear fluids – water and fruit juices. Breastfeeding infants will require more frequent feeds and may take water and fruit juice in addition. Solid food is not necessary for anyone with an acute fever and will usually be rejected anyway. (See the section on **Abdominal Complaints**, pages 202 to 217.)

Headaches 1

The first part of this chart shows the possible **causes** and **onsets of** headaches. Read down the list to find which ones are relevant to you. The symbols on the chart indicate the remedies most suitable for each variable. Once you have established the cause and onset of the particular case you are taking, and noted the possible remedies, turn to the following pages to trace the remedies that suit the other elements in your case. As you work your way through the chart, following the system of symbols, you should be able to eliminate unsuitable remedies and eventually make a final selection that matches your case as nearly as possible.

The remedy names are given in an abbreviated form in the charts. Full names are given in the key below.

REMEDY KEY

Ars.	Arsenicum album	**Nux v.**	Nux vomica
Bell.	Belladonna	**Puls.**	Pulsatilla nigricans
Bry.	Bryonia alba	**Spig.**	Spigelia anthelmia
Ferr.p.	Ferrum phosphate	**Sang.**	Sanguinaria canadensis
Gels.	Gelsemium sempervirens	**Sulph.**	Sulphur
Iris	Iris versicolor		
Lach.	Lachesis		
Lyc.	Lycopodium clavatum		
Nat. m	Natrum muriaticum		

REMEDY	Ars.	Bell.	Bry.	Ferr. p.	Gels.	Iris	Lach.	Lyc.	Nat. m.	Nux v.	Puls.	Spig.	Sang.	Sulph.
CAUSE *why symptoms appear*														
AFTER EXPERIENCING														
EMBARRASMENT					❀									
EXCITEMENT	❀													
EYESTRAIN									❀					
FEAR					❀									
GRIEF									❀					
HUMILIATION									❀					
MENTAL STRESS (ON RELAXING AFTER)						❀								
AFTER EXPOSURE TO														
COLD			❀		❀		❀					❀		
COLD (TO HEAD)		❀												
HEAT	❀													
STIMULANTS										❀				
SUN							❀					❀	❀	
WASHING IN COLD WATER			❀											
RESULTING FROM														
EXERTION	❀													
HUNGER							❀							
ICE CREAM											❀			
MISSED MEALS														❀
NIGHT WATCHING										❀				
OVEREATING											❀		❀	
OVEREXERTION										❀				
RICH FOOD													❀	
SUPPRESSED CATARRH		❀					❀							
SWEATING			❀							❀				
WINE													❀	

The illustration shows the poison nut plant, the source for Nux vomica remedy.

Headaches 2

This part of the chart shows the possible **sites of headaches** and their attendant **sensations**. Read down the list to find which ones are relevant to you. The symbols on the chart indicate the remedies most suitable for each variable. Once you have established the site and any sensations in the particular case you are taking, and noted the possible remedies, turn to the following pages to trace the remedies that suit the other elements in your case. As you work your way through the chart, following the system of symbols, you should be able to eliminate unsuitable remedies and eventually make a final selection that matches your case as nearly as possible.

The remedy names are given in an abbreviated form in the charts. Full names are given in the key below.

REMEDY KEY

Ars. Arsenicum album
Bell. Belladonna
Bry. Bryonia alba
Ferr.p. Ferrum phosphate
Gels. Gelsemium sempervirens
Iris Iris versicolor
Lach. Lachesis
Lyc. Lycopodium clavatum
Nat. m Natrum muriaticum
Nux v. Nux vomica
Puls. Pulsatilla nigricans
Spig. Spigelia anthelmia
Sang. Sanguinaria canadensis
Sulph. Sulphur

REMEDY	Ars.	Bell.	Bry.	Ferr. p.	Gels.	Iris	Lach.	Lyc.	Nat. m.	Nux v.	Puls.	Spig.	Sang.	Sulph.
ONSET *when and how symptoms appear*														
SLOWLY			•		•									
SUDDENLY		•												
VIOLENTLY		•												
BEFORE A MENSTRUAL PERIOD											•			
AT SUNRISE												•		
ON WAKING							•		•					
10-11AM									•					
1-3PM	•													
IN SPRINGTIME							•							
SITE *where on head pains appear*														
FOREHEAD	•		•	•										
FRONTAL						•								
OCCIPUT	•		•	•	•				•			•	•	
RIGHT TEMPLE						•								
RIGHT EYE									•					
SIDES				•							•			
ONE SIDE											•			
RIGHT SIDE				•									•	
LEFT SIDE							•					•		
TEMPLES											•			
RIGHT TEMPLE													•	
VERTEX				•										
PAINS EXTEND														
DOWN SPINE									•					
TO RIGHT SIDE							•							
TO ABOVE EYES												•		
TO ABOVE RIGHT EYE													•	
SENSATIONS *how the head and pains in the head feel*														
SENSATIONS AS IF														
BRAIN WILL BURST													•	

EYES PRESSED OUT													❀												
HEAD IN A VICE									❀																
SCALP CONSTRICTED						❀																			
SKULL WOULD SPLIT OPEN			❀																						
WEIGHT AND PRESSURE IN HEAD							❀																		
WEIGHT IN VERTEX										❀															
SENSATIONS GENERAL AND PARTICULAR																									
BEGINS WITH BLURRING (OF EYES)						❀																			
BLINDING				❀																					
BORING				❀																					
BURNING	❀	❀				❀				❀		❀	❀	❀											
BURNING (VERTEX)							❀																		
BURSTING		❀	❀	❀			❀						❀												
CATARRHAL				❀				❀	❀																
CHILLY	❀																								
COLD				❀				❀																	
CONGESTIVE	❀	❀			❀		❀				❀		❀												
CONGESTIVE ON WAKING			❀																						
CONGESTIVE SENSATION (MARKED)														❀											
CONSTRICTING						❀					❀			❀											
CRUSHING									❀																
DILATED (PUPILS)					❀																				
DRAWING										❀															
DRY			❀																						
DUSKY (FACE)					❀																				
ENGORGED (FACE)														❀											
FAINTS AND WEEPS (WITH PAIN)										❀															
FLUSHES OF HEAT				❀	❀																				
FULLNESS			❀	❀																					
GLAZED (EYES)					❀																				
HOT	❀	❀	❀	❀				❀			❀		❀	❀											
HOT (VERTEX)				❀										❀											
HAMMERING		❀		❀	❀				❀																
INTENSE												❀													
INTOLERABLE			❀									❀													
HEAVY		❀																							
MOTION (OF EYES PAINFUL)												❀													
MOTTLED (FACE)			❀				❀																		
NAUSEA AND VOMITING (WITH PAIN)					❀	❀																			
NEURALGIC	❀				❀					❀		❀													
PALE FACE (ALTERNATES FLUSHING)				❀			❀																		
PERIODICAL	❀								❀		❀														
PERIODICAL (EVERY 7 DAYS)														❀											
PERIODICAL (EVERY 7TH OR 3RD DAY)													❀												

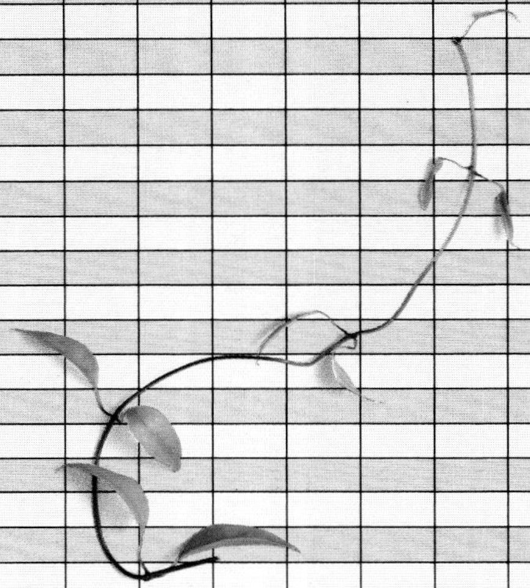

The illustration shows false jasmine, the source for the Gelsemium sempervirens remedy.

Headaches 3

This part of the chart shows the **further possible sensations** attendant on headaches, and some **modalities** (what makes the patient feel better or worse). Read down the list to find which ones are relevant to you. The symbols on the chart indicate the remedies most suitable for each variable. Once you have established the sensations and modalities of the particular case you are taking, and noted the possible remedies, turn to the following pages to trace the remedies that suit the other elements in your case. As you work your way through the chart, following the system of symbols, you should be able to eliminate unsuitable remedies and eventually make a final selection that matches your case as nearly as possible.

The remedy names are given in an abbreviated form in the charts. Full names are given in the key below.

REMEDY KEY

Ars. Arsenicum album
Bell. Belladonna
Bry. Bryonia alba
Ferr.p. Ferrum phosphate
Gels. Gelsemium sempervirens
Iris Iris versicolor
Lach. Lachesis
Lyc. Lycopodium clavatum
Nat. m Natrum muriaticum
Nux v. Nux vomica
Puls. Pulsatilla nigricans
Spig. Spigelia anthelmia
Sang. Sanguinaria canadensis
Sulph. Sulphur

REMEDY	Ars.	Bell.	Bry.	Ferr. p.	Gels.	Iris	Lach.	Lyc.	Nat. m.	Nux v.	Puls.	Spig.	Sang.	Sulph.
SENSATIONS (CONTINUED)														
PERIODICAL (EVERY 4 TO 6 WEEKS)						✿								
PIERCING										✿				
PRESSING			✿	✿			✿	✿	✿					✿
PRESSURE (BETTER FOR)			✿											
PULSATING		✿			✿		✿					✿		
PURPLE (FACE)			✿				✿							
REDNESS (FACE)		✿		✿										✿
SENSITIVE							✿							✿
SENSITIVE TO COLD (VERTEX)				✿										
SEVERE	✿													
SHARP			✿											
SHOOTING		✿										✿		
SICK	✿					✿							✿	✿
STABBING		✿	✿									✿		
STABBING (OVER EYES)			✿											
STICKING										✿				
STINGING										✿				
STITCHING				✿								✿		
SWELLING		✿												
TEARING		✿								✿		✿		
TENSION										✿				
THIRSTY			✿											
THIRSTLESS											✿			
THROBBING	✿		✿				✿	✿	✿		✿			✿
THROBBING (ON MOTION)			✿											
OVERSENSITIVE							✿							
WAVES OF PAIN	✿						✿							
DESIRES *the patient has the desire*														
TO GO TO BED									✿					
FOR HEAD TO BE COOL	✿													

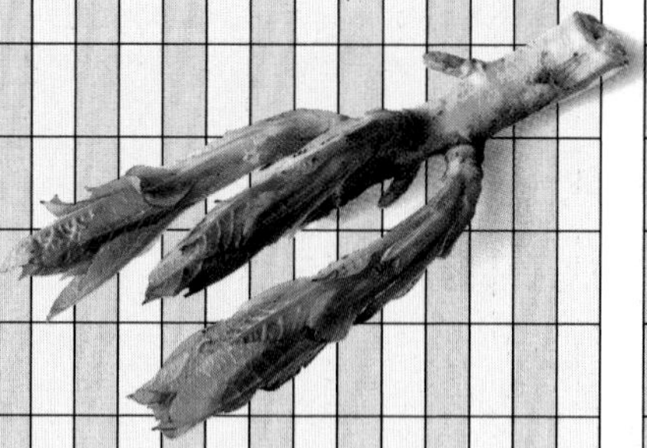

TO WRAP UP	●																								
FOR WARMTH	●																								
MODALITIES *what makes the patient or headache better or worse*																									
WORSE																									
TIME																									
12AM														●											
1-2AM	●																								
10-11AM									●																
4-8PM								●																	
12PM														●											
DAYTIME											●		●												
NIGHT													●												
TEMPERATURE AND WEATHER																									
COLD DAMP												●													
COLD DRAFT		●																							
HEAT	●						●	●		●	●														
OPEN AIR										●															
RAINY DAYS												●													
WARMTH												●													
WARM STUFFY ROOM			●																						
WARM WRAPS								●																	
MOVEMENT																									
BENDING HEAD FORWARD		●																							
COUGHING			●	●																					
EXERTION			●									●													
JAR	●	●		●										●											
MOTION	●	●		●	●							●	●	●											
MOTION (SLIGHT)			●																						
MOVING EYES										●	●														
RISING		●								●															
SITTING QUIETLY											●														
SITTING UP			●																						
STEPPING		●		●																					
STOOPING		●									●			●											
GENERAL																									
COLD DRINKS														●											
EATING			●							●		●		●											
LIGHT	●	●	●	●									●	●											
LYING		●						●			●														
NOISE	●	●		●			●	●	●			●	●												
MENTAL EXERTION												●													
REST						●																			
SLEEP (BEGINNING OF)							●																		
TOUCH		●					●																		
TOUCH (EYES)												●													

The illustration shows deadly nightshade, the source for the Belladonna remedy.

Headaches 4

This part of the chart shows the **further possible modalities** that may characterize a headache and **some concomitants** (other symptoms that come on with the headache). Read down the list to find which ones are relevant to you. The symbols on the chart indicate the remedies most suitable for each variable. Once you have established the modalities and concomitants of the particular case you are taking, and noted the possible remedies, turn to the following pages to trace the remedies that suit the other elements in your case. As you work your way through the chart, following the system of symbols, you should be able to eliminate unsuitable remedies and eventually make a final selection that matches your case as nearly as possible.

The remedy names are given in an abbreviated form in the charts. Full names are given in the key below.

REMEDY KEY

Ars.	Arsenicum album
Bell.	Belladonna
Bry.	Bryonia alba
Ferr.p.	Ferrum phosphate
Gels.	Gelsemium sempervirens
Iris	Iris versicolor
Lach.	Lachesis
Lyc.	Lycopodium clavatum
Nat. m	Natrum muriaticum
Nux v.	Nux vomica
Puls.	Pulsatilla nigricans
Spig.	Spigelia anthelmia
Sang.	Sanguinaria canadensis
Sulph.	Sulphur

REMEDY	Ars.	Bell.	Bry.	Ferr. p.	Gels.	Iris	Lach.	Lyc.	Nat. m.	Nux v.	Puls.	Spig.	Sang.	Sulph.
MODALITIES (CONTINUED)														
UNCOVERING														
VOMITING (NEURALGIA)					●									
WAKING							●							
WRAPPING UP				●										
BETTER														
COLD											●			
COLD AIR				●										
COLD APPLICATIONS				●							●			
COOL AIR								●						
COVERED UP										●				
DISCHARGE (ONSET OF)							●	●						
DRAWING HEAD BACK		●												
DRY AIR												●		
FRESH AIR											●			
HEAT (NEURALGIA)		●												
HOT DRINKS														●
LYING IN BED PROPPED UP					●									
LYING IN DARK ROOM		●												
LYING DOWN				●										
LYING HEAD HIGH												●		
MENSTRUAL PERIOD (DURING)											●			
MOTION								●						
MOTION (SLOW IN OPEN AIR)											●			
PRESSURE		●		●							●			
PRESSURE (FIRM)							●							
PRESSURE (TO HEAD)		●												
QUIET										●				
REST												●		
SLEEP									●					
STILL					●									

URINE (PASSING COPIOUS)					●																				
WARM APPLICATIONS														●											
WARM ROOM														●											
CONCOMITANTS *other symptoms that come on with the headache*																									
BACKACHE (WORSE LYING)										●															
BURNING (PALMS AND SOLES)													●												
BURNING (TONGUE TO STOMACH)						●																			
CHEEKS RED													●												
DIZZINESS				●			●																		
DIZZINESS (LOOKING DOWN)												●													
DIZZINESS (MOVING HEAD)		●																							
DIZZINESS (WORSE STOOPING)		●																							
DRYNESS OF MUCOUS MEMBRANES									●																
EXTREMITIES COLD					●																				
EYES CONGESTED			●																						
EYES GLASSY					●																				
EYES RED			●											●											
EYEBALLS SORE			●																						
FACE RED														●											
FAINTNESS													●												
FEET COLD								●																	
FEVER		●																							
GASTROENTERITIS					●																				
HEADACHE WITH EVERY ILLNESS			●																						
HUNGER								●																	
LIGHTS (FLICKERING BEFORE HEADACHE)									●					●											
MENSTRUAL PERIOD											●														
MENSTRUAL PERIOD (SUPPRESSED)											●														
NAUSEA	●				●	●	●			●			●	●											
NECK STIFF												●													
NOSEBLEED			●																						
PALPITATIONS												●													
PERSPIRATION (EASY)										●															
PULSE WEAK							●																		
PUPILS DILATED		●																							
RUSH OF BLOOD TO HEAD		●																							
SALIVA (PROFUSE)						●																			
SCALP SORE				●																					
SHOULDERS STIFF												●													
TREMBLING					●																				
URINE SCANTY					●																				
VERTIGO												●													
VISION DIM							●																		
VISION FLICKERING							●																		

The illustration shows arsenious oxide, the source for the Arsenicum album remedy.

Headaches 5

This part of the chart shows the **further possible concomitants** that may accompany a headache, any **peculiar symptoms**, and **general mental and physical symptoms** that show up. Read down the list to find which ones are relevant to you. Take particular note of any peculiar symptoms, as these are often the key to the correct homeopathic remedy for a case. The symbols on the chart indicate the remedies most suitable for each variable. By assessing the data you have collected while consulting the chart, you should now be able to make a final selection to match your case as nearly as possible.

If you are in any doubt, consult the advice panel on page 165.

The remedy names are given in an abbreviated form in the charts. Full names are given in the key below.

REMEDY	Ars.	Bell.	Bry.	Ferr. p.	Gels.	Iris	Lach.	Lyc.	Nat. m.	Nux v.	Puls.	Spig.	Sang.	Sulph.
CONCOMITANTS (CONTINUED)														
VISION (LOSS OF)							•							
VOMITING	•			•			•						•	
VOMITING OF BILE													•	•
VOMITING (SOUR)						•				•				
VOMITING AFTER SOUR FOOD											•			
ZIGZAG LINES AND FLICKERING									•					
PECULIARS *peculiar symptoms*														
CRACK IN MIDDLE OF LOWER LIP									•					
EYES FEEL TOO LARGE												•		
FRONTAL HEADACHE BETTER FOR NOSEBLEED				•										
NAUSEA AND FAINTNESS ON RISING			•											
GENERALS *symptoms that affect the whole person*														
MENTAL														
ANGER (WHEN ISOLATED)									•					
ANXIETY	•													
CHANGEABLE MOODS											•			
CLINGING											•			
DULL AND STUPID			•											•
IRRITABLE			•							•				
NERVOUS EXCITEMENT								•						
OVERSENSITIVE							•			•				
RESTLESSNESS	•													
TALKATIVE							•							
TOUCHY										•				
WEEPY											•			
WEEPY (BUT DOES NOT SHOW IT)									•					
PHYSICAL														
BRUISED FEELING ALL OVER			•											
CAN'T BEAR TOUCH OF CLOTHES							•							
CHILLY								•						
[illegible]	•									•				

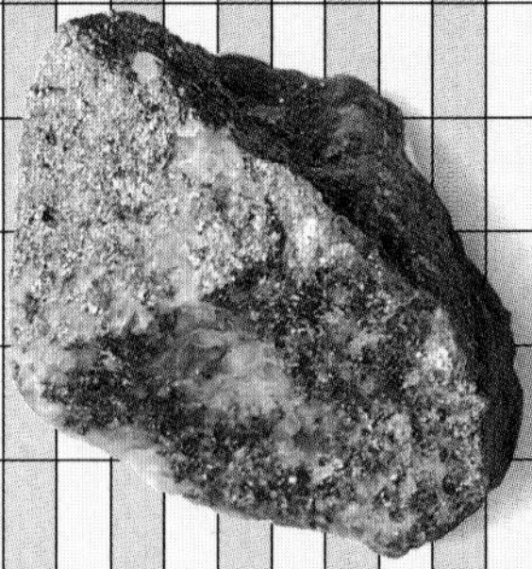

REMEDY KEY

Ars.	Arsenicum album	**Nux v.**	Nux vomica
Bell.	Belladonna	**Puls.**	Pulsatilla nigricans
Bry.	Bryonia alba	**Spig.**	Spigelia anthelmia
Ferr.p.	Ferrum phosphate	**Sang.**	Sanguinaria canadensis
Gels.	Gelsemium sempervirens	**Sulph.**	Sulphur
Iris	Iris versicolor		
Lach.	Lachesis		
Lyc.	Lycopodium clavatum		
Nat. m	Natrum muriaticum		

COLD (FEELS BETTER WHEN HEAD COLD)	✓							✓		✓															
COMPLAINTS PRECEDED BY HEADACHE			✓																						
EXHAUSTION (PROFOUND)					✓																				
HUNGRY AT 11AM														✓											
ITCHING SKIN (WORSE FOR HEAT)														✓											
JERKING		✓																							
LIMBS FEEL HEAVY					✓																				
PALLOR	✓																								
PROSTRATION	✓							✓																	
SLOW, SLUGGISH, PASSIVE			✓																						
STANDING (DISLIKES)														✓											
STILL (MUST KEEP)			✓																						
SYMPTOMS CHANGE											✓														
TIREDNESS (GREAT)					✓																				
TWITCHING		✓																							
WEAKNESS					✓																				
WITH:																									
DARK CIRCLES UNDER EYES				✓																					
PILES										✓															
REDNESS IN CHEEKS				✓																					
SALLOWNESS				✓																					
STOMACH OR LIVER TROUBLES										✓															

The illustrations show iron phosphate (top), the source for the Ferrum phosphoricum remedy; and sulphur, the source for the Sulphur remedy.

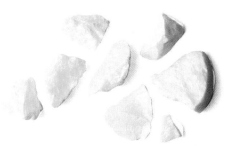

WHEN TO SEEK ADVICE

Urgently, right now!

- If the level of consciousness is affected – drowsiness, confusion, etc.
- For any severe unexpected headache.
- If there is stiffness of the neck and/or high fever, above approximately 40°C (104°F) and/or photophobia.
- If the headache follows a head injury, especially if there is drowsiness or vomiting. (See the First Aid section pages 240 to 245.)

Within 24 hours

- For headaches with any symptoms involving other parts of the nervous system, such as disturbances of sensation, especially vision and dizziness or any disturbed capacity to initiate movement, such as speech difficulty or weakness.
- If the headache is continuous with no signs of improvement over several days even if the headache is mild.

Eye Complaints 1

The first part of this chart shows the possible **causes** and **onsets** of eye problems, **which side they affect**, what the eye looks like and some **sensations** that may be felt. Read down the list to find which ones are relevant to you. The symbols on the chart indicate the remedies most suitable for each variable. Once you have established the cause and onset, side, appearance and sensations experienced in the particular case you are taking, and noted the possible remedies, turn to the following pages to trace the remedies that suit the other elements in your case. As you work your way through the chart, following the system of symbols, you should be able to eliminate unsuitable remedies and eventually make a final selection that matches your case as nearly as possible.

The remedy names are given in an abbreviated form in the charts. Full names are given in the key below.

REMEDY KEY

- **Acon.** Aconitum napellus
- **Apis** Apis mellifica
- **Arg. n.** Argentum nitricum
- **Bell.** Belladonna
- **Bry.** Bryonia alba
- **Euph.** Euphrasia officinalis
- **Hep.** Hepar sulphuris calcareum
- **Merc.** Mercurius vivus
- **Puls.** Pulsatilla nigricans
- **Rhus t.** Rhus toxicodendron
- **Sil.** Silica
- **Sulph.** Sulphur

REMEDY	Acon.	Apis	Arg. n.	Ars.	Bell.	Bry.	Euph.	Hep.	Merc.	Puls.	Rhus t.	Sil.	Sulph.
CAUSE AND ONSET HOW, *when and why symptoms appear*													
TEMPERATURE AND WEATHER													
COLD	•				•	•							
COLD (DRY)	•												
COLD DAMP WIND											•		
COLD DAMP WEATHER												•	
COLD DRY WIND	•					•		•					
EMOTIONAL													
ANGER		•											
EMOTIONAL STRESS		•											
JEALOUSY		•											
GENERAL													
FOREIGN BODIES												•	
RAPID		•											
SUDDEN	•				•								
SUPPRESSED SWEAT						•					•		
TRAUMA												•	
VIOLENT	•												
WITH A COLD									•				•
SIDE *which side symptoms appear*													
RIGHT					•								
RIGHT TO LEFT		•											
APPEARANCE *how the eyes look*													
DILATED (VEINS)						•							
DUSKY					•								
INFLAMED		•					•		•				
CONJUNCTIVA									•				
LIDS									•				

FROM TRAUMA												●													
AFTER REMOVAL OF FOREIGN BODY												●													
EDEMA OF LIDS		●																							
EDEMA OF CONJUNCTIVA		●																							
RED			●				●						●												
RED (BRIGHT)	●				●																				
REDNESS OF LIDS											●														
REDNESS OF CONJUNCTIVA						●																			
SWELLING			●		●				●																
BAG-LIKE UNDER EYES				●																					
OF CONJUNCTIVA		●	●				●				●														
CLOSES EYES											●														
MARKED AND RAPID	●																								
OF LIDS		●	●			●	●				●														
SENSATION *how the eyes and pains in the eyes feel*																									
ACHING						●																			
ACHING (VIOLENT)	●																								
BITING							●																		
BORING								●																	
BRUISED											●														
BURNING	●	●		●		●	●		●			●	●												
BURNING (INTENSE)					●																				
CLOSED SPASMODICALLY									●																
CONGESTION	●	●																							
CUTTING							●																		
DRYNESS					●		●																		
FOG OR MIST BEFORE EYES									●																
FOLLICULAR CONJUNCTIVITIS										●															
IRITIS		●									●														
ITCHING (VIOLENT, MUST RUB)							●																		
OVERSENSITIVE								●																	
PHOTOPHOBIA		●	●						●		●	●													
PRESSING						●	●																		
SAND IN EYES							●																		
SMARTING						●																			
SORE						●	●	●			●		●												
SORE AND ITCHING (LIDS)										●															
STINGING		●										●													
STITCHING						●																			
SUPPURATING (LID MARGINS)												●													

The illustration shows poison ivy, the source for the Rhus toxicodendron remedy.

Eye Complaints 2

This part of the chart shows **further sensations** that may be experienced, **any discharges** and any **peculiar symptoms**. Read down the list to find which ones are relevant to you. The symbols on the chart indicate the remedies most suitable for each variable. Once you have established the sensations experienced, identified the discharges and observed any peculiar symptoms (often a key element in homeopathic diagnosis) in the particular case you are taking, and noted the possible remedies, turn to the following pages to trace the remedies that suit the other elements in your case. As you work your way through the chart, following the system of symbols, you should be able to eliminate unsuitable remedies and eventually make a final selection that matches your case as nearly as possible.

The remedy names are given in an abbreviated form in the charts. Full names are given in the key below.

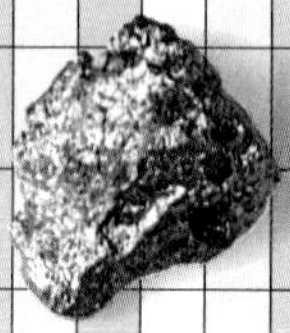

REMEDY	Acon.	Apis	Arg. n.	Ars.	Bell.	Bry.	Euph.	Hep.	Merc.	Puls.	Rhus t.	Sil.	Sulph.
SENSATIONS (CONTINUED)													
TEARING									✓				
THROBBING					✓								
TOUCH (CAN'T BEAR)						✓		✓					
ULCERATION			✓	✓					✓				✓
DISCHARGES *nature of eye discharge*													
ACRID				✓			✓		✓				
BLAND										✓			
BLOODY				✓				✓				✓	
CATARRHAL								✓					
CHEESY								✓					
COPIOUS							✓		✓		✓	✓	
GREEN									✓	✓			
MUCOUS	✓										✓		✓
OFFENSIVE								✓	✓				
PROFUSE			✓							✓			
PURULENT			✓				✓	✓			✓		
PUS													✓
STICKY (LIDS) IN MORNING											✓		
STICKY CORNEA (BETTER BLINKING)							✓						
TEARS (COPIOUS)		✓											
THICK				✓				✓		✓		✓	
THIN	✓			✓								✓	
WATERY	✓					✓	✓					✓	
YELLOW									✓	✓		✓	
PECULIARS *unusual symptoms*													
BURNING, BETTER FOR HEAT				✓									
METALLIC TASTE IN MOUTH									✓				

REMEDY KEY

Acon.	Aconitum napellus	**Puls.**	Pulsatilla nigricans
Apis	Apis mellifica	**Rhus t.**	Rhus toxicodendron
Arg. n.	Argentum nitricum	**Sil.**	Silica
Bell.	Belladonna	**Sulph.**	Sulphur
Bry.	Bryonia alba		
Euph.	Euphrasia officinalis		
Hep.	Hepar sulphuris calcareum		
Merc.	Mercurius vivus		

MODALITIES *what makes the patient or symptoms worse or better*

WORSE																									
12AM													✿												
12PM													✿												
3PM					✿																				
9PM						✿																			
MORNING											✿														
NIGHT					✿				✿																
AIR (OPEN)							✿																		
COLD					✿				✿		✿														
COLD AND DRY								✿																	
DRAFT									✿																
HEAT		✿		✿		✿			✿	✿			✿												
JAR					✿																				
LIGHT	✿				✿	✿	✿																		
MOTION					✿																				
MOVING EYEBALL						✿					✿														
PRESSURE					✿			✿																	
WARM ROOM			✿																						
WASHING EYES													✿												
WASHING IN COLD WATER				✿																					
WINDY WEATHER							✿																		
BETTER																									
COLD		✿				✿																			
COLD APPLICATIONS		✿	✿																						
DAMP								✿																	
HEAT								✿			✿														
MOTION (GENTLE)										✿															
STILLNESS					✿																				
WASHING		✿																							
WASHING IN COLD OR TEPID WATER		✿								✿															

CONCOMITANTS *other symptoms that come on with the eye complaint*

CORYZA (BLAND AND FLUENT)							✿																		
COUGH WORSE DAYTIME							✿																		
COUGH BETTER NIGHT							✿																		
DRYNESS	✿				✿																				
ERUPTION (FACE)													✿												
FEET COLD					✿																				
FOUL MOUTH									✿																

The illustration shows silicon, the source for the Silica remedy.

Eye Complaints 3

This part of the chart shows the **concomitants** that may accompany an eye problem and **general mental and physical symptoms** that show up. Read down the list to find which ones are relevant to you. The symbols on the chart indicate the remedies most suitable for each variable. By assessing the data you have collected while consulting the chart, you should now be able to make a final selection to match your case as nearly as possible.

If you are in any doubt, consult the advice panel on page 171.

The remedy names are given in an abbreviated form in the charts. Full names are given in the key below.

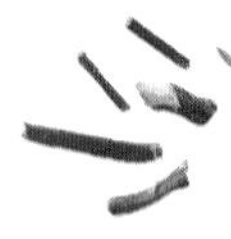

REMEDY KEY

Acon. Aconitum napellus
Apis Apis mellifica
Arg. n. Argentum nitricum
Bell. Belladonna
Bry. Bryonia alba
Euph. Euphrasia officinalis
Hep. Hepar sulphuris calcareum
Merc. Mercurius vivus
Puls. Pulsatilla nigricans
Rhus t. Rhus toxicodendron
Sil. Silica
Sulph. Sulphur

REMEDY	Acon.	Apis	Arg. n.	Ars.	Bell.	Bry.	Euph.	Hep.	Merc.	Puls.	Rhus t.	Sil.	Sulph.
CONCOMITANTS (CONTINUED)													
GLANDS ENLARGED									●				
GUMS SPONGY									●				
HEAD HOT					●								
HEADACHE						●							
HEADACHE THROBBING, CATARRHAL							●						
ITCHING SKIN (WORSE HEAT)													●
JOINT COMPLAINTS						●							
LYING DOWN AT NIGHT (WORSE)							●						
OFFENSIVE (MOUTH)									●				
PUPILS CONTRACTED	●												
RASH		●									●		
RASH (VESICULAR)													●
SALIVATION (COPIOUS)									●				
SNEEZING						●							
THIRSTLESS					●								
THIRSTY	●				●								
TONGUE FLABBY									●				
URINE SCANTY		●											
GENERALS *symptoms that affect the whole person*													
MENTAL													
ALONE (DESIRES TO BE)						●							
ANXIETY	●			●									
CLINGING, WHINING, WEEPING CHILD										●			
FEAR	●												
IRRITABLE						●		●					
MISERABLE				●									

	1	2	3	4	5	6	7	8	9	10	11	12	13	14	15	16	17	18	19	20	21	22	23	24	25
VIOLENT	●																								
PHYSICAL																									
CHILL							●																		
CHILLY				●			●	●																	
COLDS GO TO EYES									●	●			●												
COLD OPEN AIR (DESIRES)			●																						
DRY						●																			
FEVER							●				●														
FEVER DURING DAY							●																		
FRESH AIR (DESIRES)			●							●															
NOT PROLONGED AND LINGERING SYMPTOMS					●																				
RESTLESS	●			●							●														
RHEUMATIC JOINTS										●															
SHORT AND SHARP SYMPTOMS					●																				
STYES RECUR									●																
SWEAT							●																		
THIRSTLESS WITH DRY MOUTH									●																
THIRSTY				●		●																			
THIRSTY FOR SIPS ICE COLD				●																					
WEAKNESS (DISPROPORTIONATE)				●																					

The illustration shows eyebright, the source for the Euphrasia officinalis remedy.

WHEN TO SEEK ADVICE

Urgently, right now!

- If there is any deterioration or loss of vision.
- If any eye pain is severe.
- If the eye is damaged by a foreign body or chemical. Wash out liquid irritants immediately (usually copious clean water is required) and seek advice without delay.

Within 24 hours

- If there is a thick yellow or green discharge coming from the eye.
- If significant eye pain persists.
- If bright lights cause significant pain, especially if the eye is red mainly around the iris or the pupil is irregular and does not react normally to changes of light.
- If there is a rash, such as shingles, or an infection on the face close to or involving the eye in any way.

ACUTE EYE INJURY

The eyes are very vulnerable and should be treated as quickly as possible if they are accidentally injured. This is an instant guide to acute remedies which should help most cases.

- For the ill effects of bruises and other mechanical trauma, use *Arnica montana* followed by *Euphrasia officinalis*. *Euphrasia officinalis* can also be used for conjunctivitis after injury if the eyes are hot, burning and watering.

- For a black eye, use *Lachesis*, which helps blood reabsorption.

- For blunt injury, such as a squash ball in the eye, use *Symphytum*.

Ear Complaints 1

The first part of this chart shows the possible **causes and onsets** of ear problems, **any discharges, concomitant symptoms** and some modalities which make the patient better or worse. Read down the list to find which ones are relevant to you. The symbols on the chart indicate the remedies most suitable for each variable. Once you have established the cause and onset, type of discharge, attendant symptoms and any modalities in the particular case you are taking, and noted the possible remedies, turn to the following pages to trace the remedies that suit the other elements in your case. As you work your way through the chart, following the system of symbols, you should be able to eliminate unsuitable remedies and eventually make a final selection that matches your case as nearly as possible.

The remedy names are given in an abbreviated form in the charts. Full names are given in the key below.

REMEDY KEY

Acon.	Aconitum napellus
All. c.	Allium cepa
Bell.	Belladonna
Cham.	Chamomilla
Ferr. p.	Ferrum phosphoricum
Hep.	Hepar sulphuris calcareum
Lach.	Lachesis
Lyc.	Lycopodium
Merc.	Mercurius vivus
Nux v.	Nux vomica
Puls.	Pulsatilla nigricans
Sil.	Silica
Sulph.	Sulphur

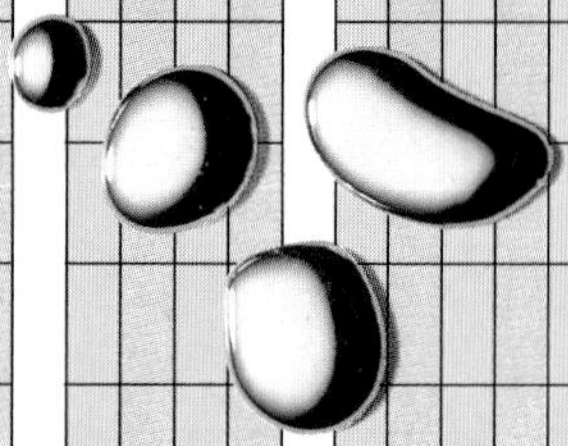

REMEDY	Acon.	All. c.	Bell.	Cham.	Ferr. p.	Hep.	Lach.	Lyc.	Merc.	Nux v.	Puls.	Sil.	Sulph.
CAUSE *why symptoms appear*													
AIR				•									
ANGER				•									
COLD	•	•	•		•			•	•	•			
COLD DRY AIR	•					•							
COLD DRY WEATHER										•			
DAMP COLD									•			•	
DRAFT			•										
EXPOSURE OF HEAD			•										
SUPPRESSED SWEAT												•	
TEMPER				•									
WIND				•									
WIND (PENETRATING)		•											
ONSET *when and how symptoms appear*													
AFTER RASH (MEASLES, ETC)											•		
COLDS													•
EVENING				•									
SUDDEN	•		•			•							
IN THROAT, MOVES TO EAR					•								
VIOLENT	•												
SIDE *which side the symptoms appear*													
LEFT							•						
LEFT TO RIGHT		•					•						
RIGHT		•						•					
RIGHT TO LEFT								•					
DISCHARGE *nature of the ear discharge*													
ACRID									•				•
BLAND											•		
BLOODY						•			•		•		•
BURNING													•
CHEESY ODOR						•							
COPIOUS													•
CURDY												•	

PURULENT		•			•	•	•				•		•												
SEPTIC							•																		
STINKING									•																
THICK						•		•	•		•	•													
WATERY												•													
YELLOW						•		•			•	•													
CONCOMITANTS *other symptoms that come on with the ear complaint*																									
CHILLY								•																	
CHILLS									•																
CHILLS (CREEPING)									•																
CORYZA ACRID WATERY		•																							
COUGH (DRY)								•																	
DIGESTION UPSET										•															
DRYNESS	•		•																						
ERUPTIONS WITH ITCHING													•												
ERUPTIONS WORSE HEAT AND WATER													•												
ECZEMA AND RASHES AROUND EARS								•																	
EYE DISCHARGES		•																							
FACE CONGESTED	•												•												
FEET COLD			•		•																				
FEVERS	•		•					•																	
GLANDS SWOLLEN								•																	
GUMS SOFT								•																	
HEAD HOT			•																						
METALLIC TASTE									•																
MOUTH MOIST AND FOUL									•																
NECK STIFF									•																
NECK SENSITIVE TO TOUCH							•																		
REDNESS			•																						
SALIVATION									•																
SWEAT OFFENSIVE									•			•													
SWEAT (UPPER PART BODY)												•													
SWEAT (HEAD)												•													
SWEAT DOES NOT RELIEVE						•																			
THIRSTLESSNESS			•																						
THIRSTY	•		•	•					•																
THROAT SORE							•																		
TONGUE FLABBY									•																
MODALITIES *what makes the symptoms or patient worse or better*																									
WORSE																									
12AM													•												
9AM				•																					
3PM			•																						
4-8PM								•																	
9-12PM				•																					
12PM													•												
MORNING										•															

The illustration shows mercury, the source for the Mercurius vivus remedy.

Ear Complaints 2

This part of the chart shows **further modalities** which affect the way the patient feels and **any general mental symptoms** manifested. Read down the list to find which ones are relevant to you. The symbols on the chart indicate the remedies most suitable for each variable. Once you have established the modalities and mental symptoms in the particular case you are taking, and noted the possible remedies, turn to the following pages to trace the remedies that suit the other elements in your case. As you work your way through the chart, following the system of symbols, you should be able to eliminate unsuitable remedies and eventually make a final selection that matches your case as nearly as possible.

The remedy names are given in an abbreviated form in the charts. Full names are given in the key below.

REMEDY	Acon.	All. c.	Bell.	Cham.	Ferr. p.	Hep.	Lach.	Lyc.	Merc.	Nux v.	Puls.	Sil.	Sulph.
MODALITIES (CONTINUED)													
WORSE													
NIGHT			•			•			•		•		
IN BED										•			
COLD			•			•		•	•				
COLD AIR				•	•								
CONSTRICTION							•						
DRAFT						•		•	•				
EXERTION					•								
HEAT							•		•		•		•
MOTION			•										
NOISE	•				•			•					
PRESSURE							•						
SLEEP (AFTER)							•						
SLEEP (ENTERING)							•						
SWEATING									•				
TOUCH			•				•						
UNCOVERING						•		•					
WAKING							•						
WARMTH	•	•											
WASHING													•
BETTER													
BEING CARRIED				•									
COOL AIR								•					
GENTLE MOTION					•						•		
HEAT			•	•		•							
STILLNESS			•										
SENSATIONS *how the ears and pains in the ears feel*													
ACHING (VIOLENT)		•											
BAD TASTE (MORNINGS)											•		
BURNING	•								•				•
BURNING (INTENSE)			•										
BURSTING						•		•					

REMEDY KEY

Acon.	Aconitum napellus	**Merc.**	Mercurius vivus
All. c.	Allium cepa	**Nux v.**	Nux vomica
Bell.	Belladonna	**Puls.**	Pulsatilla nigricans
Cham.	Chamomilla	**Sil.**	Silica
Ferr. p.	Ferrum phosphoricum	**Sulph.**	Sulphur
Hep.	Hepar sulphuris calcareum		
Lach.	Lachesis		
Lyc.	Lycopodium		

CHILLINESS WITH PAIN											●														
CONGESTED													●												
DEAFNESS								●			●	●	●												
DRYNESS WITHOUT THIRST											●														
FULLNESS				●																					
HEARING RETURNS WITH A SNAP												●													
HISSING												●													
HEAT				●																					
HYPERSENSITIVE										●															
ITCHES IN EAR					●					●															
MEATUS SENSITIVE							●																		
OPEN AIR (DESIRES)											●		●												
PAIN IN FOREHEAD TO EARS		●																							
PAINS							●																		
CUTTING	●																								
DRAWING		●																							
DEEP, DRAWING					●																				
PRESSING								●																	
SHARP				●																					
STICKING						●																			
STINGING	●								●				●												
STITCHING		●		●	●					●															
PULSATION IN EAR							●																		
PUS ALREADY FORMED						●																			
RAWNESS									●																
RINGING				●																					
ROARING				●								●													
SCREAMS WITH PAIN (CHILD)	●																								
STRANGE NOISES					●						●		●												
TEARING	●	●				●		●																	
THROBBING	●																								
THROBBING (INTENSE)	●		●																						
GENERALS *symptoms that affect the whole person*																									
MENTALS																									
ANGERED EASILY										●															
ANGRY				●																					
BITING						●																			
CHANGEABLE											●														
CLINGY											●														
CONTRARY											●														
FUSSY				●																					
IRRITABILITY	●			●						●															
KICKING						●																			
MAD				●																					
RESTLESS	●																								
SATISFIED (NEVER)				●																					

The illustration shows the deadly bushmaster snake, the source for the Lachesis remedy.

Ear Complaints 3

This part of the chart shows further **general mental symptoms** and any **general physical symptoms**. Read down the list to find which ones are relevant to you. The symbols on the chart indicate the remedies most suitable for each variable. By assessing the data you have collected while consulting the chart, you should now be able to make a final selection to match your case as nearly as possible.

For further advice consult the panel below right. Ear complaints are a particular problem with children; read page 124 to 125 for further information.

The remedy names are given in an abbreviated form in the charts. Full names are given in the key below.

REMEDY KEY

Acon.	Aconitum napellus
All. c.	Allium cepa
Bell.	Belladonna
Cham.	Chamomilla
Ferr. p.	Ferrum phosphoricum
Hep.	Hepar sulphuris calcareum
Lach.	Lachesis
Lyc.	Lycopodium
Merc.	Mercurius vivus
Nux v.	Nux vomica
Puls.	Pulsatilla nigricans
Sil.	Silica
Sulph.	Sulphur

REMEDY	Acon.	All. c.	Bell.	Cham.	Ferr. p.	Hep.	Lach.	Lyc.	Merc.	Nux v.	Puls.	Sil.	Sulph.
GENERALS (CONT)													
MENTALS (CONT)													
SCREAMING						•							
SENSITIVE				•		•				•			
WEEPING (PITIFUL)											•		
WHINING				•									
PHYSICAL													
CARRIED (MUST BE)	•												
COVERS EAR WITH HAND				•									
CHILLY						•				•			
CHRONIC EAR INFECTION												•	
COLD (EASILY)										•			
DAMAGE SINCE INFECTION											•		
DELIRIOUS			•										
DROWSY			•										
EMACIATING CHILD								•					
EUSTACHIAN CATARRH												•	
FLUSHES EASILY					•								
HOT													
HYPERSENSITIVE NERVES	•					•							
INFLAMMATION BLUE PURPLE							•						
JERKING			•										
LOW FEVER					•								
MALAISE					•								
PALE					•								
SENSITIVE TO TOUCH, PAIN COLD						•							
STARTING			•										
THIRSTY					•								
COMPARISON OF REMEDIES													
TO FINISH A CASE AFTER PULSATILLA												•	

WHEN TO SEEK ADVICE

Urgently, right now!
- If there is also drowsiness, severe headache, stiffness of the neck or severe lethargy.

Within 24 hours
- If a baby persistently pulls or rubs an ear. Frequently this indicates an ear infection. Most mild ear infections will settle in time without any treatment, but their progress should be monitored and homeopathic treatment will help them to settle more quickly.
- If the earache is severe or if any earache accompanies measles.
- Any ear discharge.
- If the bony lump behind the ear (mastoid bone) becomes tender or red.
- If the hearing is significantly and persistently impaired.

Refer to other chapters as necessary.

Nose and Sinus Complaints 1

This part of the chart shows the **possible causes and onsets** of nose and sinus problems and **some peculiar symptoms**. Read down the list to find which ones are relevant to you. The symbols on the chart indicate the remedies most suitable for each variable. Once you have established the cause and onset, and any peculiar symptoms, of the particular case you are taking, and noted the possible remedies, turn to the following pages to trace the remedies that suit the other elements in your case. As you work your way through the chart, following the system of symbols, you should be able to eliminate unsuitable remedies and eventually make a final selection that matches your case as nearly as possible.

The remedy names are given in an abbreviated form in the charts. Full names are given in the key below.

REMEDY KEY			
All.c.	Allium cepa	**Kali bi.**	Kali bichromicum
Ars.	Arsenicum album	**Merc.**	Mercurius vivus
Bry.	Bryonia alba	**Nat. m.**	Natrum muriaticum
Dulc.	Dulcamara	**Nux v.**	Nux vomica
Euph.	Euphrasia officinalis	**Puls.**	Pulsatilla nigricans
Gels.	Gelsemium sempervirens	**Rhus t.**	Rhus toxicodendron
Hep.	Hepar sulphuris calcareum	**Sil.**	Silica
Ip.	Ipecacuanha	**Sulph.**	Sulphur

REMEDY	All. c.	Ars.	Bry.	Dulc.	Euph.	Gels.	Hep.	Ip.	Kali bi.	Merc.	Nat. m.	Nux v.	Puls.	Rhus t.	Sil.	Sulph.
CAUSE *why symptoms appear*																
COLD	●		●	●												
COLD AND DAMP										●				●	●	
COLD DRY WIND			●				●					●				
COLD DRY WEATHER												●				
COLD DAMP PENETRATING WIND	●															
HOT TO COLD (CHANGE)				●												
LATER STAGES OF A COLD																●
SUDDEN WEATHER CHANGE				●												
SWEAT SUPPRESSED			●											●	●	
WARM MOIST MILD WEATHER						●										
WET (GETTING)													●		●	
ONSET *how and why symptoms appear*																
10-11AM									●							
MORNING			●													
NIGHT														●		
SPRING				●												
FALL				●												
RAPID								●								
SEVERAL DAYS AFTER EXPOSURE						●										
SLOW						●										
WITH SNEEZING									●							
TAKES COLD EASILY																●
SIDE *which side the pain appears*																
LEFT THEN RIGHT	●															
PECULIARS *peculiar symptoms*																
BLOOD VESSELS ICY AND BOILING		●														

The illustration shows bittersweet, the source for the Dulcamara remedy.

Nose and Sinus Complaints 2

This part of the chart shows **further peculiar symptoms**, characteristic **discharges** and **some sensations** experienced in nose and sinus problems. Read down the list to find which ones are relevant to you. The symbols on the chart indicate the remedies most suitable for each variable. Once you have identified any peculiar symptoms (very significant in any homeopathic diagnosis), observed the nature of the discharge and established any sensations in the particular case you are taking, and noted the possible remedies, turn to the following pages to trace the remedies that suit the other elements in your case. As you work your way through the chart, following the system of symbols, you should be able to eliminate unsuitable remedies.

The remedy names are given in an abbreviated form in the charts. Full names are given in the key below.

REMEDY KEY			
All.c.	Allium cepa	**Kali bi.**	Kali bichromicum
Ars.	Arsenicum album	**Merc.**	Mercurius vivus
Bry.	Bryonia alba	**Nat. m.**	Natrum muriaticum
Dulc.	Dulcamara	**Nux v.**	Nux vomica
Euph.	Euphrasia officinalis	**Puls.**	Pulsatilla nigricans
Gels.	Gelsemium sempervirens	**Rhus t.**	Rhus toxicodendron
Hep.	Hepar sulphuris calcareum	**Sil.**	Silica
Ip.	Ipecacuanha	**Sulph.**	Sulphur

REMEDY	All. c.	Ars.	Bry.	Dulc.	Euph.	Gels.	Hep.	Ip.	Kali bi.	Merc.	Nat. m.	Nux v.	Puls.	Rhus t.	Sil.	Sulph.
PECULIARS (CONTINUED)																
BURNING, BETTER FOR HEAT		•														
METALLIC TASTE										•						
NOSEBLEED WITH COLD								•								
ONE SIDED													•			
STRINGY MUCUS									•							
TRIANGULAR RED TIP TO TONGUE														•		
DISCHARGES *nature of discharge*																
ACRID		•				•			•	•						•
ACRID NASAL	•					•										
ACRID TEARS					•											
BLAND, FROM EYE	•												•			
BLAND NASAL					•								•			
BLOODY										•					•	
BLOODY CRUSTS				•												
BURNING																•
COPIOUS									•		•		•			
DRY CRUSTY											•					
DRY WHEN EXPOSED TO COLD									•							
EGG WHITE (LIKE)											•					
EXCESSIVE											•					
FETID									•						•	
FLUENT					•							•				
FLUENT IN WARM ROOM												•				
GREEN									•	•			•	•		
HARD CRUSTS															•	
HORRIBLE															•	
JELLY-LIKE MUCUS									•							

NOSEBLEED															❦										
OFFENSIVE							❦		❦	❦				❦											
POST NASAL											❦														
PROFUSE	❦						❦							❦											
SEVERE					❦																				
SORE CHEEKS FROM ACRID TEARS					❦																				
SORE UPPER LIP FROM DISCHARGE		❦																							
SMELLS SOUR							❦																		
SMELLS OF DECOMPOSED CHEESE							❦																		
STINKING										❦															
STRINGY									❦																
STUFFED UP												❦													
THICK			❦	❦			❦		❦	❦			❦	❦											
THIN AND ACRID (INITIALLY)										❦															
THICKER DISCHARGE AMELIORATES	❦																								
VISCID									❦																
WATER		❦				❦			❦		❦		❦												
WATERY EYE	❦		❦																						
WATERY INITIALLY							❦																		
WHITE									❦																
YELLOW				❦			❦		❦	❦			❦	❦											
SENSATIONS *how the nose and sinuses and pains in the nose and sinus feel*																									
BAD ODOR AND TASTE													❦												
BURNING	❦	❦			❦					❦						❦									
BRUISED					❦									❦											
COMPLAINTS START WITH SNEEZING, HEADACHE	❦		❦																						
COLD DRINKS CAUSE CHILL, COUGH														❦											
COLDS BEGIN IN NOSE SPREAD TO CHEST								❦																	
COLDS SETTLE IN NOSE								❦																	
CONGESTED	❦																								
CHILL 10-11AM											❦														
CHILL (VIOLENT)								❦																	
CHILLY												❦													
CHILLINESS (CREEPING)										❦															
COPIOUS FLOW IN MORNING													❦												
CORYZA WITH SNEEZING			❦																						
DRY									❦			❦													
DRY LIPS											❦														
DRY MOUTH			❦								❦														
DRY WITH PRESSURE AT ROOT OF NOSE									❦																

The illustration shows bichromate of potash, the source for the Kali bichromicum remedy.

Nose and Sinus Complaints 3

This part of the chart shows **further sensations** experienced in nose and sinus problems and **any modalities** that might make the patient better or worse. Read down the list to find which ones are relevant to you. The symbols on the chart indicate the remedies most suitable for each variable. Once you have established any sensations and observed any modalities in the particular case you are taking, and noted the possible remedies, turn to the following pages to trace the remedies that suit the other elements in your case. As you work your way through the chart, following the system of symbols, you should be able to eliminate unsuitable remedies and eventually make a final selection that matches your case as nearly as possible.

The remedy names are given in an abbreviated form in the charts. Full names are given in the key below.

REMEDY KEY

All.c.	Allium cepa
Ars.	Arsenicum album
Bry.	Bryonia alba
Dulc.	Dulcamara
Euph.	Euphrasia officinalis
Gels.	Gelsemium sempervirens
Hep.	Hepar sulphuris calcareum
Ip.	Ipecacuanha
Kali bi.	Kali bichromicum
Merc.	Mercurius vivus
Nat. m.	Natrum muriaticum
Nux v.	Nux vomica
Puls.	Pulsatilla nigricans
Rhus t.	Rhus toxicodendron
Sil.	Silica
Sulph.	Sulphur

REMEDY	All. c.	Ars.	Bry.	Dulc.	Euph.	Gels.	Hep.	Ip.	Kali bi.	Merc.	Nat. m.	Nux v.	Puls.	Rhus t.	Sil.	Sulph.
SENSATIONS (CONTINUED)																
DUST IN EYES (AS IF)					●											
FRESH AIR (DESIRES)																●
FULLNESS	●															
HOT WATER PASSING (AS IF)						●										
HUGS FIRE IN CHILL												●				
HYPERSENTIVIE TO TOUCH, PAIN, COLD							●									
LEFT TO RIGHT	●															
LIP BURNED BY NASAL DISCHARGE	●															
LIP RED AND RAW	●															
PAIN IN FACE									●				●			
HARD									●							
SEVERE													●			
ON SWALLOWING														●	●	
PRESSURE ON BONES OF FACE										●						
PRESSURE IN EYES					●											
PULSATING									●							
RAWNESS	●									●		●				
ROUGH THROAT												●				
ROUGH SCRAPING																
SHAKES ALL OVER								●								
SHOOTING IN CHEEK BONES									●							
SMARTING											●					
SMELL (LOSS OF)											●		●		●	
SNEEZING			●		●			●				●	●	●		
CAUSES BLEEDING								●								
IN COLD WIND							●									
EARLY AND INCREASES	●															

DOES NOT RELIEVE IRRITATON		✿																							
EVERY CHANGE OF WEATHER		✿																							
SORE		✿										✿		✿											
SORE INSIDE									✿																
SORE NOSTRILS					✿									✿											
STITCHING			✿																						
STUFFED UP NOSE	✿	✿		✿			✿					✿	✿			✿									
EVENING OR NIGHT								✿				✿	✿												
WITH EVERY COLD														✿											
INDOORS													✿												
COLD AIR (BETTER FOR HEAT)							✿																		
COLD AIR							✿					✿													
COLD DAMP WEATHER				✿																					
SWELLING INSIDE NOSE										✿															
SWELLING NASAL MEMBRANES					✿																				
TASTE (LOSS OF)											✿				✿										
TASTE (BITTER)											✿														
TEETH CHATTER								✿																	
THIRST ABSENT								✿																	
COLD DRINKS			✿											✿											
LARGE QUANTITIES			✿																						
THROBBING	✿																								
TICKLING BEHIND STERNUM														✿											
WATERY DISCHARGE	✿																								
MODALITIES *what makes the patient or symptoms better or worse*																									
WORSE																									
12AM																✿									
10AM-NOON											✿														
9PM			✿																						
12PM																✿									
DAY					✿																				
MORNING									✿		✿	✿													
EVENING	✿			✿										✿											
NIGHT				✿	✿				✿	✿				✿											
COLD		✿		✿			✿			✿															
COLD AIR							✿																		
COLD DAMP WEATHER				✿										✿											
DAMP								✿																	
DAMP WEATHER									✿																
DRAFT										✿		✿													

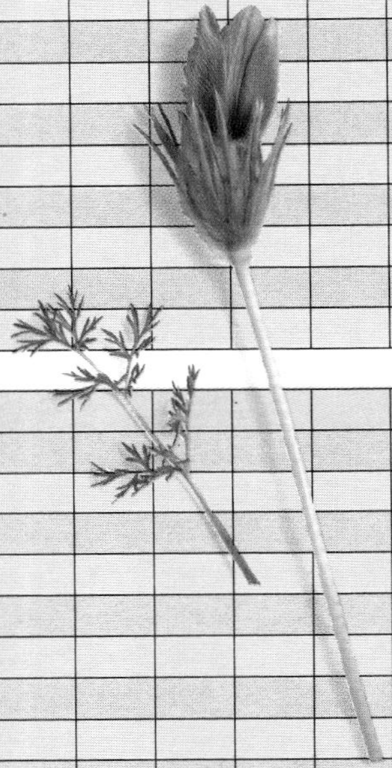

The illustration shows the wind-flower, the source for the Pulsatilla nigricans remedy.

Nose and Sinus Complaints 4

This part of the chart shows **further modalities** that might make the patient better or worse and **some concomitant symptoms** that may appear with the nose or sinus problem. Read down the list to find which ones are relevant to you. The symbols on the chart indicate the remedies most suitable for each variable. Once you have established the modalities and observed the concomitants in the particular case you are taking, and noted the possible remedies, turn to the following pages to trace the remedies that suit the other elements in your case. As you work your way through the chart, following the system of symbols, you should be able to eliminate unsuitable remedies.

The remedy names are given in an abbreviated form in the charts. Full names are given in the key below.

REMEDY KEY

All.c.	Allium cepa
Ars.	Arsenicum album
Bry.	Bryonia alba
Dulc.	Dulcamara
Euph.	Euphrasia officinalis
Gels.	Gelsemium sempervirens
Hep.	Hepar sulphuris calcareum
Ip.	Ipecacuanha
Kali bi.	Kali bichromicum
Merc.	Mercurius vivus
Nat. m.	Natrum muriaticum
Nux v.	Nux vomica
Puls.	Pulsatilla nigricans
Rhus t.	Rhus toxicodendron
Sil.	Silica
Sulph.	Sulphur

REMEDY	All. c.	Ars.	Bry.	Dulc.	Euph.	Gels.	Hep.	Ip.	Kali bi.	Merc.	Nat. m.	Nux v.	Puls.	Rhus t.	Sil.	Sulph.
MODALITIES (CONTINUED)																
WORSE (CONTINUED)																
DRY WEATHER												🏵				
FIRST MOVEMENT														🏵		
FRESH AIR											🏵					
HEAT			🏵							🏵			🏵			🏵
INDOORS	🏵															
LYING DOWN					🏵											
MOTION			🏵						🏵							
OPEN AIR					🏵											
REST														🏵		
STOOPING									🏵							
SWEATING										🏵						
UNCOVERING							🏵							🏵		
WARM ROOM												🏵	🏵			
WARMTH	🏵															
WIND					🏵											
BETTER																
COLD															🏵	
CONTINUED MOVEMENT														🏵		
COOL		🏵														
DRY															🏵	
GENTLE MOTION													🏵			
HEAT				🏵			🏵							🏵		
HEAT (EXCEPT HEAD)		🏵														
LYING DOWN (COUGH)					🏵											
MOTION				🏵												
NIGHT					🏵											

PERSPIRATION														•											
PRESSURE			•						•																
REST								•																	
STILL			•																						
SWEAT											•														
WARMTH									•																
WET WEATHER							•																		
CONCOMITANTS *other symptoms that come on with the complaint*																									
BACK STIFF				•																					
CONVALESCENCE SLOW																•									
CHILL ALTERNATES WITH HEAT												•													
CHILL (VIOLENT)								•																	
CHILL IN FEVER		•																							
CORYZA EXTENDS TO LARYNX	•				•																				
CORYZA GOES TO EARS, THROAT	•																								
COLDS GO TO CHEST								•				•													
COLDS DESCEND								•																	
COUGH ABSENT AT NIGHT					•																				
WITH BURSTING HEADACHE											•														
IN COLD WIND							•																		
DRY PAINFUL			•																						
DRY TICKLING										•															
HARD		•			•																				
TEASING						•																			
TICKLING		•				•																			
DIGESTIVE UPSET												•													
DIZZINESS									•																
ERUPTIONS CRUSTY															•										
EYES PRODUCE WATERY DISCHARGE											•														
EYES RED, SORE, WATERY			•																						
EYES SORE				•																					
EXTREMITIES COLD						•																			
FACE FLUSHED						•		•																	
FACE DUSKY, MOTTLED						•																			
GLANDS SWOLLEN														•											
HEAD HOT						•																			
HEADACHE			•																						
ACCOMPANIES MOST COMPLAINTS			•																						
CATARRHAL	•				•																				
CONGESTED	•					•																			

The illustration shows onion, the source for the Allium cepa remedy.

Nose and Sinus Complaints 5

This part of the chart shows **further concomitants** and any **general mental and physical symptoms** that may appear. Read down the list to find which ones are relevant to you. The symbols on the chart indicate the remedies most suitable for each variable. By assessing the data you have collected while consulting the chart, you should now be able to make a final selection to match your case as nearly as possible.

The remedy names are given in an abbreviated form in the charts. Full names are given in the key below.

REMEDY	All. c.	Ars.	Bry.	Dulc.	Euph.	Gels.	Hep.	Ip.	Kali bi.	Merc.	Nat. m.	Nux v.	Puls.	Rhus t.	Sil.	Sulph.
CONCOMITANTS (CONTINUED)																
HEADACHE (CONTINUED)																
VIOLENT									●							
HOARSENESS							●	●		●	●					
LIPS CHAPPED AND PEELING													●			
LIPS WITH COLD SORES											●					
LIPS ROUGH, CRACK, PEEL															●	
MOUTH ULCERS										●						
NAUSEA								●								
NAUSEA WITH CLEAN TONGUE								●								
NECK STIFF				●										●		
NOSE BLEEDING	●												●			
NOSE RED AND SWOLLEN, SHINING										●						
RAWNESS								●								
SALIVATION INCREASED										●						
SHIVERING FROM MOTION, UNCOVERING												●				
SLEEPLESS IN WARM ROOM											●					
SNEEZING		●								●	●					
SWEATING AT NIGHT WITHOUT RELIEF							●									
PROFUSE AND OFFENSIVE										●						
EASY												●				
THIRSTLESS WITH DRY MOUTH													●			
TASTE METALLIC, SWEET, SALTY, PUTRID										●						
TIRED																●
TONGUE COATED													●			
TONGUE SWOLLEN, FLABBY										●						
THROAT RED, SWOLLEN, SORE		●												●		
ULCERS OF MUCOUS MEMBRANES		●														
VISION DIM									●							

REMEDY KEY

All.c.	Allium cepa	**Kali bi.**	Kali bichromicum
Ars.	Arsenicum album	**Merc.**	Mercurius vivus
Bry.	Bryonia alba	**Nat. m.**	Natrum muriaticum
Dulc.	Dulcamara	**Nux v.**	Nux vomica
Euph.	Euphrasia officinalis	**Puls.**	Pulsatilla nigricans
Gels.	Gelsemium sempervirens	**Rhus t.**	Rhus toxicodendron
Hep.	Hepar sulphuris calcareum	**Sil.**	Silica
Ip.	Ipecacuanha	**Sulph.**	Sulphur

MENTAL																									
ALONE (DESIRES TO BE)			●								●														
ANXIOUS		●																							
CHANGEABLE													●												
COMPANY (DESIRES)													●												
DEMANDS ATTENTION, SYMPATHY													●												
DEPRESSED											●														
FEAR AT NIGHT														●											
FUSS (HATES)											●														
IRRITABLE							●																		
MILD													●												
MISERABLE		●																							
RESTLESS		●																							
RESTLESS AT NIGHT														●											
TIMID													●												
WEEPY											●		●												
PHYSICAL																									
ALWAYS TAKING COLD		●					●									●									
BURNING PAINS, BETTER FOR HEAT		●																							
CATARRH ALTERNATES JOINT PAINS									●																
CHANGEABLE SYMPTOMS													●												
CHILLY		●			●		●								●										
CHILLY IN FEVER					●																				
COLD DAMP (MUCH WORSE FOR)				●																					
CHILLS UP AND DOWN SPINE						●																			
CHILLS FROM BATH, OVERHEATING																●									
CREEPING CHILLINESS										●															
EXTREME (EVERYTHING)		●																							
FIRE (HUGS)		●																							
LONGSTANDING CATARRHS													●												
LOSS OF SMELL													●												
MOTION AGGRAVATES			●																						
OVERSENSITIVE TO COLD, TOUCH, PAIN							●																		
PAINS WORSE WITH FIRST MOTION														●											
PAINS BETTER CONTINUED MOTION														●											
PROSTRATION IN SPELLS								●																	
RECURRENT COLDS				●																					
STILL (DESIRES TO BE)			●																						
SALT (CRAVES OR DISLIKES)											●														
SENSITIVE TO DRAFT		●																							
THIRST FOR ICE COLD SIPS		●																							
TREMBLING										●															
TREMBLING AND WEAKNESS						●																			
WALK (DESIRES TO)										●															
WEAK		●													●										
WEIGHT AND TIREDNESS						●																			

The illustration shows arsenious oxide, the source for the Arsencium album remedy.

Toothache

This self-contained chart shows a comprehensive list of **symptoms, modalities and sensations** observable in the patient suffering from toothache. The remedies are assigned mainly on the basis of what makes the patient feel better or worse. Read down the list to find which ones are relevant to you. The symbols on the chart indicate the remedies most suitable for each variable. As you work your way through the chart, following the system of symbols, you should be able to eliminate unsuitable remedies and eventually make a final selection that matches your case as nearly as possible.

The remedy names are given in an abbreviated form in the charts. Full names are given in the key below.

REMEDY	Bry.	Cal. p.	Cham.	Coff.	Ign.	Kreo.	Merc.	Puls.
BITTER		•				•		
WEEPING								•
ON WAKING					•			
WORSE								
COLD		•						
COLD AIR		•					•	
COLD DRINKS							•	
EVERYTHING							•	
HOT FOOD				•				
LYING HEAD LOW								•
MOTION	•							
NIGHT			•					
SMOKING	•				•		•	
TEA, COFFEE, WINE					•			
WARM FOOD			•					
WARM DRINKS			•	•				•
WARM ROOM			•					
WARMTH	•							

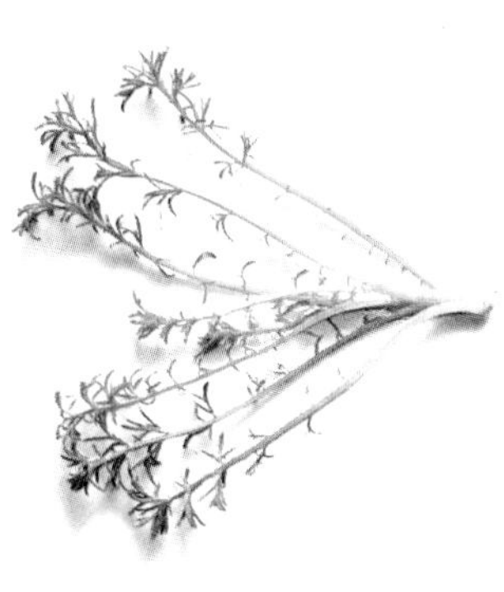

REMEDY KEY	
Bry.	Bryonia alba
Calc.p.	Calcarea phosphorica
Cham.	Chamomilla
Coff.	Coffea cruda
Ign.	Ignatia amara
Kreo.	Kreosotum
Merc.	Mercurius vivus
Puls.	Pulsatilla nigricans

REMEDY	Bry.	Cal. p.	Cham.	Coff.	Ign.	Kreo.	Merc.	Puls.
ACHING			•					
BETTER								
BITING TEETH TOGETHER				•	•			
COLD DRINKS IN MOUTH	•		•	•				•
COLD AIR	•		•					•
EATING				•				
NOTHING							•	
PRESSURE					•			•
FIRM PRESSURE	•							
WALKING OPEN AIR								•
CHANGEABLE SYMPTOMS								•
COMPANY (DESIRES)								•
DECAY RAPID						•		
GRINDS TEETH				•				
GUMS SPONGY, BLEEDING						•		
HEAD HOT			•					
IRRITABLE			•					
NERVOUS				•				
ODOR OFFENSIVE (MOUTH)							•	
PUTRID						•		
PAINS								
BURNING			•					
DRAWING							•	
RADIATE TO EAR OR TEMPLE						•		
TEARING AND STITCHING	•		•					•
PERSPIRATION							•	
TEETH CRUMBLING						•		
TONGUE COATED AND SWOLLEN		•						
SALIVATION							•	
SENSITIVE TOUCH PRESSURE		•						
TASTE SWEET METALLIC							•	

Teething in babies and young children

This self-contained chart shows a comprehensive list of **symptoms** and **modalities** which can be readily observed in a teething baby or a young child. Read down the list to find which ones are relevant to you. The symbols on the chart indicate the remedies most suitable for each variable. As you work your way through the chart, following the system of symbols, you should be able to eliminate unsuitable remedies and eventually make a final selection that matches your case as nearly as possible.

The remedy names are given in an abbreviated form in the charts. Full names are given in the key below.

REMEDY KEY

Calc. p. Calcarea phosphorica
Cham. Chamomilla
Ign. Ignatia amara
Merc. Mercurius vivus
Puls. Pulsatilla nigricans

REMEDY	Calc. p.	Cham.	Ign.	Merc.	Puls			
BITES INSIDE OF CHEEK			❦					
CAPRICIOUS		❦						
CONSTANT CARRYING RELIEVES		❦						
DECAY EARLY, RAPID	❦							
EXASPERATED (ONE BECOMES WITH CHILD)		❦						
HEAD HOT		❦						
ODOR OFFENSIVE (MOUTH)				❦				
IRRITABLE		❦						
PAIN								
ACHING		❦						
BURNING		❦						
DRAWING				❦				
STITCHING, TEARING		❦			❦			
PERSPIRATION								
PITEOUS WAILING		❦						
RELIEF DOES NOT LAST		❦						
REJECTS THING DEMANDED		❦						
SALIVATION				❦				
SNARLING CRY		❦						
SLOW DENTITION	❦							
SYMPATHY (ONE FEELS FOR CHILD)					❦			
TASTE SWEET, METALLIC				❦				
TASTE FOUL BITTER	❦							
TONGUE COATED SWOLLEN	❦							
TOOTHACHE ON WAKING			❦					
WEEPY, WHINY, CLINGY					❦			
WANTS TO BE HELD, TOUCHED					❦			

REMEDY	Calc. p.	Cham.	Ign.	Merc.	Puls.			
MODALITIES								
BETTER								
BITING TEETH TOGETHER			❦					
COLD AIR		❦						
COLD WATER (IN MOUTH)		❦						
NOTHING				❦				
PRESSURE			❦					
WORSE								
CHEWING	❦							
COLD	❦							
COLD AIR				❦				
COLD AIR ON TEETH	❦							
COLD DRINKS				❦				
EVERYTHING				❦				
NIGHT		❦						
TOUCH, PRESSURE	❦							
WARM FOOD, DRINK		❦						
WARM ROOM, BED		❦						

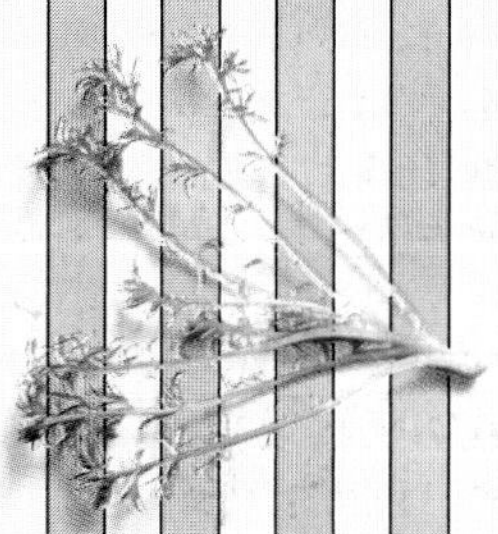

The illustration shows wild chamomile, the source for the Chamomilla remedy.

Coughs

This is a self-contained chart, listed alphabetically, to help you identify a suitable cough remedy. As coughing is also a symptom of other problems, you should also look out for concomitant symptoms.

You need to get help **urgently** if there is severe difficulty in breathing, shortness of breath, wheezing, labored, rapid or shallow breathing, the patient is confused or drowsy, if there is a marked chest pain, or if the lips, tongue or face take on a purply-bluish tint. Make sure that nothing solid has been inhaled; if there has **there is likely to be much coughing, though not always, and the coughing may cease. Help should be urgently sought.** You should also seek advice if the cough persists without improvement for a week or more and there is much weakness, tiredness and lack of energy, or if the breathing is labored or rapid with unexpected wheezing or pain.

The remedy names are given in an abbreviated form in the charts. Full names are given in the key below.

REMEDY KEY

Acon.	Aconitum napellus
Alli.c.	Allium cepa
Ant. t.	Antimonium tartaricum
Ars.	Arsenicum album
Bell.	Belladonna
Bry.	Bryonia alba
Caust.	Causticum
Dros.	Drosera rotundifolia
Dulc.	Dulcamara
Euph.	Euphrasia officinalis
Ferr. p.	Ferrum phosphoricum
Gels.	Gelsemium sempervirens
Hep.	Hepar sulphuris calcareum
Ip.	Ipecacuanha
Kali bi.	Kali bichromicum
Kali c.	Kali carbonicum
Lach.	Lachesis
Lyc.	Lycopodium clavatum
Merc.	Mercurius vivus
Nat. m.	Natrum muriaticum
Nux v.	Nux vomica
Phos.	Phosphorus
Puls.	Pulsatilla nigricans
Rhus t.	Rhus toxicodendron
Rumex.	Rumex crispus
Spong.	Spongia tosta
Sulph.	Sulphur

REMEDY	Acon.	Alli. c.	Ant. t.	Ars.	Bell.	Bry.	Caus.	Dros.	Dulc.	Euph.	Fer. p.	Gels.	Hep.	Ipe.	Kali. bi.	Kali. c.	Lach.	Lyc.	Merc.	Nat. m.	Nux v.	Phos.	Puls.	Rhus. t.	Rumex.	Spon.	Sulph.
BATHING (AFTER)																								✓			✓
COLD (WORSE)				✓		✓	✓		✓	✓	✓	✓	✓		✓	✓	✓				✓	✓		✓	✓	✓	✓
COLD DAMP WEATHER		✓	✓						✓					✓	✓	✓								✓			✓
COLD DRY WEATHER	✓						✓						✓								✓	✓			✓	✓	
COLD FOOD		✓	✓										✓						✓								
COLD SORES (WITH)				✓			✓		✓				✓	✓						✓				✓		✓	✓
CROUPY	✓	✓		✓	✓			✓				✓	✓		✓		✓					✓			✓	✓	
DAY					✓	✓				✓	✓					✓	✓	✓				✓					✓
DEEP BREATHING				✓		✓		✓			✓		✓		✓		✓	✓	✓			✓	✓		✓	✓	✓
DRINKING (WORSE)				✓		✓		✓					✓			✓	✓	✓				✓					
DRINKS COLD (WORSE)				✓							✓							✓	✓			✓		✓		✓	
DRINKS WARM (BETTER)				✓		✓												✓			✓			✓		✓	
DRY EVENING		✓		✓	✓	✓							✓		✓	✓	✓	✓	✓	✓	✓	✓	✓	✓		✓	✓
MORNING			✓			✓	✓						✓		✓	✓		✓			✓			✓			✓
NIGHT	✓			✓	✓	✓		✓					✓	✓		✓	✓	✓	✓	✓	✓	✓	✓	✓		✓	✓
MOUTH	✓		✓	✓	✓	✓	✓		✓		✓	✓			✓	✓	✓	✓	✓	✓	✓	✓	✓	✓		✓	✓
EATING (WORSE)			✓	✓		✓					✓		✓	✓	✓	✓		✓			✓	✓			✓	✓	✓
EXERTION (WORSE)																✓		✓	✓	✓	✓		✓				✓
LOOSE		✓	✓	✓		✓			✓	✓	✓		✓	✓		✓	✓	✓	✓			✓	✓				✓
MOTION (WORSE)				✓	✓	✓				✓	✓	✓			✓	✓		✓	✓		✓	✓			✓		
NIGHT (WORSE)	✓			✓	✓		✓	✓	✓			✓	✓	✓		✓	✓	✓	✓	✓		✓	✓	✓	✓	✓	✓
ONSET SLOW			✓			✓	✓				✓	✓														✓	
ONSET SUDDEN	✓				✓									✓													
OPEN AIR (BETTER)		✓				✓		✓	✓					✓									✓				✓
OPEN AIR (WORSE)	✓	✓		✓						✓	✓		✓			✓	✓	✓				✓		✓	✓		✓
PAINS IN CHEST	✓				✓	✓		✓		✓	✓				✓	✓				✓	✓	✓	✓	✓	✓	✓	
PAINS IN THROAT	✓	✓			✓	✓							✓		✓	✓	✓				✓	✓	✓			✓	
SUFFOCATING	✓		✓	✓	✓	✓	✓	✓					✓	✓		✓	✓				✓	✓	✓			✓	✓
TALKING (WORSE)					✓		✓	✓		✓	✓		✓	✓			✓		✓			✓			✓	✓	✓
THIRSTY	✓			✓	✓	✓			✓	✓							✓		✓	✓		✓		✓			✓
WARMTH (BETTER)										✓			✓		✓	✓					✓						

Throat Complaints 1

The first part of this chart shows the possible **causes and onsets** of throat complaints. Read down the list to find which ones are relevant to you. The symbols on the chart indicate the remedies most suitable for each variable. Once you have established the cause and onset of the particular case you are taking, and noted the possible remedies, turn to the following pages to trace the remedies that suit the other elements in your case. As you work your way through the chart, following the system of symbols, you should be able to eliminate unsuitable remedies and eventually make a final selection that matches your case as nearly as possible.

The remedy names are given in an abbreviated form in the charts. Full names are given in the key below.

REMEDY KEY

Acon.	Aconitum napellus	**Gels.**	Gelsemium sempervirens	**Nit. ac.**	Nitricum acidum
Apis	Apis mellifica	**Hep.**	Hepar sulphuris calcareum	**Nux v.**	Nux vomica
Arg. n.	Argentum nitricum	**Lac c.**	Lac caninum	**Phos.**	Phosphorus
Arn.	Arnica montana	**Lach.**	Lachesis	**Phyt.**	Phytolacca decandra
Ars.	Arsenicum album	**Lyc.**	Lycopodium clavatum	**Puls.**	Pulsatilla nigricans
Bell.	Belladonna	**Merc.**	Mercurius vivus	**Rhus t.**	Rhus toxicodendron
Bry.	Bryonia alba	**Merc. cy.**	Mercurius cyanatus	**Sil.**	Silcica
Carb.v.	Carbo vegetabilis	**Nat. m.**	Natrum muriaticum	**Sulph.**	Sulphur
Cham.	Chamomilla				

REMEDY	Acon.	Arg. n.	Arn.	Apis	Ars.	Bell.	Bry.	Carb. v.	Cham.	Gels.	Hep.	Lac. c.	Lach.	Lyc.	Merc.	Merc. cy.	Nat. m.	Nit. ac.	Nux v.	Phos.	Phyt.	Puls.	Rhus. t.	Sil.	Sulph.
CAUSE *why symptoms appear*																									
ANGER				✿																					
CHANGE OF AIR																									✿
COLD	✿					✿	✿																✿	✿	
COLD, DRY WIND	✿										✿								✿						
COLD WHEN OVERHEATED							✿																		
COLD TO WARM ROOM													✿												
DAMP																							✿		
DRAFT	✿																								
EMOTION				✿																					
GETTING WET																						✿		✿	
GETTING FEET WET																						✿			
JEALOUSY				✿																		✿			
TAKING COLD					✿				✿				✿		✿										
OVEREXERTION			✿																						
OVERHEATING								✿												✿					
OVERUSE OF VOICE																							✿		
SUPPRESSED SWEAT																							✿		
WEATHER CHANGE										✿										✿					✿
ONSET *when and how symptoms appear*																									
10-11AM																	✿								
EVENING									✿																
AFTER SERIES OF COLDS																								✿	
EASILY TAKES COLD					✿												✿	✿	✿						
EASILY TAKES COLD WHEN SWEATING																	✿								
LINGERING STATES																									✿
RAPID				✿																					
SEVERAL DAYS AFTER EXPOSURE										✿															

The illustration shows monk's hood, the source for the Aconitum napellus remedy.

Throat Complaints 2

This part of the chart shows **further possible onsets** of throat complaints, **some peculiar symptoms** (very important for homeopathic diagnosis) and **some modalities** which make the patient feel better or worse. Read down the list to find which ones are relevant to you. The symbols on the chart indicate the remedies most suitable for each variable. Once you have identified any peculiar symptoms and observed any modalities in the particular case you are taking, and noted the possible remedies, turn to the following pages to trace the remedies that suit the other elements in your case. As you work your way through the chart, following the system of symbols, you should be able to eliminate unsuitable remedies and eventually make a final selection that matches your case as nearly as possible.

The remedy names are given in an abbreviated form in the charts. Full names are given in the key below.

REMEDY KEY

Acon.	Aconitum napellus	**Gels.**	Gelsemium sempervirens	**Nit. ac.**	Nitricum acidum
Apis	Apis mellifica	**Hep.**	Hepar sulphuris calcareum	**Nux v.**	Nux vomica
Arg. n.	Argentum nitricum	**Lac c.**	Lac caninum	**Phos.**	Phosphorus
Arn.	Arnica montana	**Lach.**	Lachesis	**Phyt.**	Phytolacca decandra
Ars.	Arsenicum album	**Lyc.**	Lycopodium clavatum	**Puls.**	Pulsatilla nigricans
Bell.	Belladonna	**Merc.**	Mercurius vivus	**Rhus t.**	Rhus toxicodendron
Bry.	Bryonia alba	**Merc. cy.**	Mercurius cyanatus	**Sil.**	Silcica
Carb.v.	Carbo vegetabilis	**Nat. m.**	Natrum muriaticum	**Sulph.**	Sulphur
Cham.	Chamomilla				

REMEDY	Acon.	Arg. n.	Arn.	Apis	Ars.	Bell.	Bry.	Carb. v.	Cham.	Gels.	Hep.	Lac. c.	Lach.	Lyc.	Merc.	Merc. cy.	Nat. m.	Nit. ac.	Nux v.	Phos.	Phyt.	Puls.	Rhus. t.	Sil.	Sulph.
ONSET (CONTINUED)																									
SLOW							❦			❦				❦											
SUDDEN	❦					❦																			
VERY SLOW																								❦	
SITE																									
CHANGES SIDE												❦													
EXTENDS																									
LEFT												❦	❦												
LEFT TO RIGHT													❦												
RIGHT SIDE				❦		❦								❦											
RIGHT TO LEFT				❦										❦											
ROOT OF TONGUE													❦												
STITCHES INTO EAR																			❦		❦				
TO EARS											❦	❦	❦	❦											
PECULIARS *unusual symptoms*																									
ACUTE PAIN BASE OF TONGUE ON PROTRUSION																					❦				
BITTER TASTE	❦																				❦				
BURNING BETTER FOR HEAT					❦																				
COLD YET WANTS TO BE FANNED								❦																	
SWALLOW SOLIDS EASIER THAN LIQUIDS													❦												
THIRST COLD FOR DRINKS IN CHILL																	❦								
TOUCH OF OWN SKIN UNBEARABLE												❦													
UNCOVERING INCREASES PAIN, COUGH											❦														
MODALITIES *what makes the patient or throat complaint better or worse*																									
WORSE																									
12AM																									
9AM									❦																❦
10-11AM																	❦								
3PM						❦																			
4-8PM														❦											

12PM																									❦
MORNING													❦										❦		
EVENING																				❦					
NIGHT						❦			❦						❦						❦				❦
CHANGE OF WEATHER					❦												❦								
COLD					❦						❦				❦			❦	❦				❦		
COLD AIR						❦								❦											
COLD DAYS																					❦				
COLD DRINKS		❦			❦	❦								❦											
COVERING UP	❦																								
COUGHING																				❦					
DRAFT					❦										❦				❦						
DRAFT (SLIGHTEST)											❦														
DRINKING													❦												
EATING																				❦					
EMPTY SWALLOWING												❦	❦												
FATS																						❦			
HEAT				❦			❦		❦				❦		❦										❦
HEAT OF BED																					❦				
HEAT BEFORE FEVER																			❦						
HEAT (RADIANT)				❦																					
HOT DRINKS				❦																					
JAR			❦			❦																			
MOTION			❦			❦	❦																		
MOTION (FIRST)																							❦		
PRESSURE											❦														
STUFFY ROOM																						❦			
SWALLOWING																					❦				
SWEATING															❦										
TALKING																				❦					
TOUCH			❦			❦					❦							❦							
TOUCH (LIGHT)													❦												
UNCOVERING											❦								❦						
WAKING													❦												
WARM TO COLD AIR																				❦					
WARM DRINKS													❦								❦				
WARM ROOM	❦																								
WARMTH	❦	❦																				❦			
BETTER																									
BEING CARRIED									❦																
COLD				❦			❦																		
COLD DRINKS				❦								❦	❦												
CONTINUED MOTION																							❦		

Throat Complaints 3

This part of the chart shows **further possible modalities** and **some of the sensations** which may be experienced in throat complaints. Read down the list to find which ones are relevant to you. The symbols on the chart indicate the remedies most suitable for each variable. Once you have established the modalities and identified some of the sensations experienced in the particular case you are taking, and noted the possible remedies, turn to the following pages to trace the remedies that suit the other elements in your case. As you work your way through the chart, following the system of symbols, you should be able to eliminate unsuitable remedies and eventually make a final selection that matches your case as nearly as possible.

The remedy names are given in an abbreviated form in the charts. Full names are given in the key below.

REMEDY KEY

Acon.	Aconitum napellus	**Gels.**	Gelsemium sempervirens	**Nit. ac.**	Nitricum acidum
Apis	Apis mellifica	**Hep.**	Hepar sulphuris calcareum	**Nux v.**	Nux vomica
Arg. n.	Argentum nitricum	**Lac c.**	Lac caninum	**Phos.**	Phosphorus
Arn.	Arnica montana	**Lach.**	Lachesis	**Phyt.**	Phytolacca decandra
Ars.	Arsenicum album	**Lyc.**	Lycopodium clavatum	**Puls.**	Pulsatilla nigricans
Bell.	Belladonna	**Merc.**	Mercurius vivus	**Rhus t.**	Rhus toxicodendron
Bry.	Bryonia alba	**Merc. cy.**	Mercurius cyanatus	**Sil.**	Silicea
Carb.v.	Carbo vegetabilis	**Nat. m.**	Natrum muriaticum	**Sulph.**	Sulphur
Cham.	Chamomilla				

REMEDY	Acon.	Arg. n.	Arn.	Apis	Ars.	Bell.	Bry.	Carb. v.	Cham.	Gels.	Hep.	Lac c.	Lach.	Lyc.	Merc.	Merc. cy.	Nat. m.	Nit. ac.	Nux v.	Phos.	Phyt.	Puls.	Rhus t.	Sil.	Sulph.
MODALITIES (CONTINUED)																									
BETTER (CONTINUED)																									
FRESH AIR		•																							
GENTLE MOTION																						•			
HEAT					•						•												•		
HEAT (BURNING PAINS)					•																				
HEAT WITH FEVER																			•						
LYING WITH HEAD HIGH										•															
LYING PROPPED UP										•															
OPEN, COOL AIR																						•			
PRESSURE													•												
SWEAT																	•								
SWALLOWING SOLIDS													•												
WARM DRINKS					•						•	•		•									•		
SENSATIONS *how the throat and pains in the throat feel*																									
BURNING	•			•	•								•					•			•				•
BURNING LIKE COALS						•																			
BURNING (INTENSE)						•														•					
CHILLY											•							•	•		•				
CHILLS UP AND DOWN BACK										•															
CHOKING													•					•							
CHOKING FROM CLOTHES AT NECK													•												
CHOKES (AS IF WOULD)	•											•													
CLUTCHING						•																			
COLD DRINKS (DESIRES)		•																							
COLD DRINKS (BRING ON COUGH)							•																		
CONSTRICTION				•									•						•	•		•			
CONSTRICTION (SPASMODIC)						•			•																
COTTON OR VELVET (SENSATION OF)																				•					
COVERED (DESIRE TO BE)																					•				

DRAWS HEAD DOWN																		•							
DRY			•		•	•		•				•		•					•	•					
DRY (APPEARS WET)															•										
DRY MUCOUS MEMBRANES																	•						•		•
DRY PARCHED							•																		
DRYNESS (GREAT)	•					•							•		•		•								
DYSPHAGIA																		•							
EARS (PAIN GOES TO)																		•			•				
FEVER (HIGH)										•															
FOOD STICKS ON WAY DOWN																	•								
FULL, AS IF CHOKED																					•				
HEAT (CHILLY ON UNCOVERING)																			•						
HAIR (SENSATION OF)																									•
HARD COUGH					•																				
HOARSE								•																	
HUNGER (VIOLENT)																				•					
HYPERESTHESIA												•													
HUSKY												•													
LARYNX SENSITIVE TO COLD																				•					
LARYNX SENSITIVE TO TOUCH																				•					
LEMONADE (DESIRES)						•																			
LUMP (SENSATION OF)						•					•		•								•	•			•
LUMP SENSATION (ON SWALLOWING)														•			•								
MUCUS BAD TASTING								•																	
MOUTH SORE																		•							
MOUTH DRY																						•			
NONDESCRIPT PAINS							•																		
PAIN EXTENDS TO ESOPHAGUS																				•					
PAIN WITH CHILL																						•			
ON FIRST SWALLOWING																							•		
SEVERE	•												•												
PAINFUL (VERY)	•																								
PARALYTIC WEAKNESS															•										
PRESSING																									•
PLUG (PAIN AS FROM)									•																
RASPING					•																				
RAW		•		•		•		•					•	•	•	•		•	•	•					•
ROUGH	•	•	•		•														•	•	•	•			•
SCRAPING	•	•			•			•											•			•			•
SENSITIVE TO TOUCH											•	•	•												•
SEVERE PAIN									•					•											
SHUDDERING										•															
SKIN HOT										•															

The illustration shows phosphorus, the source for the Phosphorus remedy.

Throat Complaints 4

This part of the chart shows **further possible sensations** which may be experienced in throat complaints and **some of the concomitants** which may appear with them. Read down the list to find which ones are relevant to you. The symbols on the chart indicate the remedies most suitable for each variable. Once you have established the sensations and identified some of the concomitants in the particular case you are taking, and noted the possible remedies, turn to the following pages to trace the remedies that suit the other elements in your case. As you work your way through the chart, following the system of symbols, you should be able to eliminate unsuitable remedies and eventually make a final selection that matches your case as nearly as possible.

The remedy names are given in an abbreviated form in the charts. Full names are given in the key below.

REMEDY KEY

Acon.	Aconitum napellus	**Gels.**	Gelsemium sempervirens	**Nit. ac.**	Nitricum acidum
Apis	Apis mellifica	**Hep.**	Hepar sulphuris calcareum	**Nux v.**	Nux vomica
Arg. n.	Argentum nitricum	**Lac c.**	Lac caninum	**Phos.**	Phosphorus
Arn.	Arnica montana	**Lach.**	Lachesis	**Phyt.**	Phytolacca decandra
Ars.	Arsenicum album	**Lyc.**	Lycopodium clavatum	**Puls.**	Pulsatilla nigricans
Bell.	Belladonna	**Merc.**	Mercurius vivus	**Rhus t.**	Rhus toxicodendron
Bry.	Bryonia alba	**Merc. cy.**	Mercurius cyanatus	**Sil.**	Silicea
Carb.v.	Carbo vegetabilis	**Nat. m.**	Natrum muriaticum	**Sulph.**	Sulphur
Cham.	Chamomilla				

REMEDY	Acon.	Arg. n.	Arn.	Apis	Ars.	Bell.	Bry.	Carb. v.	Cham.	Gels.	Hep.	Lac. c.	Lach.	Lyc.	Merc.	Merc. cy.	Nat. m.	Nit. ac.	Nux v.	Phos.	Phyt.	Puls.	Rhus. t.	Sil.	Sulph.
SENSATIONS (CONTINUED)																									
SMARTING	✓							✓							✓						✓				
SORE		✓	✓	✓		✓		✓	✓	✓		✓		✓	✓	✓		✓	✓	✓	✓		✓		
SORE WITH EVERY COLD															✓										
SORENESS COMES ON GRADUALLY										✓															
SOMETHING STUCK (SENSATION OF)											✓							✓							
SPASMS IN THROAT	✓					✓			✓																✓
SPLINTER (SENSATION OF)											✓														
SPLINTER PAINS		✓		✓								✓	✓				✓	✓			✓			✓	✓
STINGING				✓														✓				✓			
ON SWALLOWING																								✓	
SEVERE															✓										
STITCHING																	✓								✓
STITCHES ON SWALLOWING														✓						✓					
STRANGULATED		✓																							
SWALLOW (CANNOT)	✓							✓																	
DESIRE TO													✓								✓				
DIFFICULT													✓		✓										✓
IMPOSSIBLE												✓													
PAINS WORSE																						✓			
PAINFUL	✓					✓					✓		✓		✓			✓							✓
SWELLING											✓														
SWELLING (SENSATION OF)								✓															✓		✓
TASTE BAD																						✓			
TASTE SWEET, SALT, METALLIC, FOUL															✓										
TASTES BITTER (EVERYTHING)	✓																								
TEARING	✓																								
TENSION																			✓						
THIRST FOR FREQUENT SIPS					✓																				
FOR LARGE VOLUMES							✓																		

FOR ICE COLD WATER					❀																				
VIOLENT																							❀		
GREAT	❀						❀	❀																	
AND DRYNESS (GREAT)																				❀					
DURING CHILL			❀																						
THIRSTY			❀												❀										❀
THIRSTLESS				❀		❀							❀					❀				❀			
THROBBING						❀					❀														
TICKLING																						❀			
TICKING COUGH																			❀						
TIGHTNESS																			❀						
TINGLING	❀																								
TONGUE (PAIN IN ROOT)																					❀				
PAIN ON PROTRUSION																					❀				
SWOLLEN																									
ULCERS STING AND BURN															❀										
CONCOMITANTS *other symptoms that come on with the throat complaint*																									
APPETITE POOR									❀																
BED FEELS HARD			❀																						
BODY COLD			❀																						
BODY VERY SORE			❀																						
BLEEDING								❀																	
BREATH COLD								❀																	
CAROTIDS THROBBING						❀																			❀
CATARRHAL STATES																									
CATARRH (COPIOUS)		❀									❀														
CHEESY ODOR											❀													❀	
CHRONIC																						❀		❀	
IN THROAT																									
CHILLINESS IN FEVER					❀																				
CHOKING													❀												
COLDNESS								❀																	
CONSTIPATION																			❀						
CORYZA WHITE						❀																			
WITH SNEEZING					❀							❀													
THIN BY DAY																			❀	❀					
COUGH (SUPPRESSED)																									
COUGH (TICKLING HARD)					❀																				
DELIRIUM WITH JERKING						❀																			
DIGESTIVE UPSETS																			❀						
DIGESTIVE SOURNESS																			❀						
DISCHARGES (BLAND)																						❀			

The illustration shows the poison nut plant, the source for the Nux vomica remedy.

Throat Complaints 5

This part of the chart shows **further possible concomitants** which may be experienced in throat complaints. Read down the list to find which ones are relevant to you. The symbols on the chart indicate the remedies most suitable for each variable. Once you have observed the concomitants in the particular case you are taking, and noted the possible remedies, turn to the following pages to trace the remedies that suit the other elements in your case. As you work your way through the chart, following the system of symbols, you should be able to eliminate unsuitable remedies and eventually make a final selection that matches your case as nearly as possible.

The remedy names are given in an abbreviated form in the charts. Full names are given in the key below.

REMEDY KEY

Acon.	Aconitum napellus	**Gels.**	Gelsemium sempervirens	**Nit. ac.**	Nitricum acidum
Apis	Apis mellifica	**Hep.**	Hepar sulphuris calcareum	**Nux v.**	Nux vomica
Arg. n.	Argentum nitricum			**Phos.**	Phosphorus
Arn.	Arnica montana	**Lac c.**	Lac caninum	**Phyt.**	Phytolacca decandra
Ars.	Arsenicum album	**Lach.**	Lachesis	**Puls.**	Pulsatilla nigricans
Bell.	Belladonna	**Lyc.**	Lycopodium clavatum	**Rhus t.**	Rhus toxicodendron
Bry.	Bryonia alba	**Merc.**	Mercurius vivus	**Sil.**	Silicea
Carb.v.	Carbo vegetabilis	**Merc. cy.**	Mercurius cyanatus	**Sulph.**	Sulphur
Cham.	Chamomilla	**Nat. m.**	Natrum muriaticum		

REMEDY	Acon.	Arg. n.	Arn.	Apis	Ars.	Bell.	Bry.	Carb. v.	Cham.	Gels.	Hep.	Lac. c.	Lach.	Lyc.	Merc.	Merc. cy.	Nat. m.	Nit. ac.	Nux v.	Phos.	Phyt.	Puls.	Rhus. t.	Sil.	Sulph.
CONCOMITANTS (CONTINUED)																									
PROFUSE																						•			
YELLOW GREEN								•														•			
DRYNESS															•										
FACE RED, CONGESTED	•					•																			
LATER DUSKY						•																			
PURPLE, CONGESTED													•												
FLUSHES																						•			
VERY RED IN FEVER																			•						
FEVER (HIGH)						•				•															
VIOLENT, HIGH	•																								
WITH COLD EXTREMITIES										•														•	
EVENING AND NIGHT								•																	
WITH CHILLS, WORSE HEAT				•																					
FOOD AND DRINK REGURGITATE												•		•											
FOUL ODOR																		•							
GLANDS ENLARGED, SORE						•																		•	
SWOLLEN									•				•		•						•		•		
HARD																					•				
HEAD HOT			•			•																			
CONGESTED														•											
BETTER COOL AND UNCOVERED														•											
HEAT (FLUSHES OF)																								•	
HEADACHE						•																			
PRECEDES OR ACCOMPANIES COMPLAINTS							•																		
BURSTING, CONGESTIVE							•																		
INFLAMMATION (LOW GRADE)																					•				
HIGH GRADE	•																								
LARYNGITIS WITH HOARSENESS																				•					
TOO PAINFUL TO TALK																				•					

LIMBS COLD						✽																			
MOUTH SORE BLEEDING																				✽					
OFFENSIVE															✽										
MUCUS (THICK, TENACIOUS)																					✽				
THICK IN THROAT		✽																✽							
HAWKS						✽																			
MUSCULAR WEAKNESS										✽															
NASAL DISCHARGE COPIOUS WATERY								✽																	
THICK YELLOW, GREEN OFFENSIVE															✽										
NECK STIFF																							✽		
SWOLLEN																							✽		
MUSCLES INFLAMED, TENDER													✽												
NOSE BLOCKED														✽											
ORIFICES OF BODY RED																									✽
PALLOR								✽																	
PARALYSIS												✽													
PARALYSIS OF PHARYNX													✽												
PAROTIDS SWOLLEN																								✽	
PERSPIRATION AT NIGHT											✽														
PERSPIRATION ALTERNATES DRY SKIN				✽																					
PUPILS DILATED						✽																			
QUINSY											✽				✽									✽	
RASHES (DRY, ROUGH)				✽																					
REDNESS	✽								✽																
RESTLESS			✽																						
SALIVA ACRID																		✽							
PROFUSE															✽										
STRINGY, STICKY													✽												
SWEET, SALTY, FOUL																				✽					
SKIN COLD								✽																	
SKIN DRY				✽																					
SNEEZING (MUCH)					✽	✽																			
FROM ITCHING																			✽						
SUPPURATION															✽									✽	
RIGHT TO LEFT													✽												
SWEAT (HEAD AND NECK)																								✽	
SWEAT (COLD)								✽																	
SWEAT IN WARM ROOM								✽																	
SWEATING (MARKED)															✽										
THIRSTLESS				✽																					
TIRED AND HEAVY										✽															
THROAT BLEEDS EASILY					✽																				
BLUISH RED													✽								✽	✽			
DARK RED		✽																			✽				

The illustration shows deadly nightshade, the source for the Belladonna remedy.

Throat Complaints 6

This part of the chart shows **further possible concomitants** which may be experienced in throat complaints and any **general mental symptoms** that may be observed. Read down the list to find which ones are relevant to you. The symbols on the chart indicate the remedies most suitable for each variable. Once you have established the concomitants and observed any mental symptoms in the particular case you are taking, and noted the possible remedies, turn to the following pages to trace the remedies that suit the other elements in your case. As you work your way through the chart, following the system of symbols, you should be able to eliminate unsuitable remedies and eventually make a final selection that matches your case as nearly as possible.

The remedy names are given in an abbreviated form in the charts. Full names are given in the key below.

REMEDY KEY

Acon.	Aconitum napellus
Apis	Apis mellifica
Arg. n.	Argentum nitricum
Arn.	Arnica montana
Ars.	Arsenicum album
Bell.	Belladonna
Bry.	Bryonia alba
Carb.v.	Carbo vegetabilis
Cham.	Chamomilla
Gels.	Gelsemium sempervirens
Hep.	Hepar sulphuris calcareum
Lac c.	Lac caninum
Lach.	Lachesis
Lyc.	Lycopodium clavatum
Merc.	Mercurius vivus
Merc. cy.	Mercurius cyanatus
Nat. m.	Natrum muriaticum
Nit. ac.	Nitricum acidum
Nux v.	Nux vomica
Phos.	Phosphorus
Phyt.	Phytolacca decandra
Puls.	Pulsatilla nigricans
Rhus t.	Rhus toxicodendron
Sil.	Silcica
Sulph.	Sulphur

REMEDY	Acon.	Arg. n.	Arn.	Apis	Ars.	Bell.	Bry.	Carb. v.	Cham.	Gels.	Hep.	Lac. c.	Lach.	Lyc.	Merc.	Merc. cy.	Nat. m.	Nit. ac.	Nux v.	Phos.	Phyt.	Puls.	Rhus. t.	Sil.	Sulph.
CONCOMITANTS (CONTINUED)																									
FEELS SWOLLEN													❀												
RAW IN SPOTS																❀									
RED AND PALE															❀										
RED, SHRIVELLED					❀																				
RED AND SWOLLEN						❀																			
PURPLE													❀												
ULCERATED		❀			❀																❀				
SWELLING		❀		❀							❀		❀		❀						❀				
TONGUE DRY																							❀		
COATED							❀														❀	❀	❀		
FLABBY															❀										
RED STRAWBERRY						❀																			
RED TRIANGLE TIP																							❀		
SWOLLEN				❀										❀											
THICK, YELLOW, MOIST															❀										
WHITE							❀																		
TONSILS DUSKY PURPLE											❀														❀
RED						❀				❀															
RED AND SWOLLEN						❀																			
WORSE RIGHT						❀																			
SWELLING				❀							❀							❀		❀	❀				❀
SUPPURATION											❀														❀
YELLOW PATCHES																		❀							
ULCERATION				❀																	❀				❀
ULCERS (APTHOUS)						❀	❀	❀					❀												
BLEEDING						❀											❀								
DARK, PUTRID																	❀								
DEEP													❀												
DRY, GLISTENING												❀													
LARDACEOUS BASE																									

OOZE BLACK BLOOD								●																	
PIN HEAD						●																			
RAGGED, JAGGED																	●								
RED GREY													●												
WHITE																	●								
URINE SCANTY				●																					
STRONG SMELLING																	●								
UVULA SWOLLEN				●														●		●					
EDEMA				●																					
VEINS DISTENDED																						●			
VOICE LOST		●																							
GENERALS *symptoms that affect the whole person*																									
MENTAL																									
ALONE (WANTS TO BE)			●				●																		
(CAN'T BEAR TO BE)												●													
ANXIETY	●				●																		●		
ANGERED EASILY											●														
CAPRICIOUS									●																
CLINGY																						●			
FEAR	●																								
GENTLE																						●			
HYSTERICAL												●													
IMPULSIVE		●																							
IRRITABLE							●		●		●								●				●		
MILD																						●			
NERVOUS		●																							
NIGHTMARES			●																						
NOTHING PLEASES									●																
OFFENDED EASILY																	●								
OVERSENSITIVE																			●						
PEACE (WANTS)							●																		
RESTLESSNESS	●				●																				
SAYS IS ALL RIGHT			●																						
SEES SPIDERS, SNAKES, VERMIN												●													
SENSITIVE												●					●								
TALK (DOESN'T WANT TO)			●				●																		
TEARFUL																						●			
THINKS HAS TERRIBLE DISEASE												●													
TORMENTING THOUGHTS												●													
TOUCHY											●														
TEMPER OUT OF CONTROL									●																
WANTS FUSS AND HELP																						●			
WEEPY																							●		

The illustration shows rock salt, the source for the Natrum muriaticum remedy.

Throat Complaints 7

This part of the chart shows **further possible general mental and physical symptoms** that may be observed. Read down the list to find which ones are relevant to you. The symbols on the chart indicate the remedies most suitable for each variable. By assessing the data you have collected while consulting the chart, you should now be able to make a final selection to match your case as nearly as possible.

The remedy names are given in an abbreviated form in the charts. Full names are given in the key below.

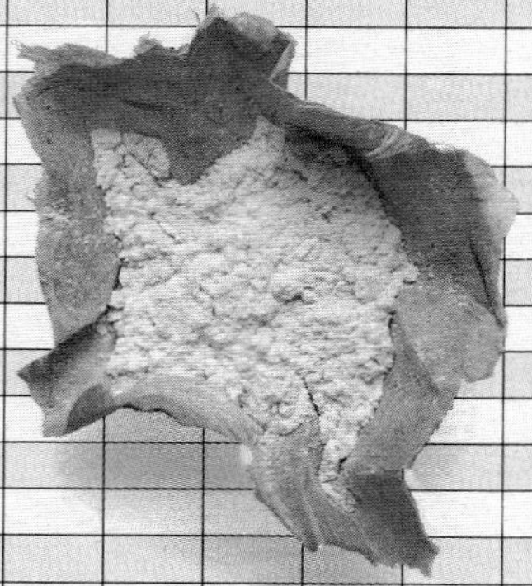

REMEDY	Acon.	Arg. n.	Arn.	Apis	Ars.	Bell.	Bry.	Carb. v.	Cham.	Gels.	Hep.	Lac. c.	Lach.	Lyc.	Merc.	Merc. cy.	Nat. m.	Nit. ac.	Nux v.	Phos.	Phyt.	Puls.	Rhus. t.	Sil.	Sulph.
GENERALS (CONTINUED)																									
PHYSICAL																									
ACHING IN BODY																					●		●		
BREAST COMPLAINTS																					●				
CHANGEABLE SYMPTOMS																						●			
CHEST (GOES TO)					●																				
CHILLY					●													●	●					●	
CHILLY, WORSE DRAFTS																								●	
CHOKING ON WAKING													●												
ON GOING TO SLEEP													●												
COLD ROOM AND AIR (DESIRES)		●																							
CONSTRICTIONS					●																				
CORYZA (RECURRENT)																		●							
COUGH DRY, HACKING					●																				
CRAMPS AND DRAWING PAINS																					●				
FACE FLUSHES				●																					
FACE FLUSHES (AFTER WINE)								●																	
FATS (LOVES)																		●							
FOLLOWS PULSATILLA WELL																								●	
FRESH AIR (DESIRES)														●											
INTENSE AND VIOLENT SYMPTOMS	●																								
LETHARGY																									●
LINGERING SORE THROAT																									●
OFFENSIVE BREATH, SWEAT, DISCHARGES																									●
ODORS															●	●									
OVERHEATS EASILY																								●	
OVERHEATING BRINGS ON COMPLAINTS								●																	
PROGRESS AND ONSET RAPID						●																			
PROSTRATE					●																				
RESTLESS																									
RESTLESSNESS MAKES PAINS WORSE																									
SALT (DESIRES)																		●							

REMEDY KEY

Acon.	Aconitum napellus	**Gels.**	Gelsemium sempervirens	**Nit. ac.**	Nitricum acidum
Apis	Apis mellifica	**Hep.**	Hepar sulphuris calcareum	**Nux v.**	Nux vomica
Arg. n.	Argentum nitricum	**Lac c.**	Lac caninum	**Phos.**	Phosphorus
Arn.	Arnica montana	**Lach.**	Lachesis	**Phyt.**	Phytolacca decandra
Ars.	Arsenicum album	**Lyc.**	Lycopodium clavatum	**Puls.**	Pulsatilla nigricans
Bell.	Belladonna	**Merc.**	Mercurius vivus	**Rhus t.**	Rhus toxicodendron
Bry.	Bryonia alba	**Merc. cy.**	Mercurius cyanatus	**Sil.**	Silicea
Carb.v.	Carbo vegetabilis	**Nat. m.**	Natrum muriaticum	**Sulph.**	Sulphur
Cham.	Chamomilla				

SENSITIVE TO PAIN									●																
HEAT															●	●					●				
COLD															●	●					●				
SENSES HYPERSENSITIVE											●														
SINKING					●																				
SORENESS BACK OF HEAD, NECK													●												
SPASMS																									
STANDING (DISLIKES)																									
STARTS AND JUMPS IN HIGH FEVER						●																			
STUPOR IN FEVER							●																		
SUFFOCATES IN WARM ROOM																									
FROM HEAT				●																	●				
SURGINGS OF BLOOD													●												●
SWEETS (DESIRES)		●																							
TAKES COLD EASILY WHEN SWEATING																	●								
THROAT (COLDS SETTLE IN)																								●	
TONSILS CHRONICALLY ENLARGED											●														
TREMBLING															●	●									
VIGOROUS HEALTH WHEN NOT SICK	●																								
WEAKNESS															●	●									
WEAKNESS (DISPROPORTIONATE)					●																			●	
WEIGHT AND TIREDNESS										●															
COMPARISON OF REMEDIES																									
NOT FOR LINGERING STATES	●					●																			
NOT VERY SICK														●											
NOT USED EARLY IN ILLNESS											●				●	●									
NOT BE REPEATED TOO OFTEN															●	●									

The illustration shows arsenious oxide, the source for the Arsenicum album remedy.

WHEN TO SEEK ADVICE

Urgently, right now!

- If the throat is so severely swollen as to cause difficulty breathing.
- If the pain is very severe with inability to swallow and much drooling.
- If there is bleeding from the mouth with measles.

Within 24 hours

- If unusual and very marked swelling occurs around the tonsils on one or both sides.
- Severe sore throats persisting more than a day or two in a young child without signs of improvement.
- If there has been a history of rheumatic fever in the past.

Refer to other chapters as necessary.

Abdominal Complaints 1

The first part of this chart shows the possible **causes and onsets** of abdominal problems and **some of the sensations** that may be experienced (note that the remedies indicated for sensations are slightly different from those for cause and onset). Read down the list to find which ones are r ant to you. The symb on the chart indicate the remedies most suitable for each variable. Once you have established the cause and onset and any possible sensations in the particular case you are taking, and noted the possible remedies, turn to the following pages to trace the remedies that suit the other elements in your case. As you work your way through the chart, following the system of symbols, you should be able to eliminate unsuitable remedies and eventually make a final selection that matches your case.

The remedy names are given in an abbreviated form in the charts. Full names are given in the key below.

REMEDY KEY	
Acon.	Aconite napellus
Ant. c.	Antimonium crudum
Ant. t.	Antimonium tartaricum
Ars.	Arsenicum album
Bell.	Belladonna
Bry.	Bryonia alba
Carb. v.	Carbo vegetabilis
Cham.	Chamomilla
Chin.	China officinalis
Coloc.	Colocynthis
Dios.	Dioscorea villosa
Dulc.	Dulcamara
Gels.	Gelsemium sempervirens
Ip.	Ipecacuanha
Lyc.	Lycopodium clavatum
Mag.p.	Magnesia phosphorica
Nat.s.	Natrum sulphuricum
Nux v.	Nux vomica
Phos.	Phosphorus
Pod.	Podophyllum peltatum.
Puls.	Pulsatilla nigricans
Sep.	Sepia
Sil.	Silica
Sulph.	Sulphur
Verat.	Veratrum album.

REMEDY	Acon.	Ant. c.	Ant. t.	Bell.	Bry.	Chin.	Coloc.	Dulc.	Gels.	Ip.	Lyc.	Mag. p.	Nat. s.	Nux v.	Phos.	Pod.	Puls.	Sep.	Sil.	Sulph.	Verat.
CAUSE *why symptoms come on*																					
ANGER							•														
ANTICIPATION									•												
CHILL				•																	
COLD					•							•									
COLD DAMP								•				•									
COLD DRINKS WHEN OVERHEATED					•																
COLD IN HOT WEATHER	•																				
COLD WHEN HEATED								•													
DRINKING WHEN OVERHEATED							•														
EMOTIONAL UPSET									•												
EXCESS STIMULANTS														•							
EATING WHAT DISAGREES		•																			
GOING FROM HOT TO COLD								•													
INDIGNATION							•														
OVEREATING					•					•				•					•		
OVERWORK														•							
PREGNANCY										•								•			
RICH FOOD							•			•							•				
SEAFOOD											•										
SOUR FOOD, FRUIT, WINE		•	•																		
STORMY WEATHER															•						
SUPPRESSED EMOTION										•											
TAKING OFFENCE							•														
WET WEATHER													•								
ONSET *when and how symptoms come on*																					
NIGHT (DIARRHEA)						•															
RAPID			•							•											
SUDDEN	•																				
SUDDEN PAINS															•						

REMEDY	Acon.	Ant. c.	Ant. t.	Ars.	Bell.	Bry.	Carb. v.	Cham.	Chin.	Coloc.	Dios.	Dulc.	Ip.	Lyc.	Mag. p.	Nat. s.	Nux v.	Phos.	Pod.	Puls.	Sep.	Sil.	Sulph.	Verat.
SENSATIONS *how the abdomen and pain in the abdomen feel*																								
ACIDS AND PICKLES (DESIRES AND BETTER FOR)		❦																						
ALL GONE WEAK																			❦					
ANGUISH WITH PAIN				❦																				
ANUS RAW							❦																	
BENDS DOUBLE																	❦							❦
BELCHING							❦							❦										
BELCHING DOES NOT RELIEVE									❦															
BLOATED									❦											❦				
BOWELS SORE									❦															
COLD SOUR THINGS (DESIRED AND VOMITED)			❦																					
COLIC	❦		❦		❦			❦		❦	❦	❦	❦		❦		❦			❦		❦		
AS IF DIARRHEA WOULD COME ON												❦												
IN INFANTS								❦							❦									
NOT BETTER FOR STOOL											❦													
VIOLENT					❦					❦														
WITH NAUSEA AND GREEN STOOL													❦											
WITH NO WIND																							❦	
CONGESTION																							❦	
CRAMPS															❦									
INTENSE															❦									
DISTENTION			❦	❦	❦	❦	❦		❦					❦	❦	❦	❦	❦			❦			
DISTENTION AFTER EATING								❦						❦										
DOUBLE UP								❦											❦					
EATING (WORSE AFTER)						❦																	❦	
EATING (NOT BETTER FOR)																					❦			
EATS MUCH																							❦	
EMPTY																		❦	❦		❦			
ERUCTATIONS (CONSTANT, LOUD)									❦															
FAINT SINKING																					❦			❦
FLATULENCE	❦		❦				❦			❦				❦	❦	❦	❦				❦	❦	❦	
GREAT											❦				❦									
FULLNESS							❦							❦		❦								
HUNGER																		❦					❦	
KICKS AND SCREAMS (CHILD)								❦																
LOATHING FOR FOOD, DRINK		❦																						
LOOSENS CLOTHING														❦										
MOUTH DRY (THIRSTLESS)																				❦				
MOUTH DRY AND BITTER											❦													
NOISY RUMBLINGS														❦										

The illustration shows the bitter cucumber plant, the source of the Colocynthis remedy.

Abdominal Complaints 2

This part of the chart shows **further sensations** that may be experienced. Read down the list to find which ones are relevant to you. The symbols on the chart indicate the remedies most suitable for each variable. Once you have established any possible sensations in the particular case you are taking, and noted the possible remedies, turn to the following pages to trace the remedies that suit the other elements in your case. As you work your way through the chart, following the system of symbols, you should be able to eliminate unsuitable remedies and eventually make a final selection that matches your case as nearly as possible.

The remedy names are given in an abbreviated form in the charts. Full names are given in the key below.

REMEDY KEY

Acon.	Aconite napellus
Ant. c.	Antimonium crudum
Ant. t.	Antimonium tartaricum
Ars.	Arsenicum album
Bell.	Belladonna
Bry.	Bryonia alba
Carb. v.	Carbo vegetabilis
Cham.	Chamomilla
Chin.	China officinalis
Coloc.	Colocynthis
Dios.	Dioscorea villosa
Dulc.	Dulcamara
Gels.	Gelsemium sempervirens
Ip.	Ipecacuanha
Lyc.	Lycopodium clavatum
Mag.p.	Magnesia phosphorica
Nat.s.	Natrum sulphuricum
Nux v.	Nux vomica
Phos.	Phosphorus
Pod.	Podophyllum peltatum.
Puls.	Pulsatilla nigricans
Sep.	Sepia
Sil.	Silica
Sulph.	Sulphur
Verat.	Veratrum album.

REMEDY	Acon.	Ant. c.	Ant. t.	Ars.	Bell.	Bry.	Carb. v.	Cham.	Chin.	Coloc.	Dios.	Dulc.	Ip.	Lyc.	Mag. p.	Nat. s.	Nux v.	Phos.	Pod.	Puls.	Sep.	Sil.	Sulph.	Verat.
SENSATIONS (CONTINUED)																								
PAINS																								
AGONIZING										✿														
BEARING DOWN																					✿			
BURNING	✿	✿		✿	✿	✿	✿	✿						✿				✿			✿		✿	✿
BURNING (BETTER FOR HEAT)				✿																				
CHANGEABLE																				✿				
CLUTCHING										✿														
COME AND GO											✿													
CONSTRICTING							✿																	
CRAMPING							✿			✿									✿					
CUTTING			✿					✿			✿	✿			✿		✿			✿				
DRAWING																				✿				
FREQUENT											✿													
FLITTING																				✿				
GNAWING														✿										
GRASPING										✿														
GRIPING					✿			✿			✿		✿		✿									✿
NIPPING, PINCHING															✿									
PAROXYSMS										✿														
RADIATING															✿									
RADIATING TO DISTANT PARTS											✿													
REAPPEAR IN DIFFERENT PLACE											✿													
RENDING																	✿							
SHARP													✿											
SHOOTING	✿										✿						✿							
STITCHING				✿		✿															✿			
TEARING										✿							✿	✿						✿
TWISTING												✿												✿

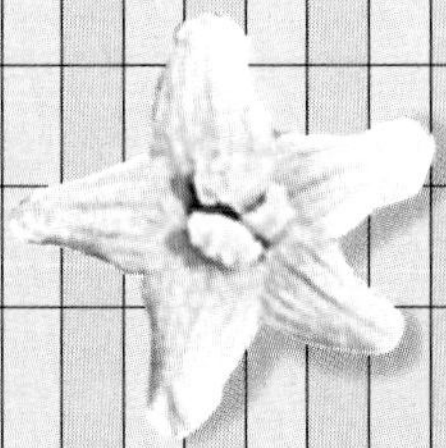

PASSING FLATUS (BETTER FOR)										✿															
PRESSURE PAIN																	✿	✿							
PRESSURE AND HEAVINESS														✿											
RECTUM SORE																			✿						
PROLAPSED																			✿						
PAINS SHOOT FROM OR TO																	✿								
PAINS SHOOT UPWARDS FROM																	✿								
RESTLESS															✿										
RUMBLINGS											✿					✿			✿	✿	✿				
RUMBLINGS AND GURGLINGS																✿									
RUMBLINGS PRECEDE STOOL																			✿						
SCAPULA (PAINS BETWEEN)													✿												
SORENESS						✿																	✿		
SORENESS FROM PRESSURE																						✿			
SPASMS IN STOMACH															✿										
STOMACH																									
ANXIETY IN			✿																						
AS IF WOULD BURST						✿																			
DISORDERED						✿	✿																		
DISTENDED		✿											✿												
OVERLOADED		✿																							
SENSITIVE TO TOUCH				✿		✿																			
SENSITIVE TO PRESSURE						✿																			
SINKING FEELING																								✿	
SENSATION OF LUMP		✿																							
SOUR							✿																		
WEIGHT IN STOMACH	✿					✿																			
WEIGHT IN STOMACH (SENSATION OF)																	✿			✿			✿		
STOOL (PAINS BEFORE)											✿														
SWEAT OFFENSIVE							✿																		
TASTE BAD																				✿					
TASTE PUTRID, BITTER																	✿								
TENESMUS													✿				✿								
TENDERNESS						✿											✿			✿					
THIRST						✿												✿							
THIRST FOR COLD SIPS				✿																					
THIRSTLESS		✿	✿																						
TONGUE CLEAN															✿										
UMBILICUS (PAINS IN)													✿												
VOMITS (AFTER PAROXYSMS)										✿															

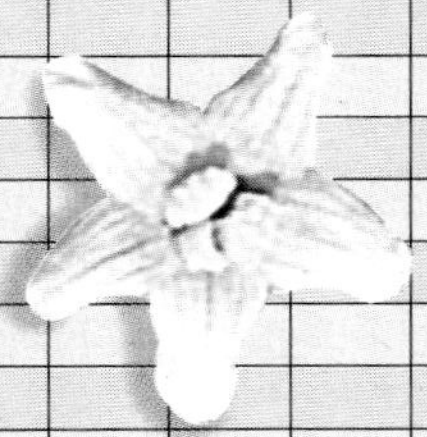

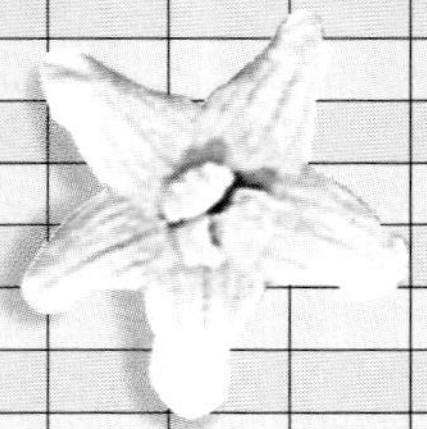

The illustration shows white bryony, the source for the Bryonia alba remedy.

Abdominal Complaints 3

This part of the chart shows **further sensations** that may be experienced. and describes the **character of diarrhea** experienced. Read down the list to find what is relevant to you. The symbols on the chart indicate the remedies most suitable for each variable. (Note that the diarrhea remedies are slightly different from those indicated for sensations.) Once you have established the sensations and identified the type of diarrhea suffered in the particular case you are taking, and noted the possible remedies, turn to the following pages to trace the remedies that suit the other elements in your case. As you work your way through the chart, following the system of symbols, you should be able to eliminate unsuitable remedies and eventually make a final selection that matches your case.

The remedy names are given in an abbreviated form in the charts. Full names are given in the key below.

REMEDY KEY

Acon.	Aconite napellus	**Coloc.**	Colocynthis	**Phos.**	Phosphorus
Ant. c.	Antimonium crudum	**Dios.**	Dioscorea villosa	**Pod.**	Podophyllum peltatum.
Ant. t.	Antimonium tartaricum	**Dulc.**	Dulcamara	**Puls.**	Pulsatilla nigricans
Ars.	Arsenicum album	**Gels.**	Gelsemium sempervirens	**Sep.**	Sepia
Bell.	Belladonna	**Ip.**	Ipecacuanha	**Sil.**	Silica
Bry.	Bryonia alba	**Lyc.**	Lycopodium clavatum	**Sulph.**	Sulphur
Carb. v.	Carbo vegetabilis	**Mag.p.**	Magnesia phosphorica	**Verat.**	Veratrum album.
Cham.	Chamomilla	**Nat.s.**	Natrum sulphuricum		
Chin.	China officinalis	**Nux v.**	Nux vomica		

REMEDY	Acon.	Ant. c.	Ant. t.	Ars.	Bell.	Bry.	Carb. v.	Cham.	Chin.	Coloc.	Dios.	Dulc.	Gels	Ip.	Lyc.	Nat. s.	Nux v.	Phos.	Pod.	Puls.	Sep.	Sil.	Sulph.	Verat.
DIARRHEA																								
ANUS (AS IF OPEN)																		●						
SORE																							●	
BURNS AND RAW																							●	
AS IF DIARRHEA WOULD COME ON																●								
BLOOD (LITTLE)																				●				
BLOODY																		●						
CHRONIC																					●			
CONSTIPATION																	●							
HARD						●																		
ALTERNATES WITH																				●				
COPIOUS									●															
CRAMPS (IN ANUS)																		●						
CUTTING PAINS IN ABDOMEN (PRECEDE)						●																		
DAY TIME						●																		
DRIVES FROM BED											●												●	
DYSENTERY WITH BLOOD AND SLIME	●																							
DYSENTERY WITH BLOODY DIARRHEA				●																				
EARLY MORNING																							●	
EMOTION (FROM)													●										●	
EXPLOSIVE																			●					
FAINTING (MAY CAUSE)																			●					
FETID																		●						
FLATULENCE							●			●									●	●				
FLATUS ONLY																●								
FOAMING														●										
FREQUENT																			●					
GUSHING																●		●	●					

HOT (FEELS)								❦																	
HOT WEATHER (DURING)																						❦			
IN INFANTS												❦													
LITTLE AND OFTEN		❦																							
LIQUID		❦																							
LUMPS		❦																			❦				
LUMPS OF WHITE MUCUS																		❦							
MORNING (EARLY)											❦					❦									
MUCUS (GRASS GREEN)								❦																	
MILK (FROM DRINKING)																					❦				
NAUSEA (BEFORE)	❦																								
NERVOUS ANTICIPATION (FROM)													❦												
ODOR PUTRID				❦																					
OFFENSIVE							❦												❦		❦		❦		
PAINLESS									❦							❦			❦						
PERSPIRATION (BEFORE)	❦																								
PROFUSE														❦				❦	❦						
PURGING (UNTIL EXHAUSTED)																								❦	
PUTRID							❦																		
RESULT OF URGING (NONE OR A LITTLE)					❦																				
SEVERE										❦															
SMELL ROTTEN EGGS								❦																	
SLIGHT														❦											
STOOLS																									
ACRID				❦																					
BLOODY							❦							❦											
BURN				❦							❦			❦				❦							
CHOPPED EGGS (LIKE)								❦																	
COLORLESS																								❦	
COPIOUS																								❦	
DRY						❦																			
GREAT MASS																								❦	
GREEN	❦							❦						❦						❦				❦	
INVOLUNTARY													❦												
JELLY LIKE																					❦				
LOOSE																				❦					
MUCUS							❦			❦						❦		❦		❦	❦				
NO TWO ALIKE												❦								❦					
SCANTY																	❦								
SLIMY														❦											

The illustration shows phosphorus, the source for the Phosphorus remedy.

Abdominal Complaints 4

This part of the chart shows **further kinds of diarrhea** experienced and describes the character of **attendant nausea and vomiting**. Read down the list to find what is relevant to you. The symbols on the chart indicate the remedies most suitable for each variable. Once you have established the the type of diarrhea suffered and the nature of the nausea and vomiting experienced in the particular case you are taking, and noted the possible remedies, turn to the following pages to trace the remedies that suit the other elements in your case. As you work your way through the chart, following the system of symbols, you should be able to eliminate unsuitable remedies and eventually make a final selection that matches your case as nearly as possible.

The remedy names are given in an abbreviated form in the charts. Full names are given in the key below.

REMEDY KEY

Acon.	Aconite napellus	**Coloc.**	Colocynthis	**Phos.**	Phosphorus
Ant. c.	Antimonium crudum	**Dios.**	Dioscorea villosa	**Pod.**	Podophyllum peltatum
Ant. t.	Antimonium tartaricum	**Dulc.**	Dulcamara	**Puls.**	Pulsatilla nigricans
Ars.	Arsenicum album	**Gels.**	Gelsemium sempervirens	**Sep.**	Sepia
Bell.	Belladonna	**Ip.**	Ipecacuanha	**Sil.**	Silica
Bry.	Bryonia alba	**Lyc.**	Lycopodium clavatum	**Sulph.**	Sulphur
Carb. v.	Carbo vegetabilis	**Mag.p.**	Magnesia phosphorica	**Verat.**	Veratrum album.
Cham.	Chamomilla	**Nat.s.**	Natrum sulphuricum		
Chin.	China officinalis	**Nux v.**	Nux vomica		

REMEDY	Acon.	Ant. c.	Ant. t.	Ars.	Bell.	Bry.	Carb. v.	Cham.	Chin.	Coloc.	Dios.	Dulc.	Gels	Ip.	Lyc.	Nat. s.	Nux v.	Phos.	Pod.	Puls.	Sep.	Sil.	Sulph.	Verat.
DIARRHEA (CONTINUED)																								
STOOLS (CONT)																								
SOFT																				•				
SOUR CURDS																						•		
YELLOW											•	•												
YELLOW MUSHY						•																		
WATERY							•					•		•						•				•
SUDDEN													•											
STRAINING																	•							
TEETHING (WITH)								•														•		
TENESMUS		•		•										•			•	•					•	
GREAT	•																							
THIN																•								
URGING TO STOOL FREQUENT				•	•					•														
EXCESSIVE										•														
INEFFECTUAL																	•							
VOMITING SIMULTANEOUS																								•
WATERY																			•					
YELLOW (BRIGHT)																			•					
NAUSEA AND VOMITING																								
APPETITE (NONE)																	•							
ALL GONE HUNGRY FEELING																					•		•	
BILIOUS			•																					
BILIOUS AND ACRID																							•	
CATARRH		•																					•	
COLD AND SOUR THINGS VOMITED			•																					
COLD DRINKS VOMITED ON BECOMING WARM IN STOMACH																		•						
COLD SWEAT								•																

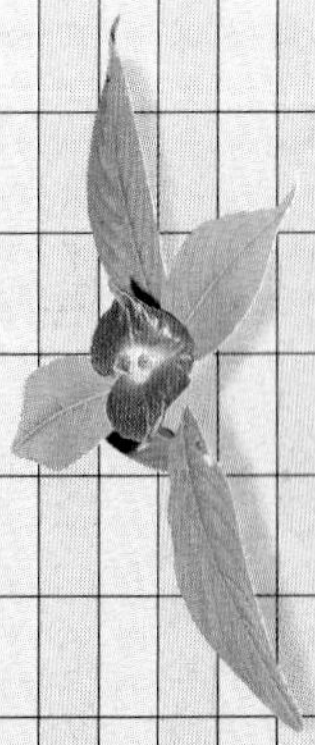

DESIRES PUNGENT, BITTER	●																								
DIARRHEA (SIMULTANEOUS)				●																				●	
EATING CAUSES UNEASINESS																	●								
EATING (WORSE FOR)																					●				
EATING (BETTER FOR)																					●				
EFFORT MUCH (TO VOMIT)																	●								
ERUCTATIONS																									
AS ROTTEN EGGS								●											●						
BILE														●											
BITTER									●							●	●								
OF BITTER FOOD																				●					
CONSTANT							●																		
EMPTY														●											
FOOD OR GAS																		●							
SOUR									●		●				●		●				●				
SOUR BURNING															●										
EVERYTHING VOMITED				●										●											
EXCESSIVE																								●	
EVENING (WORSE)																				●					
FORCIBLE																								●	
FOOD TURNS TO WIND							●																		
GAGGING			●																●						
HICCUP									●																
HUNGRY 11AM																							●		
LOATHING OF FOOD			●																						
MILK (AVERSE TO AND VOMITED)			●																						
MORNING (NAUSEA)														●							●				
MOUTH DRY (WITH THIRST)						●														●					
NERVOUS DYSPEPSIA, HEARTBURN, WATERBRASH															●										
NOTHING RELIEVES (NAUSEA)														●											
PAIN (VOMITS FROM)										●															
PAINFUL VOMITING				●																					
PUTRID BREATH								●																	
REGURGITATION							●																		
REFLUX SOUR																								●	
RUMBLINGS (NOISY)															●								●		
RETCHING	●	●	●														●								
AFTER VOMITING		●																							
VIOLENT	●		●					●																	
WITHOUT NAUSEA										●															
SALIVATION								●						●											

The illustration shows Cephaelis ipecacuanha, the source for the Ipecacuanha remedy.

Abdominal Complaints 5

This part of the chart shows further kinds of **nausea and vomiting** experienced and describes some of the **modalities** which may make the patient feel better or worse. Read down the list to find which ones are relevant to you. The symbols on the chart indicate the remedies most suitable for each variable. Once you have established the type of nausea and vomiting suffered and identified any modalities in the particular case you are taking, and noted the possible remedies, turn to the following pages to trace the remedies that suit the other elements in your case. As you work your way through the chart, following the system of symbols, you should be able to eliminate unsuitable remedies and eventually make a final selection that matches your case as nearly as possible.

The remedy names are given in an abbreviated form in the charts. Full names are given in the key below.

REMEDY KEY

Acon.	Aconite napellus	**Coloc.**	Colocynthis	**Phos.**	Phosphorus
Ant. c.	Antimonium crudum	**Dios.**	Dioscorea villosa	**Pod.**	Podophyllum peltatum.
Ant. t.	Antimonium tartaricum	**Dulc.**	Dulcamara	**Puls.**	Pulsatilla nigricans
Ars.	Arsenicum album	**Gels.**	Gelsemium sempervirens	**Sep.**	Sepia
Bell.	Belladonna	**Ip.**	Ipecacuanha	**Sil.**	Silica
Bry.	Bryonia alba	**Lyc.**	Lycopodium clavatum	**Sulph.**	Sulphur
Carb. v.	Carbo vegetabilis	**Mag.p.**	Magnesia phosphorica	**Verat.**	Veratrum album.
Cham.	Chamomilla	**Nat.s.**	Natrum sulphuricum		
Chin.	China officinalis	**Nux v.**	Nux vomica		

REMEDY	Acon.	Ant. c.	Ant. t.	Ars.	Bell.	Bry.	Carb. v.	Cham.	Chin.	Coloc.	Dios.	Dulc.	Gels	Ip.	Lyc.	Mag. p.	Nat. s.	Nux v.	Phos.	Pod.	Puls.	Sep.	Sil.	Sulph.	Verat.
NAUSEA AND VOMITING (CONTINUED)																									
STRAINING			●															●							
SUDDEN AND VIOLENT	●																								
SMELL OF FOOD COOKING (FROM)																						●			
SINKING (PIT OF STOMACH)											●														
TASTE																									
BAD (MORNING)																					●				
BITTER NAUSEATING						●																			
BITTER, SALTY									●																
BITTER (EVERYTHING)	●																								
DIMINISHED SENSE OF																					●				
SLIMY BITTER																	●								
TONGUE CLEAN														●											
SLIGHT COATING														●											
TOUCH (SENSITIVE TO)																								●	
VOMIT																									
BILE						●									●							●			
BLOOD (BRIGHT RED)	●																								
COFFEE GROUNDS															●										
MUCUS			●																			●			
SOUR																							●		
STRINGY			●																						
TENACIOUS			●																						
WHITE			●																						
WARM DRINKS RELIEVE				●																					
VOMITED				●															●						
WEAK STOMACH																							●		
ON WAKING						●																			

MODALITIES (GENERAL) *what makes patient of abdominal pains better or worse*

12AM AND 12PM																								●	
4–8PM															●										
WORSE																									
AT REST										●															
COLD				●					●						●	●		●							
DRINKING										●															
DOUBLING UP											●														
EATING						●				●					●			●					●	●	
ERUCTATIONS								●																	
EVENING																			●						
HEAT																					●				
LYING					●		●				●														
ON AFFECTED SIDE					●																				
JAR					●																				
MORNING																		●			●				
MOTION					●	●			●	●						●		●							
NIGHT																●									
OVEREATING														●											
PRESSURE					●	●	●								●					●			●		
SLIGHTEST																		●					●		
RICH FATTY FOOD																					●				
STRETCHED OUT																●									
TOUCH	●			●		●			●								●								
VOMITING (PAIN)																			●			●			
WARM THINGS																			●						
BETTER																									
APPLIED HEAT						●																			
BELCHING							●			●							●								
BENDING FORWARD					●																				
COLD																					●				
COLD THINGS																			●						
DOUBLING UP										●						●									
FLATUS										●							●								
FRESH AIR																					●				
HARD PRESSURE										●						●									
HEAT				●				●		●						●		●					●		
MOTION											●												●		
MOTION (GENTLE)																					●				

The illustration shows magnesium phosphate, found in cereal grain, the source for the Magnesia phosphorica remedy.

Abdominal Complaints 6

This part of the chart shows **further general modalities** which may make the patient feel better or worse and **modalities that affect the nature of the diarrhea and nausea and vomiting** which may present. Read down the list to find which ones are relevant to you. The symbols on the chart indicate the remedies most suitable for each variable. Once you have established the various modalities in the particular case you are taking, and noted the possible remedies, turn to the following pages to trace the remedies that suit the other elements in your case. As you work your way through the chart, following the system of symbols, you should be able to eliminate unsuitable remedies and eventually make a final selection that matches your case as nearly as possible.

The remedy names are given in an abbreviated form in the charts. Full names are given in the key below.

REMEDY KEY

Acon.	Aconite napellus	**Coloc.**	Colocynthis	**Phos.**	Phosphorus
Ant. c.	Antimonium crudum	**Dios.**	Dioscorea villosa	**Pod.**	Podophyllum peltatum.
Ant. t.	Antimonium tartaricum	**Dulc.**	Dulcamara	**Puls.**	Pulsatilla nigricans
Ars.	Arsenicum album	**Gels.**	Gelsemium sempervirens	**Sep.**	Sepia
Bell.	Belladonna	**Ip.**	Ipecacuanha	**Sil.**	Silica
Bry.	Bryonia alba	**Lyc.**	Lycopodium clavatum	**Sulph.**	Sulphur
Carb. v.	Carbo vegetabilis	**Mag.p.**	Magnesia phosphorica	**Verat.**	Veratrum album.
Cham.	Chamomilla	**Nat.s.**	Natrum sulphuricum		
Chin.	China officinalis	**Nux v.**	Nux vomica		

REMEDY	Acon.	Ant. c.	Ant. t.	Ars.	Bell.	Bry.	Carb. v.	Cham.	Chin.	Coloc.	Dios.	Dulc.	Gels	Ip.	Lyc.	Mag. p.	Nat. s.	Nux v.	Phos.	Pod.	Puls.	Sep.	Sil.	Sulph.	Verat.
MODALITIES (CONTINUED)																									
LYING																		●							
ON STOMACH										●										●					
ON ABDOMEN																				●					
PASSING STOOL																									
PRESSURE									●																
REST																		●							
RUBBING																●									
STRETCHING OUT											●														
SITTING																		●							
STANDING STRAIGHT											●														
WARM APPLICATIONS																●									
WARMTH									●						●										
WALKING																								●	
WALKING IN OPEN AIR											●														
MODALITIES (DIARRHEA)																									
WORSE																									
4AM																				●					
5AM																							●		
4-8PM														●											
AFTER MIDNIGHT				●																					
MORNING						●					●														
EVENING																	●				●				
NIGHT									●																
ACID OR TINNED FRUIT																				●					
AFTER EATING									●																
AFTER BATHING																				●					
BEGINNING MOTION						●																			
COLD DAMP WEATHER																									

KEEPING STILL																				•					
MILK																			•			•			
MOTION						•																			
SLIGHT EATING										•															
MORNING																	•								
BETTER																									
GENTLE MOTION																				•					
HEAT										•															
PASSING STOOL																		•							
MODALITIES (NAUSEA AND VOMITING)																									
WORSE																									
12AM AND 12PM																							•		
4-8PM															•										
MORNING																			•		•				
NIGHT									•																
COLD DRINKS				•																					
EATING AND DRINKING				•																					
EATING (AFTER)						•																	•		
FATTY RICH FOOD																				•					
FISH									•																
FRUIT									•																
MILK									•													•			
MOTION						•																			
OVEREATING														•											
SITTING UP						•																			
WINE									•																
WARM THINGS																			•						
BETTER																									
BELCHING							•																		
COLD THINGS																			•						
EVENING																		•							
LYING STILL AND FLAT						•																			
NAUSEA BETTER VOMITING			•																						
OPEN AIR														•											
REST														•											
CONCOMITANTS *other symptoms that come on with the abdominal complaint*																									
APPETITE LOST ON EATING															•										
INCREASES ON EATING															•										
AVERSE TO MILK																						•			
DRYNESS																				•					

The illustration shows leaves from the quinaquina tree, the source for the Cinchona officinalis remedy.

Abdominal Complaints 7

This part of the chart shows the **concomitant symptoms** thay may accompany the abdominal pain and the **general mental and physical symptoms** that may also be observed. (Note that the remedies for mental symptoms differ slightly from those indicated for concomitants.) Read down the list to find which ones are relevant to you. The symbols on the chart indicate the remedies most suitable for each variable. Once you have established the concomitants and mental and physical symptoms in the particular case you are taking, and noted the possible remedies, turn to the following pages to trace the remedies that suit the other elements in your case.

The remedy names are given in an abbreviated form in the charts. Full names are given in the key below.

REMEDY KEY

Abbr.	Remedy	Abbr.	Remedy	Abbr.	Remedy
Acon.	Aconite napellus	**Coloc.**	Colocynthis	**Phos.**	Phosphorus
Ant. c.	Antimonium crudum	**Dios.**	Dioscorea villosa	**Pod.**	Podophyllum peltatum.
Ant. t.	Antimonium tartaricum	**Dulc.**	Dulcamara	**Puls.**	Pulsatilla nigricans
Ars.	Arsenicum album	**Gels.**	Gelsemium sempervirens	**Sep.**	Sepia
Bell.	Belladonna	**Ip.**	Ipecacuanha	**Sil.**	Silica
Bry.	Bryonia alba	**Lyc.**	Lycopodium clavatum	**Sulph.**	Sulphur
Carb. v.	Carbo vegetabilis	**Mag.p.**	Magnesia phosphorica	**Verat.**	Veratrum album.
Cham.	Chamomilla	**Nat.s.**	Natrum sulphuricum		
Chin.	China officinalis	**Nux v.**	Nux vomica		

REMEDY	Acon.	Ant. c.	Ant. t.	Ars.	Bell.	Bry.	Carb. v.	Cham.	Chin.	Coloc.	Dios.	Dulc.	Gels	Ip.	Lyc.	Mag. p.	Nat. s.	Nux. v	Phos.	Pod.	Puls.	Sep.	Sil.	Sulph.	Verat.
CONCOMITANTS (CONTINUED)																									
EXTREMITIES COLD					●																				
FACE RED					●																				
FLUSHED AFTER WINE							●																		
FEBRILE STATE	●																								
HEAD HOT					●																				
HEADACHE BURSTING, CRUSHING IN VERTEX																		●							
HUNGER 11AM																			●						
LIVER PAINS																				●					
MOUTH DRY				●																					
RIGHT SIDED																●									●
SWEAT COLD ON FOREHEAD							●																		●
TONGUE COATED										●															
TONGUE CLEAN														●		●									
TONGUE WITH THICK MILKY WHITE COATING		●			●																				
THIRST FOR SIPS				●																					
THIRSTLESS																					●				
VISION DIM, DOUBLE, MISTY													●												
GENERALS *symptoms that affect the whole person*																									
MENTAL																									
ANGRY										●								●							
ANXIETY	●			●																					
AVERSION TO																									
TALK, THINK						●																			
BEING LOOKED AT		●	●																						
BEING TOUCHED			●																						
COMPANY											●														
FUSS AND SYMPATHY																						●			
CAN'T BEAR PAIN CALMLY								●																	

CLINGY, WEEPY																				●					
CHANGEABLE																				●					
DEPRESSED											●														
DESPISES EVERYTHING														●											
FEARS				●																					
HARD TO PLEASE								●																	
INDIFFERENT																					●				
IRRITABLE			●			●		●		●	●							●							
MOANS AND HOWLS								●																	
OFFENDED EASILY																		●							
OVERSENSITIVE								●										●							
PEEVISH		●																							
RESTLESS	●			●				●		●															
SENTIMENTAL		●																							
SULKY														●											
WANTS INSTANT PAIN RELIEF										●															
TO BE ALONE			●			●				●															
PEACE						●																			
PHYSICAL																									
AVERSION TO FOOD, MEAT, FAT, BREAD																					●				
AIR HUNGER							●																		
APPETITE (LITTLE)															●										
BLUE																									●
CLOTHING (INTOLERABLE)																			●					●	
COLD			●				●																		●
COLD (WORSE FOR)				●								●													
CHILLY				●			●											●							
CONGESTED														●											
CRAMPS																●									●
DIGESTON (POOR)																								●	
DIZZY										●															
DROWSY																				●					
DRAFT (WORSE FOR)					●											●									
DESIRES ALCOHOL																								●	
FAT																								●	
SWEETS																								●	
FAINTNESS										●											●			●	
FANNED (WANTS TO BE)							●																		
FACE RED	●																								
FEEBLE AND BROKEN DOWN			●																						
FEVER MARKED					●																				
FLATULENCE AND BELCHING															●										

Abdominal Complaints 8

This part of the chart shows the **further general physical symptoms** that may also be observed. Read down the list to find which ones are relevant to you. The symbols on the chart indicate the remedies most suitable for each variable. By assessing the data you have collected while consulting the chart, you should now be able to make a final selection to match your case as nearly as possible.

If you are in any doubt, consult the advice panel on page 217.

The remedy names are given in an abbreviated form in the charts. Full names are given in the key below.

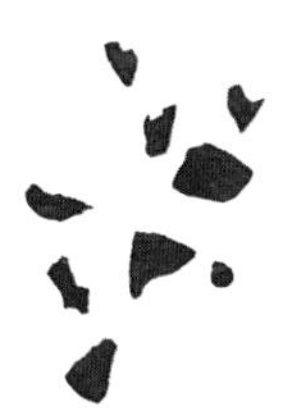

REMEDY	Acon.	Ant. c.	Ant. t.	Ars.	Bell.	Bry.	Carb. v.	Cham.	Chin.	Coloc.	Dios.	Dulc.	Gels	Ip.	Lyc.	Mag. p.	Nat. s.	Nux v.	Phos.	Pod.	Puls.	Sep.	Sil.	Sulph.	Verat.
GENERALS (CONTINUED)																									
PHYSICALS (CONTINUED)																									
FULLNESS							•								•										
HUMID WEATHER (WORSE FOR)																	•								
HEAT (WORSE FOR)																	•								
IN FLASHES																								•	
NIGHT (WORSE)				•																		•			
PALLOR			•	•			•							•											
PROSTRATION			•	•																•					
OUT OF PROPORTION				•																					
IN SPELLS														•											
PUPILS DILATED					•																				
RAPID ONSET																									•
REDNESS					•									•											
SENSITIVE NOISE, ODOR, LIGHT																		•							
SHORT SLEEP (BETTER FOR)																			•						
SLUGGISH							•																		
THIN, TENSE, CHILLY																•									
THIRSTLESS													•									•			
THIRST	•				•																				
FOR COLD WATER																				•					
SWEAT																						•			
SWEAT COLD																									•
STRETCH (DESIRE TO)																				•					
TWITCHING MUSCLES																•									
WEAK										•			•												
WEAK IF NOT EATING																									

REMEDY KEY

Acon.	Aconite napellus	**Coloc.**	Colocynthis	**Phos.**	Phosphorus
Ant. c.	Antimonium crudum	**Dios.**	Dioscorea villosa	**Pod.**	Podophyllum peltatum.
Ant. t.	Antimonium tartaricum	**Dulc.**	Dulcamara	**Puls.**	Pulsatilla nigricans
Ars.	Arsenicum album	**Gels.**	Gelsemium sempervirens	**Sep.**	Sepia
Bell.	Belladonna	**Ip.**	Ipecacuanha	**Sil.**	Silica
Bry.	Bryonia alba	**Lyc.**	Lycopodium clavatum	**Sulph.**	Sulphur
Carb. v.	Carbo vegetabilis	**Mag.p.**	Magnesia phosphorica	**Verat.**	Veratrum album.
Cham.	Chamomilla	**Nat.s.**	Natrum sulphuricum		
Chin.	China officinalis	**Nux v.**	Nux vomica		

Baby Colic

This self-contained chart shows the symptom picture for colic in babies, with symptoms listed alphabetically. It shows four of the most commonly indicated remedies with their key symptoms. If these are not successful, consult the general Abdominal Complaints charts.

If in any doubt, consult the advice panel on the right.

The remedy names are given in an abbreviated form in the charts. Full names are given in the key below.

WHEN TO SEEK ADVICE ABOUT ABDOMINAL COMPLAINTS

Urgently, right now!

- If there are significant signs of dehydration (loss of body fluids), usually from diarrhea or vomiting, especially in an infant, as shown by:
  1. Eyes appear sunken.
  2. In babies the fontanelle (soft spot on the top of the head) is sunken.
  3. Dryness of the mouth or eyes.
  4. Loss of skin tone or turgor – gently pinch up the skin which will normally snap straight back into place. If it does not then marked dehydration is present.
  5. Decreased quantity of urine being passed. It may be very strong.
- Constant repeated vomiting.
- If the vomit is bloodstained or looks like coffee grounds.
- If the stool is bloody, black or tar-like. Bleeding from the rectum with measles.
- If marked abdominal symptoms follow a head or abdominal injury, especially if vomiting follows a head injury (see First Aid Section pages 240 to 245).
- Severe pain anywhere in the abdomen.
- In children with vomiting, inconsolable screaming or lethargy.
- If there is evidence or suspicion of drugs or poisonous substances having been taken. If possible keep a sample of the substance and of the vomited material for later analysis.

Within 24 hours

- Unexpected swelling, pain or tenderness in the groin or insides of the tops of the thighs.
- For constipation with pain and or vomiting of a day or more duration.
- Abdominal symptoms in someone with diabetes may become urgent – advice should **always** be sought sooner for a person with diabetes.
- Likewise with abdominal symptoms in pregnancy – if in doubt, seek advice.
- Signs of jaundice – yellow eyes or skin, dark urine and possibly light colored stools.
- Any urinary symptoms – pains, discharge, bleeding or deposit in the urine, frequent urging, especially if the urinary symptoms are accompanied by backache or loin pains which may suggest that the kidneys are affected in some way.

Refer to other chapters as necessary.

The illustration shows charcoal, the source for the Carbo vegetabilis remedy.

REMEDY	Cham.	Coloc.	Dios.	Mag. p.
BETTER FOR BEING CARRIED	●			
DOUBLING UP		●		●
FIRM PRESSURE			●	●
HEAT	●	●	●	●
PRESSURE		●		
STRETCHING OUT			●	
DIARRHEA GREEN, ROTTEN EGGS SMELL	●			
DOUBLES UP AND SCREAMS	●			
FACE HOT, FLUSHED, SWEATS	●			
FRANTICALLY IRRITABLE	●			
HICCUPS				●
RESTLESS, IRRITABLE, ANGRY		●		
RETCHING				●
SUDDEN ONSET			●	
TEMPER INCONSOLABLE	●			
TONGUE COATED		●		
WIND OR BELCHING DOESN'T RELIEVE				●
WORSE AT NIGHT	●			
DOUBLING UP			●	

REMEDY KEY	
Cham.	Chamomilla
Coloc.	Colocynthis
Dios.	Dioscorea villosa
Mag.p.	Magnesia phosphorica

Period Pains 1

The first part of this chart lists the **possible sensations of** period pains, their **radiation pattern** and **any peculiar symptoms**. Read down the list to find which ones are relevant to you. The symbols on the chart indicate the remedies most suitable for each variable. Once you have established the sensations and any peculiar symptoms of the particular case you are taking, and noted the possible remedies, turn to the following pages to trace the remedies that suit the other elements in your case. As you work your way through the chart, following the system of symbols, you should be able to eliminate unsuitable remedies and eventually make a final selection that matches your case.

The remedy names are given in an abbreviated form in the charts. Full names are given in the key below.

REMEDY KEY

- **Bell.** Belladonna
- **Calc. f** Calcarea fluorata
- **Calc.p** Calcarea phosphorica
- **Cham.** Chamomilla
- **Cimic.** Cimicifuga racemosa
- **Cocc.** Cocculus indicus
- **Coloc.** Colocynthis
- **Con.** Conium maculatum
- **Ferr.p.** Ferrum phosphoricum
- **Kali p.** Kali phosphoricum
- **Lach.** Lachesis
- **Mag.p.** Magnesia phosphorica
- **Nux v.** Nux vomica
- **Puls.** Pulsatilla nigricans
- **Sep.** Sepia

REMEDY	Bell.	Calc. f.	Calc. p.	Cham.	Cimic.	Cocc.	Coloc.	Con.	Ferr. p.	Kali. p.	Lach.	Mag. p.	Nux v.	Puls.	Sep.
SENSATIONS *how the period pains feel*															
ACHING													❦		
BEARING DOWN	❦	❦		❦					❦						❦
HEAVY	❦		❦												
BENDING BACK (BETTER)	❦														
BEFORE AND DURING PERIOD			❦												
BREAST NIPPLE PAIN								❦							
COLIC						❦				❦		❦			
CONGESTED									❦						
CRAMP AND SORENESS (UTERUS)											❦				
CRAMPS	❦			❦		❦						❦	❦		
FLY AROUND					❦										
CRY OUT (WITH PAIN)				❦										❦	
DESIRE TO DEFECATE													❦		
DRAGGING															❦
DULL, SORE, BRUISED															❦
EASED BY															
FIRM PRESSURE												❦			
FIRM PRESSURE LOWER ABDOMEN OR BACK												❦			
HOT WATER BOTTLE												❦			
STEADY PRESSURE							❦								
HEAT							❦								
FALL OUT (AS IF EVERYTHING WOULD)	❦														❦
FLOW EXCESSIVE		❦													
GRIPING						❦									
HEAT IN PAIN	❦														
LOWER BACK AND SACRUM (PAINS)													❦		
OVARIES PAIN (LEFT)											❦				
PAINS															
BEGIN AND END SUDDENLY	❦														
COLICKY							❦			❦					
CRAMPING				❦			❦								
GREAT WITH FLOW										❦					

PRESSING	❦					❦							❦												
SHARP	❦				❦		❦																		
SHOOTING					❦																				
STITCHING								❦																	
UNENDURABLE				❦																					
VARY														❦											
PRESSING DOWN													❦												
PRESSURE PAINS									❦						❦										
SITS WITH LEGS CROSSED															❦										
SWELLING, TENDERNESS (BREAST)								❦																	
UTERUS (PAINS)		❦				❦																			
VAGINA DRY, HOT, SENSITIVE									❦																
WEIGHT AND FULLNESS										❦															
RADIATION *where pain moves to*																									
ACROSS LOWER BACK										❦															
BACK TO INNER THIGH				❦																					
TO BACK, CHEST, UPPER ABDOMEN											❦														
CRAMPS IN CALF							❦																		
DRAWING DOWN THIGHS								❦																	
EXTEND TO RECTUM													❦												
IN ALL DIRECTIONS												❦													
IN DIFFERENT PLACES														❦											
LOWER BACK (SACRUM)					❦								❦												
THIGHS		❦																							
UP AND DOWN INNER THIGH				❦																					
PECULIAR *peculiar symptoms*																									
BALL OR PLUG SENSATION															❦										
PAINS FLY AROUND					❦																				
WITH PAIN IN VERTEX									❦																
FLOW *nature of the flow*																									
BRIGHT RED	❦								❦																
CLOTTED	❦		❦		❦																				
DARK			❦	❦	❦	❦																			
DURING DAY ONLY														❦											
EARLY OR LATE										❦															
EXCESSIVE		❦																							
FLOODING		❦																							
HEAVY	❦		❦																						
IRREGULAR					❦					❦				❦											
LATE			❦											❦											
LESS FLOW, MORE PAIN											❦														
LONG LASTING													❦												
MORE FLOW, MORE PAIN					❦																				
PROFUSE				❦	❦	❦							❦												
SCANT								❦							❦										
STRONG SMELLING										❦															
THIN										❦															

The illustration shows deadly nightshade, the source for the Belladonna remedy

Period Pains 2

This part of the chart describes the **character of the menstrual flow** experienced and shows **any concomitants** that may accompany the pain, **any modalities** that make the patient better or worse and **general mental and physical symptoms**. Read down the list to find which ones are relevant to you. The symbols on the chart indicate the remedies most suitable for each variable. By assessing the data you have collected while consulting the chart, you should now be able to make a final selection to match your case as nearly as possible.

For further advice consult the panel on the right.

The remedy names are given in an abbreviated form in the charts. Full names are given in the key below.

REMEDY KEY			
Bell.	Belladonna	**Kali p.**	Kali phosphoricum
Calc. f	Calcarea fluorata	**Lach.**	Lachesis
Calc.p	Calcarea phosphorica	**Mag.p.**	Magnesia phosphorica
Cham.	Chamomilla	**Nux v.**	Nux vomica
Cimic.	Cimicifuga racemosa	**Puls.**	Pulsatilla nigricans
Cocc.	Cocculus indicus	**Sep.**	Sepia
Coloc.	Colocynthis		
Con.	Conium maculatum		
Ferr.p.	Ferrum phosphoricum		

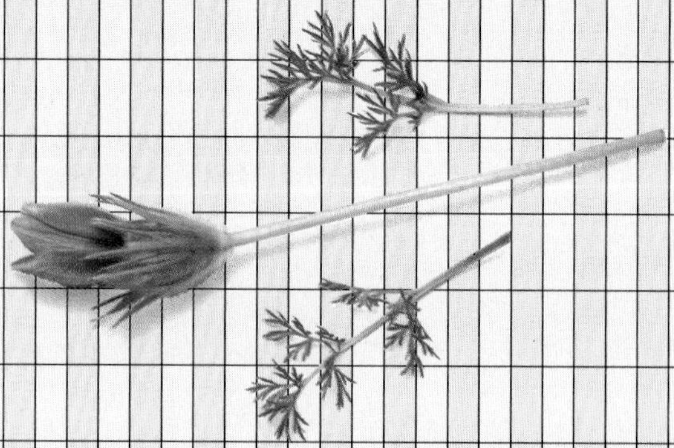

REMEDY	Bell.	Calc. f.	Calc. p.	Cham.	Cimic.	Cocc.	Coloc.	Con.	Ferr. p.	Kali. p.	Lach.	Mag. p.	Nux v.	Puls.	Sep.
CONCOMITANTS *other symptoms that come on with the period pains*															
ABDOMEN BLOATED						●									
BACKACHE		●	●								●			●	
BETTER PRESSURE, HEAT												●			
BREASTS HARD, KNOTTY LUMPS			●												
HEAVY, SWOLLEN								●							
CRAMPS CALF							●								
CRAMPS ALTERNATE DIZZINESS							●								
COLD HANDS AND FEET	●														
DIARRHEA														●	
FACE FLUSHED	●			●					●						
FAINTING													●	●	
HEADACHE	●										●			●	
THROBBING			●												
DULL										●					
JOINTS (RHEUMATIC PAINS)			●												
NAUSEA													●	●	
PILES						●									
PULSE RAPID									●						
SEXUAL DESIRE INCREASED			●												
SWEAT WITH CRAMPS				●											
THIGH PAINS MOVE UP AND DOWN					●										
TONGUE CLEAN												●			
TONGUE COATED							●								
URGE TO DEFECATE OR URINATE (CONSTANT)												●			
VERTIGO			●					●			●				
VOMITING									●					●	
WEAKNESS						●									
MODALITIES *what makes patient or symptoms better or worse*															
WORSE															
BEFORE AND DURING PERIOD	●														
BENDING FORWARD	●														
BREATHING						●									
CHANGE OF WEATHER			●												
COLD AND DRAFTS												●			

WHEN TO SEEK ADVICE

Urgently, right now!

- If the pain is unusually severe.
- If a period has been missed and there is a possibility of pregnanc.
- When severe or unusual pains develop with or without any blood flow.

Within 24 hours

- Significant bleeding between periods even without pains.
- Recurrent minor, unexplained bleeding between periods.
- Any uncharacteristic vaginal discharge, especially if accompanied by lower abdominal pain or fever.
- If sores develop on, in or near the genitals.
- If you have had sex with someone who is known to have a sexually transmissable disease such as gonorrhoea, syphilis, or chlamydia.

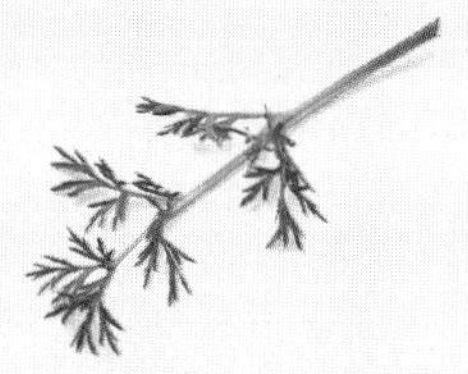

The illustration shows the wind-flower, the source for the Pulsatilla nigricans remedy

JAR	•														
MOVEMENT	•				•	•									
NIGHT				•			•								
RIDING IN CAR						•									
STANDING															•
STOOL			•												
SUPPRESSED ANGER							•								
TIGHT CLOTHING AT WAIST											•				
URINATING			•												•
WALKING	•														•
WARM ROOM														•	
BETTER															
AS SOON AS FLOW BEGINS											•				
BENDING BACK	•														
BENDING DOUBLE														•	
DOUBLING UP							•						•		
CROSSING LEGS															•
HEAT							•					•			
OPEN AIR														•	
PRESSURE FIRM							•								
PRESSURE STEADY	•						•					•			
STRAIGHTENING UP	•														
VIGOROUS EXERCISE															•
WARMTH				•											
GENERALS *symptoms that affect the whole person*															
MENTAL															
AGITATION					•										
CRAVES COMPANY															•
CRITICAL AND FAULT FINDING				•									•		
EASILY STARTLED								•							
INTOLERANCE TO PAIN				•	•										
TO TOUCH	•														
IRRITABLE AND ANGRY				•			•			•			•	•	
SEXUAL DESIRE INCREASES (BEFORE)			•												
(AFTER)										•					
WEEPY										•				•	
PHYSICAL															
CHILLY													•		
CONGESTION		•							•						
EXHAUSTED						•		•							
FLUSHING									•						
HOT, NEEDS FRESH AIR											•				
PALE										•					
PALPITATIONS								•							•
RESTLESS				•			•								
SENSITIVITY	•			•	•					•			•		
SINKING			•												
VENOUS RELAXATION		•													
WEAK			•			•		•							

Cystitis 1

The first part of this chart shows the possible **causes and onsets** of cystitis, the **character of the urine passed** and **some of the sensations** that may be experienced. Read down the list to find which ones are relevant to you. The symbols on the chart indicate the remedies most suitable for each variable. Once you have established the cause and onset, observed the urine and identified some sensations of the particular case you are taking, and noted the possible remedies turn to the following pages to trace the remedies that suit the other elements in your case. As you work your way through the chart, following the system of symbols, you should be able to eliminate unsuitable remedies and eventually make a final selection that matches your case as nearly as possible.

The remedy names are given in an abbreviated form in the charts. Full names are given in the key below.

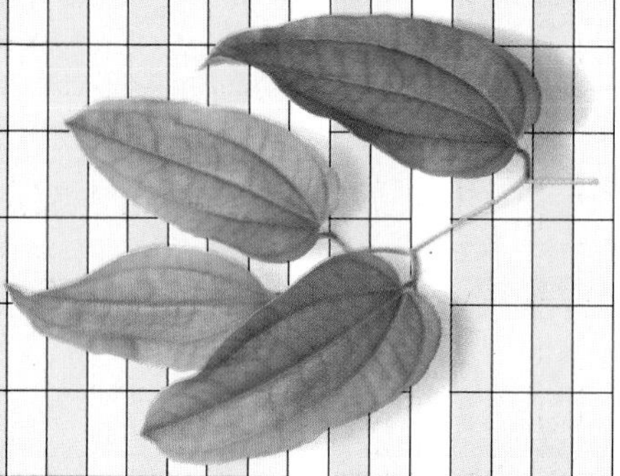

REMEDY	Apis	Canth.	Caust.	Ferr. p.	Kali. m.	Kali. p.	Lyc.	Mag. p.	Merc.	Nat. m.	Nux v.	Puls.	Sars.	Staph.	Sulph.
CAUSE *why symptoms appear*															
CHILL													❀		
COLD			❀	❀											
COLD WET WEATHER													❀		
EXCESS (EATING, ALCOHOL, COFFEE)											❀				
EXCITEMENT						❀									
INDIGNATION														❀	
OVEREXERTION				❀											
OVERWORK						❀									
SUPPRESSED EMOTIONS														❀	
WET (FEET)												❀			
WET AND COLD (GETTING)												❀			
WORRY						❀									
ONSET *when and how symptoms appear*															
RAPID TO SERIOUS STATE		❀													
SLOW				❀											
SITE *where the pains are felt*															
BLADDER	❀	❀				❀		❀		❀					
BLADDER (NECK OF)		❀		❀											
URETHRA		❀		❀		❀			❀				❀	❀	❀
URETHRA (OPENING OF)													❀		
URINE *nature of the urine*															
BEER (LIKE)															❀
BLOODY	❀	❀							❀	❀	❀	❀			
COLOR NORMAL				❀											
CLEAR				❀											
DARK					❀			❀	❀						
DARK OR LIGHT			❀												
DEPOSIT DIRTY GREY-GREEN													❀		
EXCESSIVE QUANTITY				❀											
FLAKY														❀	

REMEDY KEY

Apis	Apis mellifica	**Nat. m.**	Natrum muriaticum
Canth.	Cantharis	**Nux v.**	Nux vomica
Caust.	Causticum	**Puls.**	Pulsatilla nigricans
Ferr.p.	Ferrum phosphoricum	**Sars.**	Sarsaparilla
Kali m.	Kali muriaticum	**Staph.**	Staphisagria
Kali p.	Kali phosphoricum	**Sulph.**	Sulphur
Lyc.	Lycopodium clavatum		
Mag. p.	Magnesia phosphorica		
Merc.	Mercurius vivus		

OFFENSIVE													❦												
MILKY						❦	❦																		
MUCUS								❦					❦		❦										
PALE GREEN													❦												
PUS															❦										
RED SAND IN							❦			❦															
SCANTY	❦			❦																					
SEDIMENT			❦										❦												
SMELLS FOUL															❦										
SUPPRESSED				❦																					
THICK WHITE MUCUS					❦																				
TURBID							❦						❦												
WHITE SAND WITH MUCUS													❦												
YELLOW						❦																			
SENSATIONS *how the pains feel*																									
CHILD CRIES BEFORE URINATING							❦																		
CLEAR MUCOUS DISCHARGE										❦															
CONCENTRATES TO HOLD URINE												❦													
DESIRE TO URINATE																									
CONSTANT	❦	❦																							
FREQUENT	❦		❦								❦				❦										
INEFFECTUAL			❦				❦				❦		❦												
LYING ON BACK												❦													
SEVERE		❦																							
SOON RETURNS			❦																						
STANDING UP (BETTER)													❦												
URGENT		❦									❦				❦										
INCONTINENCE AT NIGHT							❦						❦												
FROM NERVOUS DISABILITY						❦																			
IN SLEEP							❦					❦													
SLIGHT											❦														
INVOLUNTARY URINATION														❦											
NECK BLADDER (PAIN)											❦														
NIGHT (WORSE)															❦										
PAIN																									
BURNING	❦	❦	❦	❦		❦		❦	❦	❦	❦	❦		❦	❦										
CRAMPING								❦				❦													
CUTTING		❦			❦	❦	❦	❦		❦			❦												
EXTREME		❦																							
PRESSING	❦						❦				❦														
SEVERE	❦	❦											❦												
SHOOTING								❦																	
SMARTING	❦											❦													
SORE, SHARP					❦																				

The illustration shows Smilax officinalis, the source for the Sarsaparilla remedy.

Cystitis 2

This part of the chart shows **further sensations** that may be experienced in cystitis, and some of the **concomitant symptoms** that may accompany the pain. Read down the list to find which ones are relevant to you. The symbols on the chart indicate the remedies most suitable for each variable. Once you have established the sensations and identified some of the concomitants in the particular case you are taking, and noted the possible remedies, turn to the following pages to trace the remedies that suit the other elements in your case. As you work your way through the chart, following the system of symbols, you should be able to eliminate unsuitable remedies and eventually make a final selection that matches your case as nearly as possible.

The remedy names are given in an abbreviated form in the charts. Full names are given in the key below.

REMEDY KEY

Apis	Apis mellifica
Canth.	Cantharis
Caust.	Causticum
Ferr.p.	Ferrum phosphoricum
Kali m.	Kali muriaticum
Kali p.	Kali phosphoricum
Lyc.	Lycopodium clavatum
Mag. p.	Magnesia phosphorica
Merc.	Mercurius vivus
Nat. m.	Natrum muriaticum
Nux v.	Nux vomica
Puls.	Pulsatilla nigricans
Sars.	Sarsaparilla
Staph.	Staphisagria
Sulph.	Sulphur

REMEDY	Apis	Canth.	Caust.	Ferr. p.	Kali. m.	Kali. p.	Lyc.	Mag. p.	Merc.	Nat. m.	Nux v.	Puls.	Sars.	Staph.	Sulph.
SENSATIONS (CONTINUED)															
PAIN (CONTINUED)															
STABBING		●													
STINGING	●														
STITCHING				●			●								
UNBEARABLE													●		
PRESSURE DULL, HEAVY (BLADDER)							●								
SPASMS (BLADDER)								●							
STRAINING	●														
SUPPORTS ABDOMEN WITH HANDS							●								
TENESMUS AT CLOSE URINATING													●		
URGING	●														
CONSTANT								●	●						
FREQUENT							●							●	
INTOLERABLE		●													
IRRESISTIBLE				●											
PAINFUL								●						●	
SEVERE												●			
UNCONTROLLABLE								●							
WITHOUT EFFECT												●			
URGENCY		●													
SUDDEN															●
URINE															
COPIOUS												●			
DRIBBLES					●							●	●		●
FLOODS BED AT NIGHT													●		
IN DROPS	●	●													
LARGE AMOUNTS						●				●					
PASSED VERY SLOWLY									●						
SCANTY	●								●						
SMALL AMOUNTS	●		●						●						

AFTER EVERY DRINK				✿																					
FREQUENT					✿																				
IN SLEEP			✿																						
MORE NIGHT THAN DAY							✿																		
PAIN AFTER										✿				✿											
AT END OF													✿												
BEFORE								✿			✿														
BETTER WHEN														✿											
CONTINUOUS		✿				✿									✿										
DURING		✿									✿			✿	✿										
LAST DROPS	✿																								
WHILE COUGHING			✿							✿		✿													
WORSE NOT URINATING								✿						✿											
URETHRA (PAIN IN)												✿													
(ITCHING IN)						✿					✿														
WAITS LONG FOR LITTLE RESULT			✿				✿																		
WEAKNESS IN SPHINCTER MUSCLES						✿																			
CONCOMITANTS *other symptoms that come on with cystitis*																									
ABDOMEN SENSITIVE TO TOUCH	✿																								
COLD (FOLLOWS A)															✿										
CONSTIPATION			✿																						
COUGH (CAUSES URINE TO SPURT)				✿																					
FLATULENCE, BLOATED							✿																		
KIDNEY INFLAMMATION	✿	✿											✿												
KIDNEY PAINS					✿																				
RECTAL SPASMS			✿																						
RENAL COLIC							✿																		
THIRSTLESS	✿																								
TONGUE WHITE-GREY COATING						✿																			
URETHRA BLEEDING						✿																			
SWELLING AROUND	✿																								
URGE TO DEFECATE (WITH PAIN)											✿														
URINE CORROSIVE								✿																	
CAUSES ITCHING AND INFLAMMATION								✿																	
ACRID, CAUSES SORENESS														✿	✿										
PECULIARS *unusual symptoms*																									
ITCHING AT ORIFICE OF URETHRA			✿																						
PAINS WORSE NOT URINATING								✿																	
BETTER BEGINNING URINATION								✿																	
SENSATION DROP URINE ROLLING IN URETHRA														✿											
MODALITIES *what makes the patient or the cystitis better or worse*																									
WORSE																									
COLD DRINKS		✿																							
COLD AND DRAFTS											✿														

The illustration shows the honey bee, the source for the Apis mellifica remedy.

Cystitis 3

This part of the chart shows **further concomitants** that may accompany cystitis, and some of **the peculiar symptoms, modalities** that make the patient feel better or worse and **any general mental or physical symptoms**. Read down the list to find which ones are relevant to you. The symbols on the chart indicate the remedies most suitable for each variable. By assessing the data you have collected while consulting the chart, you should now be able to make a final selection to match your case as nearly as possible.

For further advice consult the panel on the right.

The remedy names are given in an abbreviated form in the charts. Full names are given in the key below.

REMEDY KEY

Apis	Apis mellifica
Canth.	Cantharis
Caust.	Causticum
Ferr.p.	Ferrum phosphoricum
Kali m.	Kali muriaticum
Kali p.	Kali phosphoricum
Lyc.	Lycopodium clavatum
Mag. p.	Magnesia phosphorica
Merc.	Mercurius vivus
Nat. m.	Natrum muriaticum
Nux v.	Nux vomica
Puls.	Pulsatilla nigricans
Sars.	Sarsaparilla
Staph.	Staphisagria
Sulph.	Sulphur

REMEDY	Apis	Canth.	Caust.	Ferr. p.	Kali. m.	Kali. p.	Lyc.	Mag. p.	Merc.	Nat. m.	Nux v.	Puls.	Sars.	Staph.	Sulph.
MODALITIES (CONTINUED)															
HEAT	●														
LYING ON BACK												●			
MENSTRUAL PERIOD (DURING)													●		
MOTION, WALKING														●	
NIGHT	●								●						●
NOT URINATING									●						
STANDING UP (URGING)				●											
URINATION															
AFTER		●				●									
AT START OR END									●						
BEFORE		●							●						
DURING		●	●			●					●		●		●
END OF													●		
JUST AFTER										●					
BETTER															
BEGINNING URINATION									●						
BENDING DOUBLE								●							
COLD	●														
HEAT AND PRESSURE								●							
LYING ON BACK											●				
RIDING IN CAR							●								
WHEN URINATING													●		
GENERALS *symptoms that affect the whole person*															
MENTAL															
AFFECT OF															
ABUSE														●	
ASSAULT														●	
RAPE														●	
VIOLATION														●	
ANGER NOT EXPRESSED														●	
CHANGEABLE MOODS												●			

IRRITABLE												●														
NERVOUS, SENSITIVE, PALE					●																					
NERVOUS WEAKNESS							●																			
OFFENDED EASILY															●											
RESTLESS, UNEASY, DISTRESSED			●																							
SENSITIVE												●			●											
TOUCHY, WEEPY													●													
PHYSICAL																										
CHILLY												●														
DEBILITATED, WORN OUT							●																			
DOUBLES UP AND SCREAMS			●																							
FIRST STAGES OF CYSTITIS					●																					
FLUSHES EASILY (FACE)					●																					
FOLLOWS FERRUM PHOSPHORICUM						●																				
HEAT AND STUFFINESS (AVERSE)													●													
HOT, WANTS COOL AIR		●																								
INTENSE, VIOLENT, RAPID PAINS			●																							
MOVE ABOUT (DESIRE TO)						●																				
NO PAIN, THICK WHITE MUCUS			●																							
SWELLING		●																								
THIRST (GREAT)			●																							
THIRSTLESS													●													
WEAKNESS, PROSTRATION (MARKED)							●																			

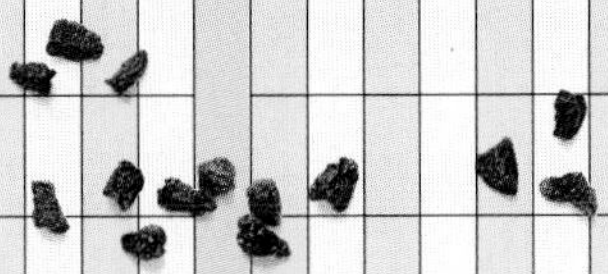

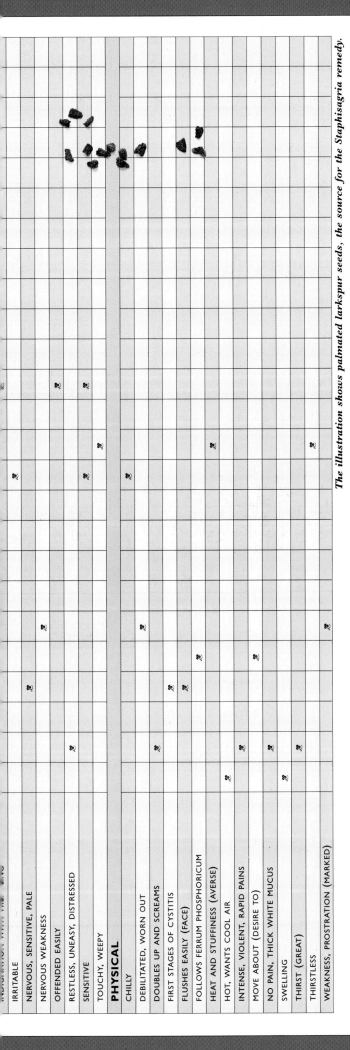

The illustration shows palmated larkspur seeds, the source for the Staphisagria remedy.

WHEN TO SEEK ADVICE

Urgently, right now!

- If there is a fever and inflammation of the kidneys. This causes pain in the kidney area (the loins). They lie on either side of the spine above the waist. If you place your hands on your hips with your fingers pointing backwards and then move them an inch or two higher over the bottom of the rib cage they will cover the loins.
- If there are rigors – bouts of cold and violent shivering and shaking.

Within 24 hours

- If any of the symptoms are severe.
- If there is a significant fever, above 38.4°C (101°F)
- If there is a significant amount of blood in the urine. It may be pink, red or a muddy-brown like tea (with milk in).
- If there is vomiting or a significant headache.
- If swelling of the hands, face or ankles develops.
- All males with cystitis should seek the advice of their health care practitioner, particularly if it is recurrent. It may be an indication of other problems in the urinary tract, some of which could potentially be serious in the long term.

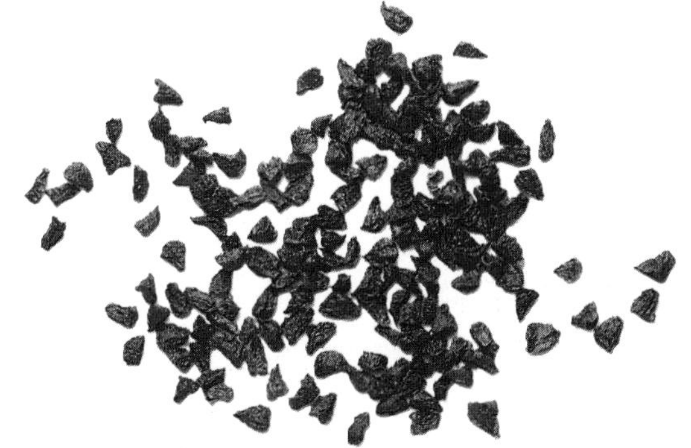

Children's Illnesses 1

The first part of this chart lists, in alphabetical order, the **physical and mental symptoms** of MEASLES together with any **concomitants or peculiars**. Read down the list to find which ones are relevant to you. The symbols on the chart indicate the remedies most suitable for each variable. Once you have identified some of the symptoms in the particular case you are taking, and noted the possible remedies, turn to the following pages to trace the remedies that suit the other elements in your case. As you work your way through the chart, following the system of symbols, you should be able to eliminate unsuitable remedies and eventually make a final selection that matches your case as nearly as possible. For when to seek advice, see sections on **Fevers** (pages 140 to 156) and **Headaches** (pages 157 to 165). This measles chart can also be used for adult cases.

The remedy names are given in an abbreviated form in the charts. Full names are given in the key below.

REMEDY KEY

Acon.	Aconitum napellus
Apis	Apis mellifica
Ars.	Arsenicum album
Bell.	Belladonna
Bry.	Bryonia alba
Camph.	Camphora officinarum
Carb.v.	Carbo vegetabilis
Euph.	Euphrasia officinalis
Ferr.p.	Ferrum phosphoricum
Gels.	Gelsemium sempervirens
Kali bi.	Kali bichromicum
Merc.	Mercurius vivus
Puls.	Pulsatilla nigricans
Rhus t.	Rhus toxicodendron
Sulph.	Sulphur

REMEDY	Acon.	Apis	Ars.	Bell.	Bry.	Camph.	Carb. v.	Euph.	Ferr. p.	Gels.	Kali. bi.	Merc.	Puls.	Rhus. t.	Sulph.
MEASLES															
AIR, COOL OPEN (DESIRES)													●		
FRESH (DESIRES)						●									
ANXIETY			●												
ANXIOUS AND FEARFUL	●														
APATHETIC, DROWSY										●					
BESOTTED LOOK										●					
BETTER															
COLD					●										
HEAT				●											
OPEN AIR (NOSE, EYES)								●							
STILL					●										
BREATH OFFENSIVE												●			
CATARRH BURNING, STINGING															●
CHANGEABLE SYMPTOMS AND MOODS													●		
CHEST PARTICULARLY AFFECTED					●										
STITCHES					●										
TEARING PAINS					●										
CHILLS AND HEAT										●					
CHILLS UP AND DOWN BACK										●					
CHILLY (DISLIKES HEAT)													●		
COLD (VERY)						●									
CONSTIPATION					●										
CONVALESCENCE SLOW															●
CORYZA FLUENT BLAND								●							
WATERY, BURNS LIP										●					
COUGH								●							
DRY AND CROUPY	●														

DRY AT NIGHT, LOOSE DAY													●												
DRY, HARD, PAINFUL					●																				
HARSH AND CROUPY										●															
RATTLING											●														
DELIRIOUS		●	●	●	●																				
DELIRIUM (MILD)														●											
DIARRHEA			●																						
DIARRHEA AFTER FEVER													●												
PROFUSE						●																			
DIGESTIVE UPSETS													●												
DISCHARGES THICK, YELLOW, BLAND						●																			
OFFENSIVE AND EXHAUSTING			●										●												
DROWSY				●																					
DRYNESS				●																					
DRYNESS OF MOUTH AND MUCOUS MEMBRANES					●																				
DESIRES COLD DRINKS														●											
DISLIKES DISTURBANCE											●														
EAR ACHE												●	●												
EFFUSIONS		●																							
EXTREMITIES COLD				●			●																		
EYE (OR EYES)																									
ACHING AND RED	●				●																				
ACRID, WATERY, PURULENT DISCHARGE								●																	
BRIGHT AND RED								●																	
INFLAMED AROUND		●						●																	
LINGERING COMPLAINTS													●												
EYELIDS SWOLLEN, ULCERATED												●													
FACE																									
DUSKY							●																		
PALE					●																				
PINCHED LOOK						●																			
SWOLLEN				●																					
SWOLLEN AND DARK RED										●															
FANNED (WANTS TO BE)							●																		
FEET HOT (STICKS THEM OUT OF BED)															●										
FEVER								●																	
GRADUAL										●															
HIGH		●		●																					
NO HIGH FEVER													●												
HEAD HOT				●			●																		
HEADACHE																									
CONGESTIVE							●																		

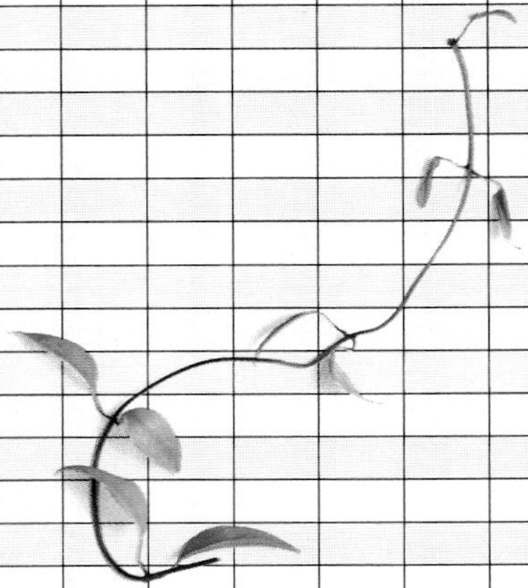

The illustration shows false jasmine, the source for the Gelsemium sempervirens remedy.

Children's Illnesses 2

This part of the chart lists, in alphabetical order, more of **the physical and mental** symptoms of MEASLES together with **any concomitants or peculiars**. Read down the list to find which ones are relevant to you. The symbols on the chart indicate the remedies most suitable for each variable. By assessing the data you have collected while consulting the chart, you should now be able to make a final selection to match your case as nearly as possible. For when to seek advice see sections on **Fevers** (pages 140 to 156) and **Headaches** (pages 157 to 165). This measles chart can also be used in adult cases.

The remedy names are given in an abbreviated form in the charts. Full names are given in the key below.

REMEDY	Acon.	Apis	Ars.	Bell.	Bry.	Camph.	Carb. v.	Euph.	Ferr. p.	Gels.	Kali bi.	Merc.	Puls.	Rhus. t.	Sulph.
MEASLES (CONTINUED)															
HEADACHE (CONTINUED)															
DULL HEAVY										●					
FRONTAL					●										
INTENSE								●							
OCCIPITAL										●					
THROBBING				●				●							
HEAT (DISLIKES)													●		
ALTERNATES CHILL							●								
HEAVY AND TIRED										●					
HIGH-PITCHED CRY		●													
KICKS OFF COVERS						●									
LIE STILL (DESIRES TO)					●										
LIPS INFLAMED		●													
LYMPH GLANDS ENLARGED							●				●				
MOTIONLESS										●					
NASAL DISCHARGE CLEAR	●														
THICK, YELLOW, STRINGY											●				
NAUSEA AFTER FEVER													●		
NOTICEABLE EDEMA		●													
ONSET SUDDEN	●			●											
SLOW										●					
PAINS STINGING		●													
PHOTOPHOBIA	●							●							
PRESSURE AT ROOT OF NOSE											●				
PROSTRATION			●												●
RASH								●							
DRY, HOT, BURNING												●		●	
FAILS TO APPEAR		●				●									●

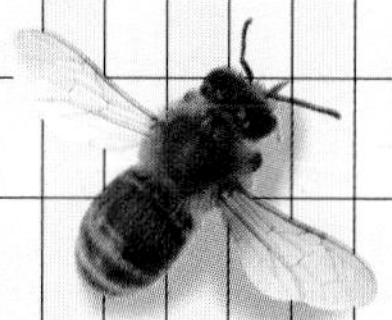

REMEDY KEY

Acon.	Aconitum napellus
Apis	Apis mellifica
Ars.	Arsenicum album
Bell.	Belladonna
Bry.	Bryonia alba
Camph.	Camphora officinarum
Carb.v.	Carbo vegetabilis
Euph.	Euphrasia officinalis
Ferr.p.	Ferrum phosphoricum
Gels.	Gelsemium sempervirens
Kali bi.	Kali bichromicum
Merc.	Mercurius vivus
Puls.	Pulsatilla nigricans
Rhus t.	Rhus toxicodendron
Sulph.	Sulphur

ITCHING														●											
NOT RELIEVED BY SCRATCHING														●											
STINGS AND BURNS															●										
WORSE FOR WATER AND WASHING															●										
RESTLESSNESS	●													●											
RESTLESSNESS (GREAT)			●																						
RESTLESS SLEEP	●																								
SKIN ITCHING, BURNING	●																								
BURNING RED				●																					
HOT, FLUSHED DUSKY RED															●										
SLEEPLESS				●																					
SNEEZING										●															
SORE LIMBS AND BODY					●																				
SORENESS														●											
STITCHES IN CHEST	●																								
STUPOROUS		●												●											
SWELLINGS		●																							
TASTE BITTER					●																				
TEARS STREAMING HOT, BURNING								●																	
TEARFUL, IRRITABLE		●																							
TEMPERATURE ERRATIC													●												
THIRST	●			●	●										●										
THIRSTLESS		●								●			●												
THROAT SORE				●						●															
TIRED AND WEAK										●					●										
TONGUE SWOLLEN, HEAVILY COATED												●													
TWITCHING (MUSCLES)					●																				
TWITCHING AND JERKING				●																					
URINE SCANTY		●																							
USE EARLY IN ILLNESS	●								●																
WANTS TO GO HOME IN DELIRIUM					●																				
WEEPY, CLINGY													●												
WORSE																									
AT REST														●											
HEAT OF BED															●										
JAR				●																					
LIGHT				●																					
MOTION					●																				
MOVEMENT					●																				
NIGHT														●											
NOISE				●																					
PRESSURE				●																					
RASH SUPPRESSED		●			●			●																	

The illustration shows the honey bee, the source for the Apis mellifica remedy.

Children's Illnesses 3

This part of the chart lists, in alphabetical order, the **physical and mental symptoms** of MUMPS together with **any concomitants or peculiars**. Read down the list to find which ones are relevant to you. The symbols on the chart indicate the remedies most suitable for each variable. Once you have identified some of the symptoms in the particular case you are taking, and noted the possible remedies, turn to the following pages to trace the remedies that suit the other elements in your case. As you work your way through the chart, following the system of symbols, you should be able to eliminate unsuitable remedies and eventually make a final selection that matches your case as nearly as possible. For when to seek advice see sections on **Fevers** (pages 140 to 156) and **Headaches** (pages 157 to 165). This mumps chart can also be used in adult cases.

The remedy names are given in an abbreviated form in the charts. Full names are given in the key below.

REMEDY KEY

Acon.	Aconitum napellus
Apis	Apis mellifica
Ars.	Arsenicum album
Bell.	Belladonna
Bry.	Bryonia alba
Carb.v	Carbo vegetabilis
Jab.	Jaborandi
Lach.	Lachesis
Lyc.	Lycopodium clavatum
Merc.	Mercurius vivus
Phyt.	Phytolacca decandra
Puls.	Pulsatilla nigricans
Rhus t.	Rhus toxicodendron

REMEDY	Acon.	Apis	Ars.	Bell.	Bry.	Carb. v.	Jab.	Lach.	Lyc.	Merc.	Phyt.	Puls.	Rhus. t.
MUMPS													
ALONE (CANNOT BEAR TO BE)		✽											
(WANTS TO BE)					✽								
ANXIETY			✽										
BREAST, OVARIES, TESTICLES AFFECTED			✽			✽	✽				✽	✽	
CHILLINESS			✽										✽
COLD (SENSITIVE TO)													✽
COLD OR COOL THINGS (DESIRES)		✽											
CONSTIPATION				✽									
DAZED				✽									
DELIRIOUS				✽									
DRY MOUTH							✽						
DRYNESS				✽									
EXTREMITIES COLD				✽									
EYES GLASSY AND WILD								✽					
EYELIDS SWOLLEN		✽											
FACE PALE (AND SKIN)											✽		
PALE AND COLD					✽								
PUFFED AND PITTED		✽											
RED AND SWOLLEN				✽				✽					
FEVER HIGH				✽									
GLANDS													
ENLARGED EVERYWHERE												✽	
HARD AND TENDER										✽			
PAINS IN				✽							✽		
PAROTIDS HOT				✽									
SWOLLEN, INFLAMED											✽		✽
SWOLLEN ON LEFT SIDE								✽					
WORSE FOR TOUCH								✽					
SUBMANDIBULAR STONY, HARD											✽		
ENLARGED							✽			✽			
INFLAMED, SWOLLEN											✽		
TENSION (SENSATION OF)											✽		

SUBMAXILLARY ENLARGED							❦						❦												
HEAD HOT				❦																					
HEADACHE THROBBING				❦																					
HEAT (DESIRES)				❦																					
INFLAMMATION				❦																					
IRRITABLE					❦																				
JAWS STIFF							❦																		
LATER STAGES OF FEVER										❦		❦													
LEFT SIDE MORE AFFECTED								❦					❦												
LIMBS ACHING, SORE													❦												
LIPS DRY					❦																				
COLD SORES													❦												
MOTION (SLIGHT) CAUSES PAIN					❦																				
MOUTH DRY												❦													
MARKED EDEMA		❦																							
ODOR FOUL										❦															
ONSET SUDDEN	❦																								
RAPID AND VIOLENT				❦																					
OPEN AIR (DESIRES)												❦													
(BETTER FOR)	❦																								
PAINS BURNING, STINGING		❦																							
SHOOT TO EARS ON SWALLOWING											❦														
PUPILS DILATED				❦																					
RASH FINE AND SMOOTH				❦																					
REDNESS		❦		❦																					
RESTLESSNESS (GREAT)	❦												❦												
RIGHT SIDE AFFECTED MORE				❦						❦															
RIGHT TO LEFT SIDE									❦																
SALIVATION COPIOUS							❦			❦															
LIKE WHITE OF EGG							❦																		
SWALLOWING DIFFICULT				❦				❦			❦														
SWELLING		❦																							
SWEAT PROFUSE							❦			❦															
AT NIGHT										❦															
CLAMMY			❦																						
COLD ON FOREHEAD						❦																			
COMES AND GOES		❦																							
OFFENSIVE										❦															
TALKING DIFFICULT							❦																		
TASTE FOUL, METALLIC, SWEET										❦															
BAD												❦													
THIRST	❦																								
COPIOUS				❦	❦																				
GREAT	❦																								
INTENSE							❦																		

The illustration shows deadly nightshade, the source for the Belladonna remedy.

Children's Illnesses 4

This part of the chart lists, in alphabetical order, more of **the physical and mental symptoms** of MUMPS together with **any concomitants or peculiars**, and some of the symptoms for CHICKEN POX. Read down the list to find which ones are relevant to you. The symbols on the chart indicate the remedies most suitable for each variable. By assessing the data you have collected while consulting the mumps chart, you should now be able to make a final selection to match your case as nearly as possible. Once you have identified some of the symptoms in the particular chicken pox case you are taking, and noted the possible remedies, turn to the following pages to trace the remedies that suit the other elements in your case. For when to seek advice see sections on **Fevers** (pages 140 to 156) and **Headaches** (pages 157 to 165). These mumps and chicken pox charts can also be used in adult cases.

The remedy names are given in an abbreviated form in the charts. Full names are given in the key below.

REMEDY KEY

Acon.	Aconitum napellus	**Lyc.**	Lycopodium clavatum
Apis	Apis mellifica	**Merc.**	Mercurius vivus
Ant. t.	Antimonium tartaricum	**Phyt.**	Phytolacca decandra
Ars.	Arsenicum album	**Puls.**	Pulsatilla nigricans
Bell.	Belladonna	**Rhus t.**	Rhus toxicodendron
Bry.	Bryonia alba		
Carb.v	Carbo vegetabilis		
Jab.	Jaborandi		
Lach.	Lachesis		

REMEDY	Acon.	Apis	Ars.	Bell.	Bry.	Crarb. v.	Jab.	Lach.	Lyc.	Merc.	Phyt.	Puls.	Rhus. t.
MUMPS (CONT)													
THIRST (CONTINUED)													
DRY BURNING													•
FOR SIPS			•										
FOR COLD WATER					•								
THIRSTLESS				•									
THROBBING								•					
THROAT													
BURNING				•									
DRY AT BACK							•						
DRY, ROUGH											•		
SORE								•					
SPASMS				•									
TONSILS SWOLLEN							•						
TONGUE FURRED							•						
SWOLLEN										•			
HEAVILY COATED, YELLOW AND WHITE												•	
TWITCHINGS AND STARTINGS				•									
WARM ROOM (WORSE)	•											•	
WARM THINGS TO DRINK (DESIRES)									•				
AMELIORATE									•				
WEEPY, CLINGY CHILD												•	
WETS BED				•									
WEAKNESS (SEVERE)			•										
WORSE													
COLD WET WEATHER											•		•
COLD WINDS													•
HEAT		•											
LYING DOWN IN												•	
HEAT OF BED		•									•		
LEAST TOUCH, PRESSURE		•						•					
NIGHT											•	•	•
TOUCH				•									

REMEDY	Ant. t.	Ars.	Bell.	Merc.	Puls.	Rhus. t.		
CHICKEN POX								
BETTER IN OPEN AIR					✿			
BREATH OFFENSIVE				✿				
BRONCHITIS	✿							
CHILLINESS		✿						
COUGH (RATTLING)	✿							
DISCHARGES IRRITATE				✿				
DROWSY BUT CAN'T SLEEP			✿					
DRYNESS					✿			
ERUPTIONS (LARGE PUS-FILLED)		✿		✿		✿		
OPEN SORES		✿		✿				
FACE RED, FLUSHED			✿					
FEVER					✿			
FEVER (LOW)					✿			
GLANDS IN NECK SWOLLEN				✿				
HEADACHE SEVERE			✿					
ILL HUMORED	✿							
ITCHING		✿			✿			
INTENSE						✿		
WORSE FOR SCRATCHING						✿		
AT NIGHT						✿		
REST						✿		
WHEN WARM					✿			
LYMPH NODES ENLARGED					✿			
MOANS	✿							
NAUSEA AND GAGGING	✿							
NEVER COMFORTABLE								
PAINS BURNING		✿						
BETTER FOR HEAT		✿						
BETTER FOR HOT APPLICATIONS		✿						
RASH COMES ON SLOWLY	✿							
PUSTULAR OR BLUE	✿							
RESTLESS						✿		
SALIVATION PROFUSE				✿				
SKIN COLD	✿							
HOT VERY			✿					
SORE				✿				
SLEEP DIFFICULT						✿		
SPUTUM WHITE	✿							
SWEAT LIGHT					✿			
OFFENSIVE				✿				

REMEDY	Ant. t.	Ars.	Bell.	Merc.	Puls.	Rhus. t.		
CHICKEN POX								
SWEAT (CONT)								
PROFUSE				✿				
THIRST, LITTLE					✿			
TONGUE WHITE	✿							
THICKLY COATED	✿							
TOUCH (CAN'T BEAR)	✿							
TWITCHING AND STARTING			✿					
VESICLES SUPPURATE				✿				
WEEPY, CLINGY CHILD					✿			
WHINES AND COMPLAINS	✿				✿			
WORSE								
AFTER MIDNIGHT		✿						
FOR COLD		✿		✿				
FOR HEAT				✿	✿			
AT NIGHT				✿	✿			

The illustration shows tartar emetic, the source for the Antimonium tartaricum remedy.

Breastfeeding problems

This self-contained chart lists, in alphabetical order, some of the more common problems encountered during breastfeeding. It covers problems with nipples, breasts and milk supply, and indicates the most helpful remedies. Of course, breastfeeding is more often than not a trouble-free bonding between mother and baby and should not be viewed as a potential illness. If there are minor problems, homeopathy can help. None of the remedies will hurt the baby.

Some of the remedies indicated in this chart are very specific to breastfeeding and do not feature anywhere else in this book. They are *Castor equi*, made from hard tissue taken from the 'thumbnail' (below the fetlock) of the horse, *Hydrastis canadensis*, made from Golden Seal and *Lac defloratum*, made from skimmed cow's milk.

The remedy names are given in an abbreviated form in the charts. Full names are given in the key below.

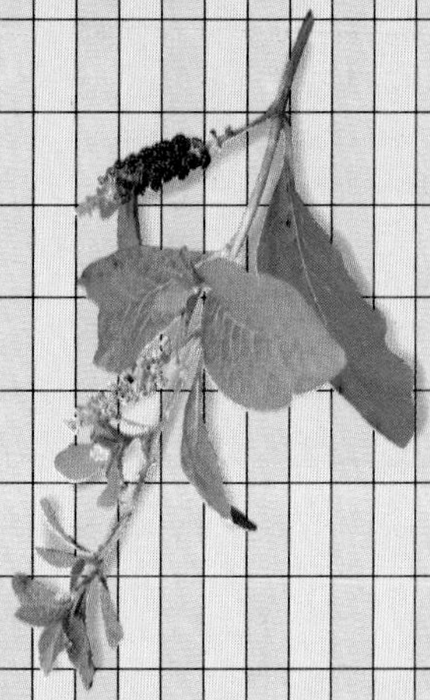

REMEDY KEY			
Arn.	Arnica montana	**Lac d.**	Lac defloratum
Bell.	Belladonna	**Merc.**	Mercurius vivus
Bry.	Bryonia alba	**Phyt.**	Phytolacca decandra
Calc.	Calcarea carbonica		
Cast. eq.	Castor equi	**Puls.**	Pulsatilla nigricans.
Con.	Conium maculatum		
Hep.	Hepar sulphuris calcareum		
Hydr.	Hydrastis canadensis		

REMEDY	Arn.	Bell.	Bry.	Calc.	Cast. eq.	Con.	Hep.	Hydr.	Lac d.	Merc.	Phyt.	Puls.
BREASTFEEDING												
ABSCESS FORMING											•	
BREASTS BRIGHT RED AND HOT		•										
HARD AND HEAVY											•	
INFLAMED (CONSOLIDATED MILK)			•									
LUMPS (HARD)											•	
RED STREAKS		•										
SUPPORTED (MUST BE)			•									
TENDER (VERY)		•										
DRY UP MILK (HELPS TO)												•
HEAT INTENSE							•					
INCREASES MILK SUPPLY				•					•			
NIPPLE ABRASIONS								•				
CRACKED					•							
FISSURED											•	
RETRACTED							•				•	
SENSITIVE					•							
SORE					•						•	
ONSET RAPID			•									
PAINS BURNING			•									
INTENSE											•	
LEFT TO RIGHT						•						
RADIATING											•	
STITCHING, TEARING			•									
THROBBING		•										
SUPPURATION BEGUN							•					
WORSE FOR JAR		•										
MOVEMENT			•									
TOUCH (LEAST)		•										
HEAT, COLD, EVERYTHING										•		

Travel Sickness

This self-contained chart lists, in alphabetical order, the **physical and mental symptoms** of travel sickness together with any **concomitants or peculiars**. Read down the list to find which ones are relevant to you. The symbols on the chart indicate the remedies most suitable for each variable. By assessing the data you have collected while consulting the chart, you should be able to make a final selection to match your case as nearly as possible. See also sections on **Headaches** (pages 157 to 165) and **Abdominal Complaints** (pages 202 to 217).

The Chinese have used Ginger (stem or root) for nausea for over 2,000 years. In its crystallized form or as ginger cookies it may also help combat travel sickness. In adults, *Nux vomica* may also help (see page 98).

The remedy names are given in an abbreviated form in the charts. Full names are given in the key below.

REMEDY	Cocc.	Petr.	Sep.	Staph.	Tab.
BELCHING (SOUR)			•		
BETTER LYING DOWN	•				
CLOSING EYES					•
FANNING					•
FRESH AIR			•		
FRESH AIR (NAUSEA)					•
OPEN AIR					•
QUIET AND DARK					•
BODY COLD					•
DIZZINESS	•	•			•
BETTER FRESH AIR					•
EATS (WANTS TO WITH THE PAIN)		•			
EMPTINESS	•	•	•		
FAINT, EMPTY, WEAK	•				
FOOD (AVERSE TO)	•				
HEADACHE (OCCIPITAL)		•			
WITH NAUSEA			•		
WORSE BENDING DOWN			•		
MOVING ABOUT			•		
HOLLOWNESS (SENSATION OF)	•				
HUNGRY FEELING		•			
INDIGNATION "UP TIGHT"				•	
LIE DOWN (MUST)	•				
NAUSEA	•	•	•	•	•
NAUSEA IN WAVES	•				
NUMBNESS, BODY PARTS GONE TO SLEEP	•				
PAIN IN STOMACH		•			
PALLOR					•
SALIVATION EXCESSIVE		•			

The illustration (top) shows American nightshade, the source for the Phytolacca remedy.

REMEDY	Cocc.	Petr.	Sep.	Staph.	Tab.
SICK HEADACHE	•				
SINK AWAY (AS IF WOULD)	•				
SINKING IN STOMACH			•		
SWEAT (PROFUSE, COLD)					•
TALK (TOO WEAK TO)	•				
VERTIGO		•			
VOMITING	•				
VOMITING OF BILE			•		
WORSE					
COLD	•				
EATING	•		•		
FRESH AIR	•	•			•
MORNINGS			•		
MOVEMENT	•		•		•
STUFFY ROOM					•
THINKING ABOUT FOOD			•		
WARMTH					•

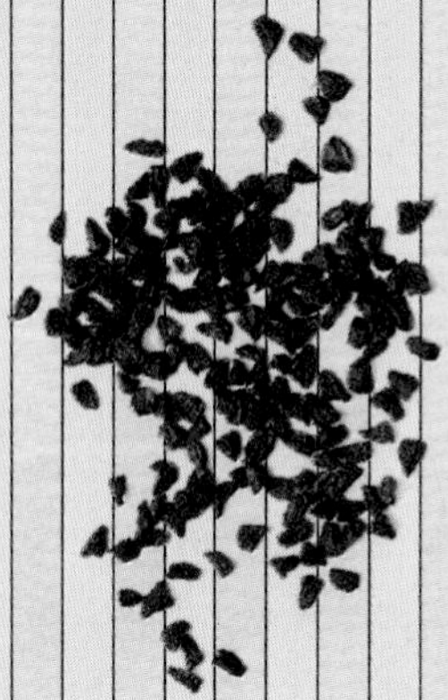

The illustration shows palmated larkspur seeds, the source for the Staphisagria remedy.

REMEDY KEY

Cocc. Cocculus indicus
Petr. Petroleum
Sep. Sepia
Staph. Staphisagria
Tab. Tabacum

Constitutional conditions

Chronic diseases reflect the state of health at a much deeper level than the simple acute illnesses whose treatment is outlined in this book. They are by their very nature more complex, particularly in the Western world where health disorders often reflect the complexity of our lifestyles and the variety of stresses we experience. It is not uncommon to find the pattern of health changing every few years in response to a stressful environment. For example, as a child someone may experience only colds and sore throats, in their teens headaches may occur, their twenties may bring abdominal pains, and in their thirties a diagnosis of irritable bowel syndrome is made. This sequence of events, if unchanged, could progress to other more serious conditions. At each stage the person is becoming more ill and, although the previous 'disease' disappeared, it was not cured. It merely changed its form and became manifest in a different area. Looked at as a whole it can be seen to be the same 'disease' throughout life.

The hierarchy of symptoms

The assessment of a patient being treated constitutionally involves looking at their health on all levels, including physical, mental and emotional. Since there is an intelligent system at work in each person, it follows that if discomfort or dysfunction is necessary in order to maintain harmony within the system as a whole then the disease will manifest in the least important parts possible thus preserving the higher functions of the person for as long as possible. Therefore, it becomes apparent that there is a hierarchy of symptoms and disease.

Among the most important functions are the mental faculties, without which a person could no longer lead a useful life. It takes little thought to see that someone who is physically crippled and confined to a wheelchair may still lead a very full life if their mental and higher faculties are in good order whereas a physically fit but totally demented person has little left to give and little capacity to receive except for physical care and a little love.

Within each realm there is a hierarchy so, in very general terms, in the physical sphere a skin rash or a cold is of minor significance whereas a heart, lung or brain disease is much more serious. Diseases of joints, muscles and gut lie somewhere in the middle. In the emotional field, minor anger and irritability are less deep than fears and phobias and mentally, a little forgetfulness is less significant than delusions or confusional states.

Palmated larkspur seeds, the source for the **Staphysagria** *remedy.*

SOME CONSTITUTIONAL CONDITIONS

Arthritis	**Hiatus hernia**	Pre-menstrual syndrome
Asthma	**Irritable bowel syndrome**	Raynaud's phenomenon
Athlete's foot	Leg ulcers	Ringworm
Bronchitis	Menstrual irregularity	Shingles
Eczema	**Migraines**	Squint
Endometriosis	M.E.	Tinnitus
Glandular fever	Nasal polyps	Verruca
Glue ear	Parasitic infections	**Warts**
Hemorrhoids (piles)	**Peptic ulceration**	

Those printed in **bold type** have acute episodes. They can often be helped with remedies which can be found from the information in this book. If in doubt about a particular condition, consult your health care practitioner.

The shifting focus of disease

This is a very brief view of the type of assessment that is made during constitutional treatment. The focus of a patient's illness, in relation to the hierarchy, is assessed and monitored. To be sure that a patient is truly regaining their health, it is of no value just to know that the symptoms of the complaint have been relieved; rather, the focus of the disease has to be seen to be shifting into less important areas, that is, moving down the hierarchy. If someone 'recovers' from their arthritic condition but later develops a heart condition then, in reality, they never recovered at all but the focus of their disease shifted.

Such connections are occasionally recognized in orthodox medicine where there is not a long time delay between one complaint developing and the next, though the significance of the link between diseases is frequently missed. For example, it is well known that asthma and eczema are linked but what is frequently overlooked is the way that a person's asthma can be bad at a time when their eczema is quiet and their eczema can be its worst when the asthma is quiet. This natural sequence of events is frequently obscured when the condition is treated without taking the person's overall constitution into account.

Treating acute symptoms

While chronic conditions require full constitutional treatment they often have an acute element. For instant an arthritis may flare up on a particular joint for a few days or a hiatus hernia may cause acute heartburn or vomiting. This acute element is even more apparent in recurrent illness such as migraine, hay fever or period pains. The acute episodes of such illnesses can be treated in a manner similar to simple acute illnesses.

It may well be possible to use this book to find remedies that will give relief from whatever pain or discomfort each time it occurs but it will not prevent the pain from recurring next time. The curative treatment of chronic and recurrent conditions should only be undertaken by a qualified homeopathic practitioner.

PREGNANCY

PREGNANCY is a wonderful time to have constitutional homeopathic treatment because changes can happen much more quickly and simply than at other times, resulting in a healthier more energetic body that will perform its functions with greater ease. If you are pregnant, or planning to be, consult a homeopathic practitioner; do not prescribe for yourself or pregnant friends.

When giving birth, however, there are some remedies that you can safely take yourself. The following remedies are intended to assist the body with some of the hold-ups that may occur in the natural birthing process whether or not you are having constitutional treatment. The remedies in the 200M and 10M potencies are only available in specialist pharmacies.

Early labor
If the contractions come and go and labor is not properly established, take one dose of *Pulsatilla* 200 every two hours until the contractions either stop, or labor will start properly. In either case take no more.

Established labor
Once the progress is definitely under way take one dose only of *Caulophyllum* 10M.

Exhaustion
The process is becoming laborious and progress is very slow. Take one dose of *Kali phos.* 12x every 15 minutes.

The baby at birth
If the baby shows any signs of shock or fright, or if he or she stays purple for too long then give one dose of *Aconite* M in liquid potency. If the baby is still attached by the cord to the mother, then she may take it.

Bleeding
If there is any sign of overbleeding after the birth, give one dose only of *Ipecacuanha* 200. The brisker the bleeding, the quicker it should stop.

Immediately after the birth
Give the new mother one dose of *Arnica* 200 every three hours for three doses only. Start as soon as the delivery is complete. It will help the body to recover quickly from any stretching, bruising or damage that it may have sustained.

The next day
Take one dose of *Bellis perennis* M. each day for three days from the day after the birth to help the mother's organs to regain their natural places.

First aid remedies/1

Homeopathy is very useful in minor accidents requiring first aid. The following section is divided into categories of accident, arranged alphabetically for easy reference. Within each category, the recommended remedies are listed in alphabetical order. A quick reference index of the remedies is shown on the right. A list of suggested remedies for a homeopathic first aid box is given on page 135.

At the end of the section, guidelines are given to help you decide when you need to call in expert advice. Clearly your own knowledge, experience and circumstances will all play a part in your decision.

INDEX TO FIRST AID REMEDIES

- The most important remedies are shown in bold.
- For emergency advice see pages 246 to 247.

BITES AND STINGS
Apis, ***Led.***, ***Nat. m.***, *Staph.*, *Urt. u.*

BRUISES
Arn., *Bellis.*, *Hyper.*, *Lach.*, *Led.*, *Ruta.*, *Symph.*

BURNS
Cal., *Canth.*, *Caust.*, *Phos.*, *Urt. u.*

CUTS AND SCRAPES
Cal., *Hyper.*, *Staph.*

DISLOCATED JOINTS
Arn., *Ruta.*

EYE TRAUMA
Euphr., *Lach.*, ***Symph.***

FRACTURES
Arn., *Bry.*, *Calc. p.*, *Eup. per.*, *Sil.*, ***Symph.***

HEAD INJURIES
Arn., *Kali. phos.*, *Nat. sulph.*

PUNCTURE WOUNDS
Apis, *Hyper.*, ***Led.***

SEPSIS
Lach.

SHOCK
Arn.

SPRAINS AND STRAINS
Arn., *Bellis.*, *Bry.*, *Calc. p.*, *Led.*, ***Rhus. t.***, *Ruta.*

SUN AND HEAT STROKE
Bell., *Cupr.*, *Glon.*

BITES AND STINGS

Apis. Marked redness, swelling, heat and pain. Pains worse for heat. Often needed in urticaria (nettle rash) which develops after a bite or sting (see *Urtica urens* also).

Apis

Ledum. Number one remedy for bee stings. Swelling, redness, stinging and pricking pains. Part feels cold, yet is ameliorated by cold applications.

Natrum mur. Very good remedy for bee and wasp stings. The remedy can even be made into a paste and applied directly to the sting.

Staphysagria. Especially good in children who get mosquito bites which become large and irritating.

Urtica urens. For people with hives (nettle rash or urticaria). It is a combination of *Apis*, *Ledum* and *Calendula*.

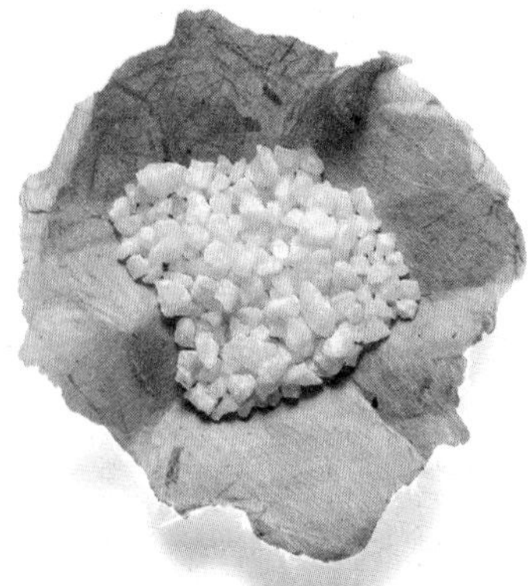

Natrum muriaticum

BRUISES

Arnica. Anywhere. The number one remedy. Sore, bruised, aching.

Bellis per. For deep injuries to muscles and joints when Arnica does not seem to be working well enough.

Hypericum. Severe. Crushed parts, especially sentient parts (see CUTS AND SCRAPES), with the same excruciating, shooting pains and great sensitivity to touch. Pain like this after a fall on the coccyx. Spinal concussion.

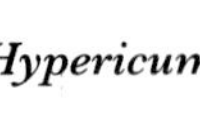

Hypericum

Lachesis. Black eyes. Aids blood reabsorption. Worse for heat, better for cold, as above.

Ledum. Black eyes or severe bruises. Bruises that feel cold and numb. Cold to touch and better for cold applications.
Ruta. Bruises of the periosteum of bones (it lies on the surface of bones and is easily injured where the bones lie just beneath the skin, for example, elbow, shin or kneecap). Sore, bruised, lame feelings.
Symphytum. In trauma to a cartilage or periosteum (the lining of a bone) especially near to the skin where pain is excessive and *Ruta* has not relieved within 24 hours. Blunt injury to the eyeball.

BURNS

Calendula. For redness without blistering, that is, first degree burns, it is the number one remedy. It is also used to dress second degree burns (blisters without skin loss) once the blisters have broken leaving an open sore (see CUTS AND SCRAPES).
Cantharis. For blistering burns, that is, second degree burns, it is the number one remedy. After the blisters have broken dress locally with *Calendula* tincture.
Causticum. The number one remedy in third degree burns, that is, the full thickness of the skin has been lost. These are serious burns requiring medical attention and often skin grafting. *Causticum* is also of use in old burns that do not resolve and if there are any ill effects of burns – other conditions that have developed from the burn itself or coincided with the burn though not apparently directly connected with it.
Phosphorus. Electrical burns or shocks.
Urtica urens. Minor burns without blistering (first degree burn).

Causticum

Ruta

Other preparations recommended for minor burns include Nelson's Burn Ointment and Pakua, a preparation which aids healing in all sorts of injuries where the skin is damaged.

CUTS AND SCRAPES

Calendula. Use the tincture topically in a dilution of 1:25 with sterile or boiled water instead of an antiseptic to clean and dress shallow wounds. Good for excessive pain. In clean cuts with stinging pains. Torn lacerations. As a mouthwash after dental extraction. Treats and prevents suppuration. (Obtain and use *Calendula* cerate or ointment in episiotomies, where it is very soothing.) Do not use if deep sepsis (infection) is present because *Calendula* promotes rapid healing which will seal the sepsis in.
Hypericum. Use in deep cuts with much pain and hypersensitivity to any touch. Lacerated fingers. Use in injury to sentient parts – fingers, toes, anus, spine, coccyx, palms, soles, teeth. Pains characteristically shoot from the site of injury and often there is great stiffness. Excruciating pain, intolerable, shooting.
Staphysagria. In clean cuts. Injuries from sharp instruments with stinging and smarting. Lacerations, use after operations. Indicated if the patient feels worse for motion, better for heat and better for pressure.

Calendula

DISLOCATED JOINTS

Arnica. The number one remedy. May need *Rhus tox.* or another remedy to follow after the joint has been reduced (put back in place).
Ruta. For repeated easy dislocation of joints after they have been relocated.

First aid remedies/2

EYE TRAUMA

Euphrasia. For the ill-effects of bruises and other mechanical trauma, after *Arnica.* Conjunctivitis after injury; the eyes are hot, burning and watering. Soreness. Generally feels better in the open air, except the eyes which stream. It can also be most soothing when used in an eyebath. Sterile eye drops can be purchased for this purpose.

Lachesis. Black eyes. Aids blood reabsorption. Worse for heat, better for cold, as above.

Symphytum. Blunt injury to the eyeball such as when a tennis or squash ball hits the eye.

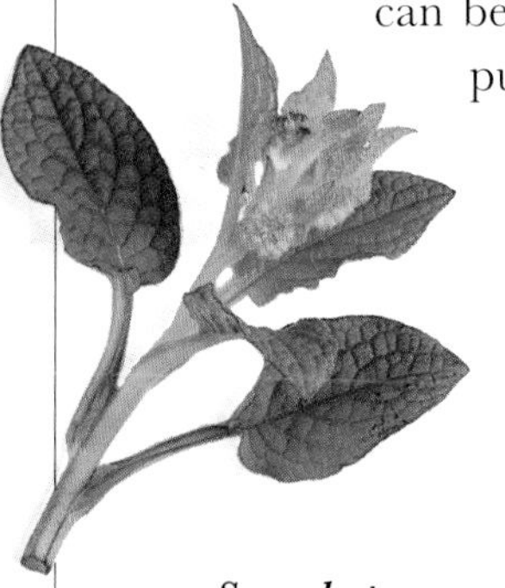

Symphytum

FRACTURES

Arnica. Helps with the shock, bruising and swelling. Often the first remedy needed because of the shock, which is the main indication. Local area very tender.

Bryonia. Sometimes in fractured ribs with worse pain in movement, must keep absolutely still and may even lie on the affected side in order to keep it from moving.

Calc. phos. Aids the nutrition of bones. May be of use if someone is malnourished or the bones are not healing (non-union).

Eup. perf. Main symptom is pain without so much bruising as would make one give *Arnica.*

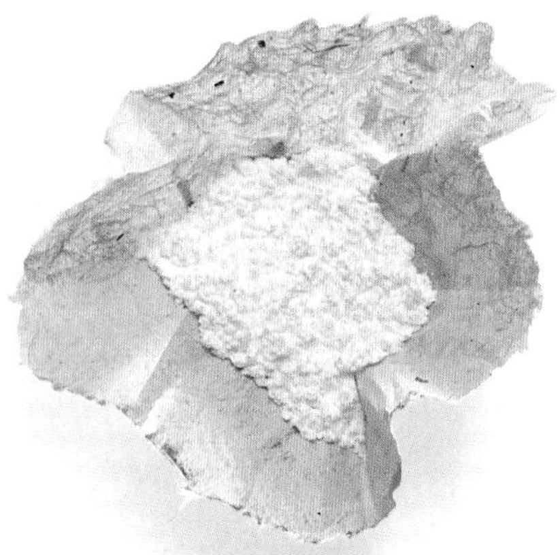

Calcarea phosphorica

Silica. May be of use if a small chip has come off a bone.

Symphytum. The number one remedy. Use only after the bones have been set. Also may be of use in cases of non-union of a fracture. *Calc. phos.* may be needed after it. Irritating, pricking, stitching sharp pain in the point of the fracture.

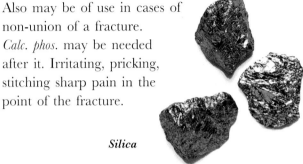

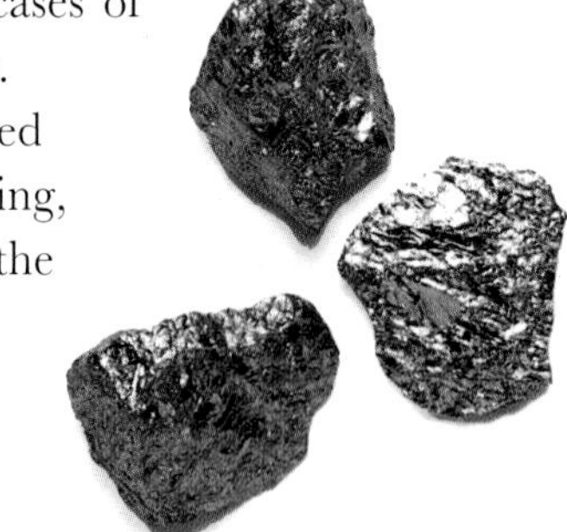

Silica

HEAD INJURIES

Please take special note of the section at the end of this chapter on when to seek advice.

Arnica. For the shock and/or the bruising – the number one remedy.

Kali phos. When there is weakness and exhaustion after a head injury.

Natrum sulph. With a headache, especially a crushing, gnawing pain in the occiput. Drowsiness, photophobia, buzzing or pain in the top of the head (vertex). (*Note:* Medical advice should be sought for such injuries with drowsiness or photophobia.) Better for cold air. This remedy may come in useful if there are any ill-effects after a head injury, even as far as a change in personality but expert assistance should be sought in such cases.

PUNCTURE WOUNDS

Apis. They feel warm or hot with stinging pains and better for cold applications. Much swelling at the site.

Apis

Hypericum. With the same excruciating, intolerable shooting pains in sentient parts (see CUTS AND SCRAPES).

Ledum. Number one remedy. Redness, swelling and throbbing pains. When the wound feels cold to touch but is better after cold applications.

SEPSIS

Lachesis. Suppuration (pus formation) after injury, sloughing, hemorrhage. This remedy has an affinity for the blood and circulation. Bad effects of poisoned wounds. An incredible sepsis remedy. Skin cold and clammy. Worse in a heated room, better for touch. Better in cold air or being slowly fanned, better once discharge has started.

SHOCK

Arnica. The number one remedy. Usually is the first remedy needed in any accident or injury.

SPRAINS AND STRAINS

Arnica. Muscles, ligaments or joints. After overexertion of muscles; pulled muscles with pain and stiffness; number one remedy for muscles. After overexertion or straining of ligaments and joints when there is considerable swelling, bruising and inflammation around the joint. Often *Rhus toxicodendron* or another remedy is needed to follow before complete resolution occurs.

Bellis perennis. Good with deep injuries to muscles and joints when *Arnica* does not seem to be working well enough.

Bellis perennis

Bryonia. Ligaments and joints. When the pain is worse for the slightest movement and continued motion only makes it worse still. Some swelling.

Calcarea Phosphorica Where nutrition is a problem causing healing to be slow and prolonged. It may be used to supplement the action of the indicated remedy in such anemic or malnourished people.

Ledum. Affecting fibrous tissues and joints, especially of ankles when parts feel cold or numb and are better for cold applications.

Rhus tox. Ligaments and muscles: of muscles, due to overexertion, after the most acute symptoms have gone or when pain is worse for

FOUR MAJOR REMEDIES

Arnica. Use in bruises and shock. The sore, bruised, aching feeling makes the patient restless; always having to change position. Worse for touch; does not want anyone to come near him. He may say he is all right when he is not. In severe injury or in head injury he may lapse in and out of consciousness. It should be plain that cases such as this require urgent, expert medical attention for which *Arnica* is no substitute, even though it may well help.

Arnica

Calendula. Has an affinity with soft tissue conditions. Excessive pain is most characteristic. It helps clot formation and keeps a wound clean.

Ledum. Generally chilly and cold but the patient desires the cold. This remedy has an affinity for fibrous tissues, joints and tendons.

Rhus tox. The grand characteristics of this remedy are the worse from first movement and better for continued movement and better for heat and worse for cold. It has a strong affinity for fibrous tissues hence its use in conditions affecting joints, ligaments and the stage of healing when fibrous scar tissue is laid down after the initial inflammation has begun to settle.

Rhus toxicodendron

First aid remedies/3

initial motion and better from continued motion and better for heat; of ligaments and joints, where it is the number one remedy. Pains and stiffness are worse for initial motion, better for continued motion and better for heat. For complaints coming on after exertion or overlifting. It often follows that there is not a clear Rhus tox. picture. Sore, lame and bruised. Paralytic rigidness as if broken.

SUN AND HEAT STROKE

Belladonna. Fever. Throbbing headache, bright-red face, stupor. Burning of the skin greater than with Glonoin. Headache better bending the head backwards, better for sitting silently, better with head covered.

Cuprum. Heat exhaustion. Cramping marks out this remedy. Stupor with jerking of muscles and even convulsions may occur. Profuse, clammy sweat, great weakness even to the point of collapse. Faintness, pallor, coldness of the body, nausea, a rapid pulse.

Belladonna

Glonoin. Sunstroke, fever, throbbing headache, red face, stupor. Less burning of the skin than in Belladonna and the patient is worse for bending head backwards, worse for cold applications, better uncovered and in the open air, better for pressure.

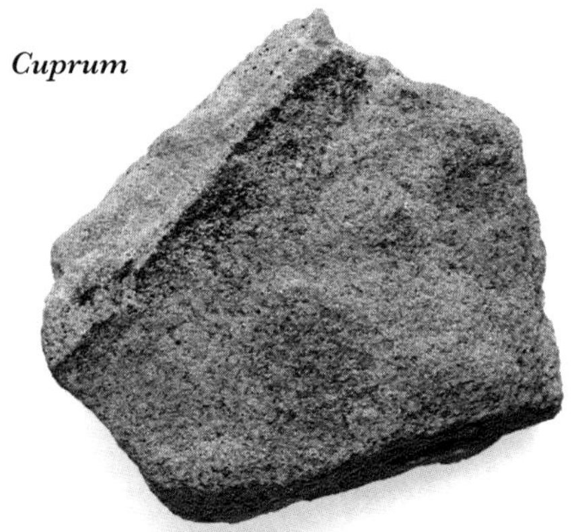

Cuprum

URGENTLY, RIGHT NOW!

If there is loss or impairment of consciousness or confusion after any form of trauma.

BITES AND STINGS

- In bites and stings if the creature is known to be poisonous or the person is known to react badly to such bites or stings.
- If after a bite or sting the conscious level is impaired or if swelling is severe and rapid especially if it affects the mouth and throat or if breathing becomes difficult.

BURNS

- In burns – any third degree burn (see below), any second degree burn (blistering and loss of the top surface of the skin – very sore and painful) occurring on sensitive skin (face, hands, genitals) or second degree burn larger than a hand size occurring anywhere else. In electrical burns remember to isolate the power before touching the person, otherwise pull them off using some non-conductive material such as rubber, plastic or dry wood. Third degree burns involve the full thickness of the skin and are likely to be less tender than first or second degree burns so do not be fooled into underestimating the severity of a serious burn by the lack of pain. Do not dress or interfere with severe burns until expert help is available but do treat the shock. Other remedies may be needed later.

HEAD INJURIES FOLLOWED BY

1. Any impairment of consciousness, from being drowsy and lethargic to total unconsciousness.
2. Unexpected irritability.
3. Any sign of neurological (nervous system) disturbance, such as slurred speech, visual abnormality (double, blurred, etc.), weakness or difficulty when moving the limbs, pupils of different sizes, numbness, fits or convulsions.
4. Vomiting.
5. Loss of a clear or a blood-stained, watery fluid from the nose or ear.

When to seek advice

HEAT AND SUNSTROKE

- In heat exhaustion (when the person has the symptoms of mild shock – cold, clammy, pale, tired, nausea, raised heart rate, they may also have muscle cramps) if the level of consciousness is affected (drowsy and dull) or they do not show signs of increasing strength and vitality after an hour of cool rest.
- In sunstroke. This is a medical emergency because the body's temperature regulating mechanism has been overloaded and has failed. The skin is hot, red and often dry. There are signs of impaired consciousness or confusion and even convulsions. Take whatever steps are possible to cool the body below 102°F (48.9°C) as quickly as possible whilst awaiting expert help.

HEMORRHAGE OR BLEEDING

- Hemorrhage (bleeding). Obviously the severity of the wound and the bleeding will dictate the degree of urgency and need for help.

JOINTS AND MUSCLES

- Any joint injury with loss of the full range of movement of the joint, albeit painful!
- If the injured part is distorted, deformed or unstable in any way.
- Intense pain or spasm of the surrounding muscles which may suggest a fracture.
- If there is marked swelling or bleeding under the skin.
- Coldness, blueness, or numbness of the injury, or the part beyond the injury, suggesting damage to the blood or nervous supply of that area.

NECK OR BACK INJURY

- If a fracture or serious neck or back injury is suspected. Do not move the person until expert help is available.

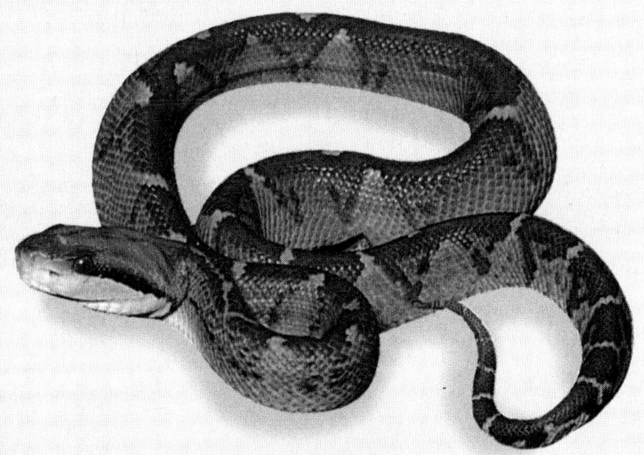

The bushmaster snake, the source of the* Lachesis *remedy.

PUNCTURE WOUNDS

- Deep puncture wounds or animal bites anywhere.
- Lacerations and puncture wounds to the following areas should be treated with great caution as there are vital organs, blood vessels and nerves close to the surface – the face, neck, chest, abdomen, and back.
- If a wound appears to involve a joint, most commonly the knee.

SHOCK

For signs of shock – pale, sweaty, faint or weak with cold limbs and a rapid, weak pulse.

WITHIN 24 HOURS

- If a wound becomes infected as shown by increasing pain, swelling and redness, particularly if the inflammation runs from the wound in red streaks towards the body (lymphangitis). There may be suppuration.
- All animal bites should be examined by your health practitioner. His advice should also be sought for all puncture wounds and lacerations regarding any measures needed to avoid tetanus.
- Any unexpected impairment of use of the injured part, such as being unable to bear weight on an injured leg or limited and painful use of a wrist after a fall, especially in a child. Refer to other chapters as necessary.

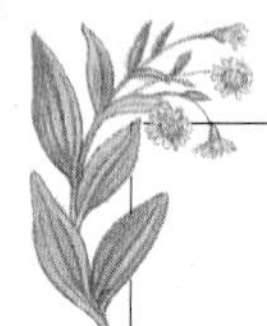

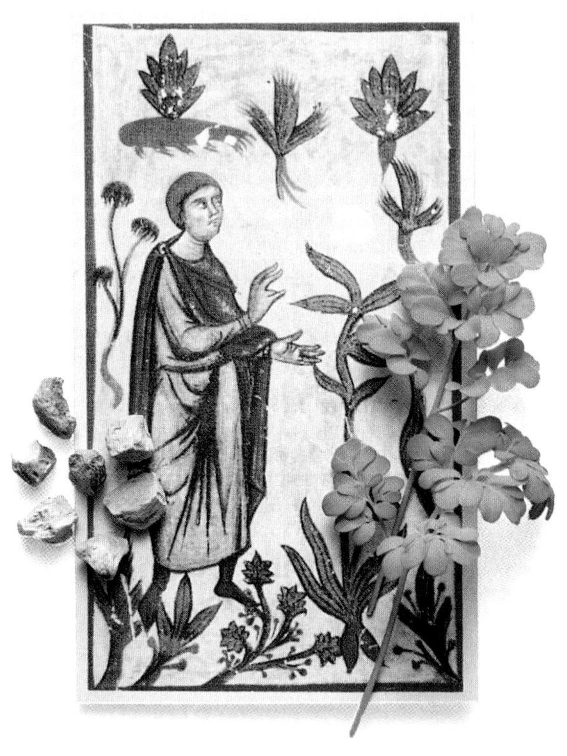

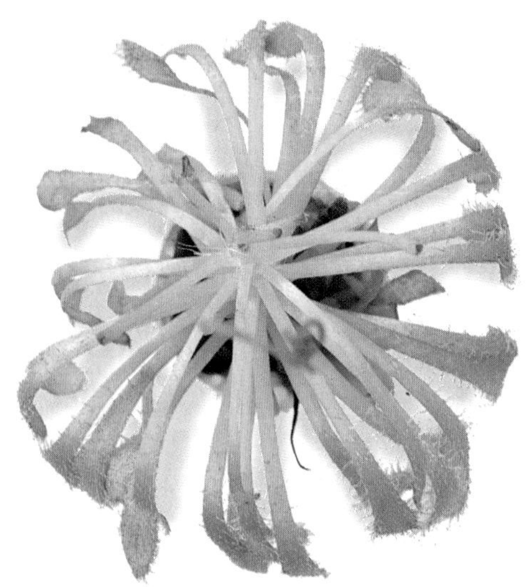

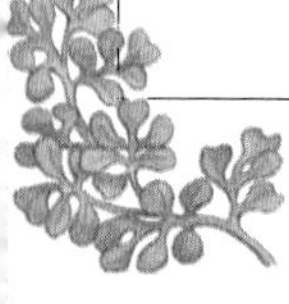

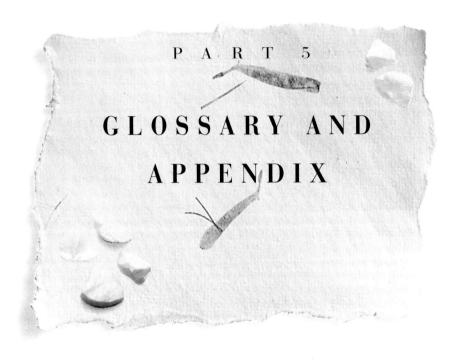

PART 5

GLOSSARY AND APPENDIX

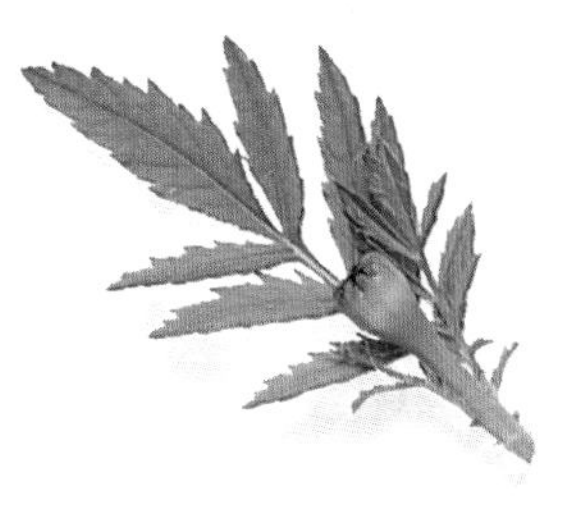

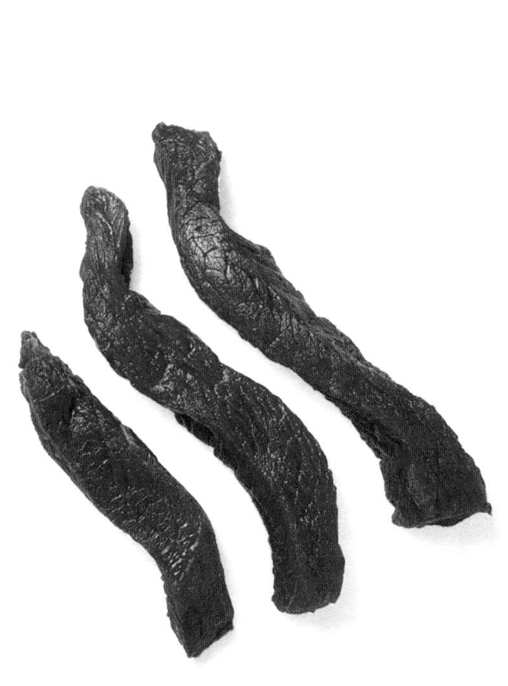

Glossary/1

Defining your Pain

In homeopathy, great attention is paid to the kind of pain experienced, and patients are encouraged to describe their pain sensations as accurately as possible, using everyday words, so that the correct remedy can be selected. Here are some of the terms most commonly used to characterize pain.

- **Burning:** a sensation of burning heat in joints or muscles or on skin
- **Splinter-like**: sharp, piercing pain confined to very small area
- **Sticking**: sharp pain as if pointed object has penetrated the body
- **Stitching:** sharp cramping pain in a small area as if the body has been caught up or pinched
- **Tearing**: pain that runs along the body, as if part of it is being torn away from the rest

Abdomen: the part of the body lying between chest and pelvis

Abscess: localized collection of pus caused by suppuration in a tissue or organ

Acrid: irritating, excoriating, bitter

Acute: of sudden onset and brief duration

-algia (suffix): 'pain in . . .' for example, *arthralgia*, pain in joints

Amenorrhea: absence of menses (periods)

Angina pectoris: severe pain in the lower chest, usually on left side

Aphthous: blistering or flaking on mucous membrane

Basilar headache: headache at base of head

Bilious: containing bile (bitter, dark yellow/green pigments)

Blepharitis: inflammation of eyelid margins

Candida: *Candida albicans*, fungus affecting mucous membranes and skin; causes thrush

Carotid artery: one of the main pairs of arteries in the front of the neck

Catarrh: discharge of mucus from inflamed mucous membranes

Chicken pox: acute infectious disease caused by a virus, with malaise, fever, and characteristic rash (red elevated vesicles or blisters which crust over and come in crops)

Chronic: persisting for a long time, a state showing no change or very slow change

Coccyx: little bone at base of the spine

Colic: acute but intermittent abdominal pain that gradually increases and then decreases

Concomitant: a symptom coming at the same time as, but not directly related to, the main complaint

Concussion: violent shock or blow to brain; may cause vertigo, nausea, loss of consciousness

Congestion: abnormal accumulation of blood

Constipation: abnormally infrequent or difficult bowel movements

Cornea: transparent front part of eye

Coryza: profuse discharge from mucous membranes of nose – 'common cold'

Cramp: painful spasmodic muscular contraction

Croup: inflammatory condition of larynx and trachea, usually of children, with laryngeal spasm, breathlessness, and difficult, noisy breathing

Cystitis: inflammation of the bladder

Delirium: a confused excited state marked by incoherent speech, illusion, hallucinations, and disorientation

Diarrhea: frequent evacuation of loose (watery) stools

Discharge: an excretion or substance evacuated from the body

Dysentery: inflammation of large intestine with evacuation of liquid and bloody stools, and tenesmus

Dyspepsia: indigestion

Dysphagia: difficulty swallowing

Dyspnea: labored or difficult breathing

Eczema: an inflammatory disease of skin with redness, itching, soreness, and sometimes discharge

Edema: abnormal accumulation of fluid in tissues which often 'dents' when depressed with a finger

Emaciation: excessive, wasted leanness

Engorgement: excessive fullness of any organ

Enuresis: involuntary bedwetting while asleep

Episiotomy: cut made in the vulva during childbirth supposed to prevent tearing

Eructations: oral ejection of gas or air from stomach (belching)

Eruption: skin lesions or rash (not due to external injury)

Eustachian tube: canal from middle ear to back of throat (nasopharynx)

Excoriate: to remove an area of skin

Expectorate: to eject phlegm from air passages

Exudate: inflammatory material deposited in tissues or oozed out on tissues surfaces

Febrile: feverish

Feces: excrement, stools

Fetid: having a rank, disagreeable smell

Fever: elevation of body temperature above normal 36.8°C (98.4°F)

Fibrous tissue: common connective tissue of body

Flatus (flatulent): gas or air in stomach or intestines; wind coming up or going down

Follicular: pouch-like

Gastritis: inflammation of stomach

Generals: symptoms relating to the whole person that can be expressed 'I am . . .' (compare with '**Particulars**')

Genitalia: organs of reproduction

Glands: refers to lymph nodes unless otherwise stated

Hawking: forceful coughing up of phlegm from throat

Hemorrhage: escape of blood from a ruptured blood vessel

Hemorrhoids: piles, anal varicose veins

Hyperesthesia: sensations abnormally increased

Hyperventilation: abnormally deep, rapid or prolonged breathing

Induration: abnormally hardened area of inflamed skin

Infection: multiplication of pathogenic (disease producing) micro-organisms within the body

Inflammation: protective tissue response to injury or destruction of body cells characterized by heat, swelling, redness, and usually pain

Iritis: inflammation of iris (in the eye)

-itis (suffix): 'inflammation of . . .' for example, *arthritis*, inflammation of joints

Jaundice: yellowness of skin and eyes from bile pigments

Laceration: wound; torn flesh

Lactation: secretion of milk from mammary glands

Lardaceous: having the appearance of lard; a fatty, greasy appearance

Laryngitis: inflammation of larynx

Larynx: part of the top of the trachea containing vocal cords

Lassitude: weariness and disinclination to exert or interest oneself

Leucorrhea: mucous discharge from the vagina

Ligament: band of tough fibrous tissue connecting two bones at a joint (or supporting an organ of the body)

Lochia: discharge from uterus and vagina after childbirth

Loquacious: excessively talkative

Lymph nodes: small masses of specialized tissue in lymphatic system that filter off foreign particles; can often be felt in neck, armpits, groin, when enlarged through disease

Malaise: feeling of unease, discomfort or being unwell

Mania: mental derangement marked by excitement, hyperactivity, hallucination, and sometimes violence

Glossary/2

Mastitis: inflammation of the breast

Materia medica: branch of science dealing with the origins and properties of remedies

Measles: acute, infectious disease caused by a virus characterized by a fever, skin rash, and inflammation of air passages and conjunctival membranes

Menses: (Latin = months) – discharge of blood and tissue debris at monthly period

Mentals: symptoms relating to the mental state, mood and ideas

Micturation: involuntary leakage of urine during coughing, laughing, or muscular effort

Modality: factor which makes symptoms better or worse

Mucous membranes: surface-linings of body that secrete mucus

Mumps: acute infection of parotid salivary gland causing swelling of face and neck, and occasionally affecting other organs

Nasal: of the nose

Nausea: feeling of sickness

Neuralgia: affection of nerves (often in head and neck) causing intense, intermittent pain

Nystagmus: continuous involuntary rolling or oscillation of eyeballs

Occipital: relating to back of the head

Ovaries: egg-producing organs in female pelvis

Pallor: paleness

Paresis: partial paralysis or weakness of muscles

Parotid gland: salivary gland within cheek in front of ear

Paroxysm: fit of disease of sudden onset and termination

Particulars: symptoms relating to a part of the person, that can be expressed 'My . . .' (compare with '**Generals**')

Patulous: widely spread apart

Peculiars: strange, rare and peculiar symptoms which relate to the individual and are not common in the illness

Periosteum: tough membrane covering bones

Phlegm: thick, shiny mucus produced in respiratory passage

Photophobia: intolerance of light

Picture: collection of symptoms which characterize a remedy or a patient with their illness

Piles: Hemorrhoids, anal varicose veins

Placenta previa: condition which can occur during pregnancy when the placenta grows so low in the uterus that it blocks the entry to the cervix and the birth canal

Plethoric: appearance indicating excessive supply of blood, usually used in connection with a ruddy complexion

Pleurisy: inflammation of pleura (membranes covering lungs and lining chest cavity) causing a sharp pain in chest when breathing

Pneumonia: acute inflammation of lung

Potency: 'strength' of a homeopathic remedy

Prostration: overwhelming physical fatigue or extreme weakness

Ptosis: drooping of eyelids

Pulse: heartbeat felt in an artery

Pupil: black circle of eye in center of iris (of eye)

Purulent: containing pus

Putrid: rotten, suppurating

Pyemia: septic infection of the blood characterized by abscesses in different parts of the body

Quinsy: abscess behind tonsil

Rectum: last part of bowel before anus

Regurgitation: return of stomach contents into mouth

Respiratory: relating to breathing

Retching: ineffectual, involuntary efforts to vomit

Rheumatic fever: acute febrile disease with pain and inflammation of joints, which can affect the heart

Rheumatic pain: pain in joints and muscles, worse in cold and damp

Saliva: digestive secretion of salivary glands in mouth

Salpingitis: inflammation of the salpynges (in the Eustachian or Fallopian tubes)

Scarlet fever: acute infectious disease characterized by fever and a rash of thickly set red spots followed by scaling or flaking skin

Sciatica: neuralgia of sciatic nerve causing pain down back of thigh and leg

Secretions: substances produced by cells and discharged for use elsewhere in the body

Septic: putrefying due to presence of pathogenic (disease-producing) bacteria

Shingles: an acute disease caused by the chicken pox virus and characterized by extremely sensitive vesicles on an area of skin limited by its nerve supply

Shock: sudden and disturbing mental or physical impression; also a state of collapse characterized by pale, cold, sweaty skin, rapid, weak, thready pulse, faintness, dizziness, and nausea

Spasms: sudden, violent involuntary muscular contractions

Sphincter: ring of muscle closing a body orifice

Sputum: mucus coughed up from chest

Sternum: breastbone

Stitch: sudden sharp pain especially in side of body

Stool: feces

Stupor: dazed, drowsy, stupid, and helpless state

Submaxillary gland: salivary gland beneath lower jaw

Suppurate: to fester and secrete pus

Symptoms: perceived changes in or impaired function of body or mind indicating presence of disease or injury

Tendons: tough fibrous tissue connecting muscles to other parts, usually bones

Tenesmus: painful and ineffectual urge to pass a stool

Testicles: male sperm-producing organs lying in the scrotum behind the penis

Thrush: fungal infection of the throat or vagina

Tissue salt: inorganic compound essential to the growth and function of the body's cells

Tonsils: pair of small lymph nodes inside mouth on either side of root of tongue; protect throat but liable to become infected themselves

Topically: local application of cream, ointment, tincture or other medicine

Trachea: wind-pipe

Trauma: physical injury or wound; also unpleasant and disturbing experience causing psychological upset

Trigeminal nerve: nerve which divides into three and supplies mandibular (jaw), maxillary (cheek), and ophthalmic (eye), and forehead areas

Ulcer: open sore on internal or external body surface caused by sloughing of necrotic (dead) tissue

Umbilicus: 'belly button', site of attachment of umbilical cord

Urethra: the tube down which urine passes from the bladder to outside

Urinary tract: bladder and passages that conduct the urine from the bladder

Urticaria: hives; nettle rash; pale or red elevated patches accompanied by severe itching

Uvula: soft, conical fleshy mass hanging centrally from soft palate at back of the mouth

Vertex: top-most part of the head

Vertigo: dizziness and sensation of rotation

Vesicles: small, round, elevated blisters containing clear, watery fluid

Waterbrash: return of sour, watery liquid from stomach into mouth

Whooping cough: infectious disease characterized by coryza, bronchitis, and violent spasmodic cough

Wry neck: stiff neck causing deformity and contortion; torticollis

Bibliography and Addresses

A Short Bibliography

There are many books to choose from reflecting the different approaches to homeopathy and the levels to which it can be studied. Some are home prescribing guides, others explore the subject further. The books are listed in alphabetical order of author's names.

Home prescribing guides

Castro, Miranda, *The Complete Homoeopathy Handbook,* Macmillan, 1990
– *Homoeopathy for Mother and Baby,* Macmillan, 1992

Chappell, Peter, *Emotional Healing with Homoeopathy: A Self-help Manual* Element Books, Shaftesbury, 1994

Cummings, Stephen, and Ullman, Dana, *Everybody's Guide to Homoeopathic Medicines,* Victor Gollancz, 1990

Garion-Hutchings, Nigel and Susan, *The New Concise Guide to Homoeopathy,* Element Books, Shaftesbury, 1993

Hayfield, Robin, *Homoeopathy for Common Ailments,* Gaia Books, 1991

Panos, Maesimund, and Heimlich, J, *Homoeopathic Medicine at Home,* Corgi Books, 1980

Pratt, Dr Noel, *Homoeopathic Prescribing,* Beaconsfield Publishers, 1985

Smith, Trevor, *Homoeopathic Medicine: A Doctor's Guide to Remedies for Common Ailments,* Thorsons Publishers, 1986

Speight, Phyllis, *Homoeopathic Treatment for Children,* Health Science Press, 1983

Wells, Henrietta, *Homoeopathy for Children,* Element Books, Shaftesbury, 1993

Further Reading

The books listed here are not home prescribing guides, but take the subject further and provide stimulating reading.

Blackie, Dr Margery, *The Challenge of Homoeopathy,* Unwin Paperbacks, 1981
– *Classical Homoeopathy,* Beaconsfield Publishers, 1990

Bodman, Dr Frank, *Clinical Homoeopathy: Insights into Homeopathy,* Beaconsfield Publishers, 1990

Borland, Dr Douglas, *Homoeopathy in Practice,* Beaconsfield Publishers, 1982

Coulter, Harris, *Homoeopathic Science and Modern Medicine,* North Atlantic Books, 1981

Gemmell, Dr David, *Everyday Homoeopathy,* Beaconsfield Publishers, 1987

Herscu, Paul, *The Homoeopathic Treatment of Children,* North Atlantic Books, 1991

Julian, Dr O A, *Materia Medica of New Homoeopathic Remedies,* Beaconsfield Publishers, 1984

Koehler, Gerhard, *The Handbook of Homoeopathy: Its Principles and Practice* Thorsons Publishers, 1986

Morrison, Roger, *Materia Medica,* Hahnemann Clinic Publishing, Albany, California, 1993

Sankaran, Rajan, *The Spirit of Homoeopathy,* Rajan Sankaran Publisher, Bombay, India, 1991

Shepherd, Dorothy, *Homoeopathy in Epidemic Diseases,* Health Science Press, 1967
– *The Magic of the Minimum Dose,* Health Science Press, 1973
– *More Magic of the Minimum Dose,* Health Science Press, 1974

Vithoulkas, George, *Homoeopathy: Medicine of the New Man,* Arco Publishing Inc., 1983
– *The Science of Homoeopathy,* Thorsons Publishers Ltd, 1993

Wright Hubbard, Dr Elizabeth, *Homoeopathy as Art and Science,* Beaconsfield Publishers, 1990

Useful Addresses

These are listed in alphabetical order under countries

Professional Associations

USA

American Foundation for Homeopathy
1508 S. Garfield
Alhambra, CA 91801 USA

American Institute of Homeopathy
1585 Glencoe St, Ste 44
Denver, CO 80220-1338 USA

Foundation for Homeopathic Education and Research
2124 Kittredge Street
Berkeley, CA 94704 USA

Homeopathic Council for Research and Education
50 Park Avenue
New York, NY 10016 USA

Homeopathic Medical Society of New Mexico
122 Dartmouth
Albuquerque, NM 87106 USA

Homeopathic Medical Society of the State of Pennsylvania
Henshaw Health Center
10 Skyport Rd
Mechanicsburg, PA 17055 USA

International Foundation for Homeopathy
2366 Eastlake Avenue E, Ste 301
Seattle, WA 98102, USA

National Center for Homeopathy
801 North Fairfax St, Ste 306
Alexandria, VA 22314 USA

New York Homeopathic Medical Society
110-56 71st Avenue, Ste 1-H
Forest Hills, NY 113751 USA

Ohio State Homeopathic Medical Society
800 Compton Rd, Ste 24
Cincinnati, OH 45231 USA

Southern Homeopathic Medical Association
10418 Whitehead Street
Fairfax, VA 22030 USA

Australia and New Zealand
Australian Institute of Homeopathy
21 Bulah Close
Berdwra Heights
NSW, Australia 2082

Institute of Classical Homoeopathy
24 West Haven Drive
Tawa, Wellington, New Zealand

Canada
Canadian Society of Homeopaths
87 Meadowlands Drive West
Nepean,
Ontario, K2G2R9, Canada

UK
British Homoeopathic Association
27a Devonshire Street
London
W1N 1RJ, UK

The Society of Homoeopaths
2 Artisan Road
Northampton
NN1 4HU, UK

France
Societé Medical de Biotherapie
62 rue Beaubourg
75003 Paris, France

Centre d'Etudes Homoeopathiques de France
228 Boulevard Raspail,
75014 Paris, France

Teaching Establishments

USA

John Bastyr College of Naturopathic Medicine
1408 NE 45th St
Seattle, WA 98105, USA

Foundation for Homeopathic Education and Research
5916 Chabot Crest
Oakland, CA 94618, USA

UK
College of Homeopathy
26, Clarendon Rise
London SE13 6JR, UK

Faculty of Homoeopathy
Royal London Homeopathic Hospital
Great Ormond Street
London WC1N 3HR, UK

The Hahnemann Society
Humane Education Centre
Avenue Lodge
Bounds Green Road
London N22 4EU, UK

London College of Classical Homoeopathy
Morley College
61 Westminster Bridge Road
London SE1 7HG, UK

Midlands College of Homoeopathy
186 Wolverhampton Street
Dudley
West Midlands, DY1 3AD, UK

Northern College of Homoeopathic Medicine
Swinburn House
Swinburn Street
Gateshead NE8 1AX, UK

The Small School of Homoeopathy
Out of the Blue Lane
North Street, Cromford
Derbyshire DE4 3RG, UK

Homeopathic Hospitals

USA
Hahnemann Medical Clinic
1918 Bonita Street
Berkeley, CA 94704, USA

UK
Glasgow Homoeopathic Hospital
1000 Great Western Road
Glasgow G12, UK

The Royal London Homoeopathic Hospital
Great Ormond Street
London WC1N 3HR, UK

Pharmacies and Suppliers
USA
American Association of Homeopathic Pharmacies
PO Box 2273
Falls Church
Virginia, VA 22042, USA

Boericke and Tafel Inc.
1011 Arch Street
Philadelphia, PA 19107, USA
and
2381-T Circadian way
Santa Rosa, CA 95407, USA

The Homeopathic Pharmacopeia Convention of the United States
1500 Massachusetts Avenue NW
Washington, DC 20005, USA

Luyties Pharmaceutical Co
4200-T Laclede Avenue
St Louis, MO 6318-2815, USA

Standard Homeopathic Co
204 T W 131st St
Los Angeles, CA 90061-1618, USA

Australia
Martin and Pleasance
PO Box 4
Collingwood
Victoria, 3066 Australia

UK
Ainsworth's Homoeopathic Pharmacy
38 New Cavendish Street
London W1M 7LH, UK

Buxton and Grant
176 Whiteladies Road
Bristol BS8 2XU, UK

Freeman's Pharmaceutical and Homoeopathic Chemists
7 Eaglesham Road
Clarkston, Glasgow, UK

Galen Homoeopathics
Lewell Mill
West Stafford
Dorchester
Dorset DT2 8AN, UK

Helios Homoeopathic Pharmacy
92 Camden Road
Tunbridge Wells
Kent TN1 2QP, UK

The Homeopathic Supply Co.
Fairview
4 Nelson Road
Sheringham
Norfolk NR26 8BU, UK

A. Nelson & Co. Ltd.
73, Duke Street
London
W1M 6BY, U.K.

Weleda (UK) Ltd.
Heanor Road
Ilkeston
Derbyshire DE7 8DR, UK

Index

Acknowledgments

PICTURE CREDITS

A-Z Botanical Collection: 52T
A-Z/Michael R. Chandler: 117
A-Z/Anthony Cooper: 48B
A-Z/David Indges: 101
A-Z/TGJ Rayner: 73

Bruce Coleman/Eric Crichton: 88T
Bruce Coleman/Michael Fogden: 89T
Bruce Coleman/Michael P. Price: 58T

Courtesy of the Hahnemann House Trustees: 15T, 17T, 17C, 19, 20T, 31BL, 32BL
from The Homoeopathic Trust's reprint of *Flora Homoeopathica*: 80, 111

e.t. Archive/Musée Versailles: 29T

Harry Smith Horticultural Photographic Collection: 46B, 69T, 71, 78, 90T
Smith/Polunin Collection: 67,116; Smith/Stainton Collection: 69B

Images Colour Library: 14TR, 24T, 27BR

The Mansell Collection: 20B

Oxford Scientific Films/Deni Brown: 91
OSF/Michael Fogden: 89B
OSF/David Fox: 38TL
OSF/Michael P. Godomski: 72T
OSF/Terry Heathcote: 33BR
OSF/Margaret Miller/Photo Researchers Inc.: 88B
OSF/Tom Ulrich: 39TL

Science Photo Library/Jean-Loup Charvet: 16B

Weleda (UK), Specialist Manufacturer of Licensed Homoeopathic Medicines: 33BL

All studio photography and jacket by Guy Ryecart

Special thanks to The Royal Botanic Gardens, Kew, London; The Chelsea Physic Garden, London; Countryside Companions, Baumber, Lincolnshire, UK; Suffolk Herbs, Kelvedon, Essex, UK; also to Sarah Bentley and David Squires.